BASIC CLINICAL REHABILITATION MEDICINE

BASIC CLINICAL REHABILITATION MEDICINE

Edited by

MEHRSHEED SINAKI, M.D.

Consultant, Department of Physical Medicine and Rehabilitation, Mayo Clinic and Mayo Foundation

Associate Professor of Physical Medicine and Rehabilitation, Mayo Medical School
Rochester, Minnesota

1987
B.C. DECKER INC • Toronto • Philadelphia

Publisher

B.C. Decker Inc
3228 South Service Road
Burlington, Ontario L7N 3H8

B.C. Decker Inc
320 Walnut Street
Suite 400
Philadelphia, Pennsylvania 19106

Sales and Distribution

United States and Possessions	**The C.V. Mosby Company** 11830 Westline Industrial Drive Saint Louis, Missouri 63146
Canada	**The C.V. Mosby Company, Ltd.** 5240 Finch Avenue East, Unit No. 1 Scarborough, Ontario M1S 4P2
United Kingdom, Europe and the Middle East	**Blackwell Scientific Publications, Ltd.** Osney Mead, Oxford OX2 OEL, England
Australia	**Harcourt Brace Jovanovich** 30–52 Smidmore Street Marrickville, N.S.W. 2204 Australia
Japan	**Igaku-Shoin Ltd.** Tokyo International P.O. Box 5063 1-28-36 Hongo, Bunkyo-ku, Tokyo 113, Japan
Asia	**Info-Med Ltd.** 802–3 Ruttonjee House 11 Duddell Street Central Hong Kong
South Africa	**Libriger Book Distributors** Warehouse Number 8 "Die Ou Looiery" Tannery Road Hamilton, Bloemfontein 9300
South America (non-stock list representative only)	**Inter-Book Marketing Services** Rua das Palmeriras, 32 Apto. 701 222-70 Rio de Janeiro RJ, Brazil

Basic Clinical Rehabilitation Medicine ISBN 1-55664-030-7

Library of Congress catalog card number: 87-70436

10 9 8 7 6 5 4 3 2 1

CONTRIBUTORS

JON B. CLOSSON, M.D.

Consultant, Department of Physical Medicine and Rehabilitation, Mayo Clinic and Mayo Foundation; Instructor in Physical Medicine and Rehabilitation, Mayo Medical School, Rochester, Minnesota

JANET M. COGOLI, M.D.

Formerly, Senior Resident Associate, Department of Physical Medicine and Rehabilitation, Mayo Clinic and Mayo Foundation, Rochester, Minnesota. Present Address: Our Lady of Lourdes Medical Center, Camden, New Jersey

ROBERT W. DEPOMPOLO, M.D.

Consultant, Department of Physical Medicine and Rehabilitation, Mayo Clinic and Mayo Foundation; Assistant Professor of Physical Medicine and Rehabilitation, Mayo Medical School, Rochester, Minnesota

ROLLAND P. ERICKSON, M.D.

Consultant, Department of Physical Medicine and Rehabilitation, Mayo Clinic and Mayo Foundation; Assistant Professor of Physical Medicine and Rehabilitation, Mayo Medical School, Rochester, Minnesota

GAIL L. GAMBLE, M.D.

Consultant, Department of Physical Medicine and Rehabilitation, Mayo Clinic and Mayo Foundation; Instructor in Physical Medicine and Rehabilitation, Mayo Medical School, Rochester, Minnesota

E. LYLE GROSS, M.D., F.R.C.P.(C)

Formerly, Senior Associate Consultant, Department of Physical Medicine and Rehabilitation, Mayo Clinic and Mayo Foundation; Instructor in Physical Medicine and Rehabilitation, Mayo Medical School, Rochester, Minnesota. Present Address: Clinical Instructor, Department of Rehabilitation Medicine, University of Alberta Hospitals, Edmonton, Alberta, Canada

TONI J. HANSON, M.D.

Consultant, Department of Physical Medicine and Rehabilitation, Mayo Clinic and Mayo Foundation; Instructor in Physical Medicine and Rehabilitation, Mayo Medical School, Rochester, Minnesota

JAMES F. MALEC, Ph.D.

Consultant, Section of Psychology, Mayo Clinic and Mayo Foundation; Assistant Professor of Psychology, Mayo Medical School, Rochester, Minnesota

MALCOLM C. McPHEE, M.D.

Consultant, Department of Physical Medicine and Rehabilitation, Mayo Clinic and Mayo Foundation; Associate Professor of Physical Medicine and Rehabilitation, Mayo Medical School, Rochester, Minnesota

JOHN L. MERRITT, M.D., F.A.C.P.

Consultant, Department of Physical Medicine and Rehabilitation, Mayo Clinic and Mayo Foundation; Associate Professor of Physical Medicine and Rehabilitation, Mayo Medical School, Rochester, Minnesota

MARK M. MITROS, M.D.

Senior Associate Consultant, Department of Physical Medicine and Rehabilitation, Mayo Clinic and Mayo Foundation; Instructor in Physical Medicine and Rehabilitation, Mayo Medical School, Rochester, Minnesota

KEVIN P. MURPHY, M.D.

Resident in Physical Medicine and Rehabilitation, Mayo Graduate School of Medicine, Rochester, Minnesota

DAVID L. NASH, M.D.

Consultant, Department of Physical Medicine and Rehabilitation, Mayo Clinic and Mayo Foundation; Instructor in Physical Medicine and Rehabilitation, Mayo Medical School, Rochester, Minnesota

STEPHEN F. NOLL, M.D.

Consultant, Department of Physical Medicine and Rehabilitation, Mayo Clinic and Mayo Foundation; Instructor in Physical Medicine and Rehabilitation, Mayo Medical School, Rochester, Minnesota

JOACHIM L. OPITZ, M.D.

Consultant, Department of Physical Medicine and Rehabilitation, Mayo Clinic and Mayo Foundation; Associate Professor of Physical Medicine and Rehabilitation, Mayo Medical School, Rochester, Minnesota

JANE L. REIMAN, M.D.

Consultant, Department of Physical Medicine and Rehabilitation, Mayo Clinic and Mayo Foundation; Assistant Professor of Physical Medicine and Rehabilitation, Mayo Medical School, Rochester, Minnesota

DANIEL E. ROHE, Ph.D.

Consultant, Section of Psychology, Mayo Clinic and Mayo Foundation; Assistant Professor of Psychology, Mayo Medical School, Rochester, Minnesota

ROBERT R. SAWTELL, M.D.

Consultant, Department of Physical Medicine and Rehabilitation, Mayo Clinic and Mayo Foundation; Assistant Professor of Physical Medicine and Rehabilitation, Mayo Medical School, Rochester, Minnesota

ANN H. SCHUTT, M.D.

Consultant, Department of Physical Medicine and Rehabilitation, Mayo Clinic and Mayo Foundation; Associate Professor of Physical Medicine and Rehabilitation, Mayo Medical School, Rochester, Minnesota

STEVEN G. SCOTT, D.O.

Consultant, Department of Physical Medicine and Rehabilitation, Mayo Clinic and Mayo Foundation; Assistant Professor of Physical Medicine and Rehabilitation, Mayo Medical School, Rochester, Minnesota

MEHRSHEED SINAKI, M.D.

Consultant, Department of Physical Medicine and Rehabilitation, Mayo Clinic and Mayo Foundation; Associate Professor of Physical Medicine and Rehabilitation, Mayo Medical School, Rochester, Minnesota

G. KEITH STILLWELL, M.D., Ph.D.

Emeritus Consultant, Department of Physical Medicine and Rehabilitation, Mayo Clinic and Mayo Foundation; Emeritus Professor of Physical Medicine and Rehabilitation, Mayo Medical School, Rochester, Minnesota

GUDNI THORSTEINSSON, M.D.

Chairman, Department of Physical Medicine and Rehabilitation, Mayo Clinic and Mayo Foundation; Assistant Professor of Physical Medicine and Rehabilitation, Mayo Medical School, Rochester, Minnesota

PREFACE

The first class of Mayo Medical School, composed of 40 students, began its studies in September 1972. These young men and women of high enthusiasm and intellect are carefully selected from many applicants. It was not until the academic year of 1974–1975 that those students began their rotation through the Department of Physical Medicine and Rehabilitation. Since then, our Department has not been the same. Their remarkable desire to learn and their inquisitiveness have enhanced our staff members' enthusiasm for educating and have enriched our academic lives. Some of these students have joined us as residents and colleagues and have furthered our cause for practice, education, and research. The original lecture series for the medical students was developed by Gordon M. Martin, M.D., chairman of the Department at that time. During the subsequent few years, the course was further strengthened through the efforts of Gudni Thorsteinsson, M.D., then chairman of the undergraduate committee for the Department of Physical Medicine and Rehabilitation, before he passed his responsibilities to me in 1980. Several members of our Department taught various topics. Gradually, the lectures and handouts were revised and a syllabus was developed. G. Keith Stillwell, M.D., and Malcolm C. McPhee, M.D., succeeding department chairmen, provided much encouragement.

The idea of preparing this book was crystallized after repeatedly being told by many of our students that we should write a book that they could use for the course. The material presented in the lecture series formed the basis of this book. It is aimed at medical students. Because excellent extensive books are available that contain detailed information on various subjects of rehabilitation, lengthy discussions have been avoided to enable the reader to grasp the concepts for rehabilitation of commonly encountered problems without elaborate reading. In addition to medical students, this book will be useful to junior residents in the field of physical medicine and rehabilitation and to physicians and residents in other fields.

I thank my colleagues in the Department of Physical Medicine and Rehabilitation for their support, for their enthusiastic teaching of the medical students, and for making the preparation of this book possible. My special gratitude goes to Roy S. Rogers III, M.D., Associate Dean for Academic Affairs of the Mayo Medical School, for his contagious enthusiasm, encouragement, and support over the years and to Mr. Jack E. Uhlenhopp, Administrative Assistant of the Mayo Medical School, for his many efforts and help. My thanks go also to members of the Section of Publications. I am deeply indebted to the efforts of LeAnn Stee for her skillful editorial work and her constructive advice. I particularly thank Roberta J. Flood for her assistance in meeting deadlines and facilitating production of the book, and my appreciation goes to Mary Jane Badker, editorial assistant, and to Dorothy Tienter, proofreader, for their efforts. I gratefully acknowledge the interest and advice of Mr. Brian C. Decker, publisher.

Mehrsheed Sinaki, M.D.

CONTENTS

1 Current Concepts and Practical Aspects of Physical Medicine and Rehabilitation 1
Mehrsheed Sinaki
G. Keith Stillwell

2 History Taking and Evaluation of Patients 4
Rolland P. Erickson
Toni J. Hanson
Malcolm C. McPhee

3 Psychologic Aspects of Disability 12
James F. Malec

4 Sexuality and Disability 22
Daniel E. Rohe

5 Examination of Joints 30
John L. Merritt
Mehrsheed Sinaki

6 Therapeutic Heat and Cold 63
G. Keith Stillwell

7 Therapeutic Electricity 67
Gudni Thorsteinsson

8 Ambulatory Aids 71
David L. Nash

9 Prostheses and Orthoses 80
Rolland P. Erickson
Malcolm C. McPhee

10 Lymphedema 96
G. Keith Stillwell

11 Rehabilitation After Stroke 101
Mehrsheed Sinaki

12 Traumatic Brain Injury 116
Robert W. DePompolo

13 Cerebral Palsy 124
Ann H. Schutt

14 Myopathies 135
Stephen F. Noll

15 Acute Polymyositis 144
Janet M. Cogoli
Mehrsheed Sinaki

16 Neuropathic Disease 149
Jon B. Closson

17 Motor Neuron Disease 153
Mehrsheed Sinaki

18 Parkinsonism 165
Gail L. Gamble
Mehrsheed Sinaki

19 Multiple Sclerosis 175
E. Lyle Gross
Mehrsheed Sinaki

20 Spinal Cord Injury 182
Mark M. Mitros
Joachim L. Opitz

21 Bladder Retraining 194
Joachim L. Opitz
Mark M. Mitros

22 Examination and Treatment of Patients With Back and Neck Pain 207
Robert R. Sawtell

23 Spinal Osteoporosis 215
Mehrsheed Sinaki

24 Arthritis 225
John L. Merritt

25 Hand Disabilities 240
Jane L. Reiman

26 Tension Myalgia 246
Mehrsheed Sinaki

27 Athletic Rehabilitation 251
Steven G. Scott

28 Geriatric Rehabilitation 265
Kevin P. Murphy
Mehrsheed Sinaki

1 CURRENT CONCEPTS AND PRACTICAL ASPECTS OF PHYSICAL MEDICINE AND REHABILITATION

Mehrsheed Sinaki, M.D.
G. Keith Stillwell, M.D., Ph.D.

The primary goal of rehabilitation medicine is the achievement of maximal independence for handicapped persons by using the organized efforts of knowledgeable personnel in the health sciences and social service areas.

DEFINITIONS

The scope and aims of rehabilitation have been conveyed by investigators in the field. Krusen[1] defined the field as follows.

> Physical medicine and rehabilitation involves the medical examination and evaluation of the disabilities of handicapped patients, the prescription and medical supervision of physical and occupational therapy and other forms of therapy, the training of the handicapped person in ambulation and self-care and medical supervision and coordination of other rehabilitation procedures.

Krusen[1] described rehabilitation as follows.

> Rehabilitation involves treatment and training of the patient to the end that he may attain his maximal potential for normal living physically, psychologically, socially and vocationally.
>
> Rehabilitation is a creative procedure which includes the cooperative efforts of various medical specialists and their associates in other health fields to improve the physical, mental, social and vocational aptitudes of persons who are handicapped, with the ob-

> jective of preserving their ability to live happily and productively on the same level and with the same opportunities as their neighbors.

The goal of rehabilitation is to decrease the dependence of the handicapped or disabled person by developing, to the greatest extent possible, the abilities needed for adequate functioning in the individual's situation.

In rehabilitation medicine, a patient's abilities rather than disabilities are stressed. "Rehabilitation medicine is the use of all methods of diagnosis and treatment which will restore the disabled individual to as nearly normal as possible."[2]

Rehabilitation should involve the progressive transition from the rehabilitation facility to home, to work, and into the community; this transition should be smooth and planned and engineered with care, foresight, and knowledgeable effort.

During recent years, medical schools have increasingly recognized the importance of physical medicine and rehabilitation, and free-standing rehabilitation centers and hospital-based rehabilitation facilities and programs have proliferated. Also, increases in the aging population and serious disabling injuries have enhanced the need for physical medicine and rehabilitation.

The team approach used in the field of physical medicine and rehabilitation involves all medical specialties. Resources of available, cooperating, trained personnel are more important than the facility. Each team is based on the individual patient's requirements. Desirable rehabilitation-oriented personnel include internists, physiatrists, neurologists, orthopedists, pediatricians, psychiatrists, speech pathologists and therapists, rehabilitation nursing personnel, physical therapists, occupational therapists, social service workers, psychologists, the patient's family, clergy, insurance carriers, vocational counselors, vocational placement services, and specialized personnel for deficits such as blindness, deafness, and mental retardation.

In the United States, associations of physicians interested in physical therapeutics date as far back as 1890 and have as their surviving descendant the American Congress of Rehabilitation Medicine. Its membership is not limited to physicians. The other principal professional organization, whose membership is limited to physiatrists, is the American Academy of Physical Medicine and Rehabilitation, founded in 1938. A smaller group, the Association of Academic Physiatrists, provides, among other functions, liaison with the Association of American Medical Colleges.

Historically, Frank H. Krusen, M.D., is regarded as the father of physical medicine, and Howard A. Rusk, M.D., was the foremost leader in the expansion of medical rehabilitation during and after World War II. The American Board of Physical Medicine was established in 1947; "rehabilitation" was added to the name in 1949.

Several disease-oriented organizations have rehabilitation as a major concern, such as the American Academy for Cerebral Palsy and Developmental Medicine, the American Spinal Injury Association, and the Muscular Dystrophy Association. The National Rehabilitation Association is principally concerned with state and federal vocational rehabilitation programs.

REFERENCES

1. Krusen FH. The scope of physical medicine and rehabilitation. In: Handbook of physical medicine and rehabilitation. 2nd ed. Philadelphia: WB Saunders, 1971:1–13.
2. Gullickson G Jr, Licht S. Definition and philosophy of rehabilitation medicine. In: Licht S, ed. Rehabilitation and medicine. Baltimore, Maryland: Waverly Press, 1968:1–14.

2 HISTORY TAKING AND EVALUATION OF PATIENTS

Rolland P. Erickson, M.D.
Toni J. Hanson, M.D.
Malcolm C. McPhee, M.D.

As with other facets of medicine, the cornerstone of rehabilitation medicine is a thorough and useful evaluation[1] of the patient. For patients who are hospitalized in a rehabilitation unit for comprehensive care, a complete general medical workup is necessary to manage the common medical problems encountered by the physiatrist serving as primary physician. The disability cannot be isolated from preexisting and concurrent general medical problems.

In addition, certain aspects of the rehabilitation evaluation go beyond the traditional medical workup.[2] Activities of daily living are those endeavors that are accomplished on a daily basis in order to maintain personal independence. The abilities to eat, bathe, groom, toilet, turn in bed, rise, sit, lie, transfer (from bed to chair, chair to toilet, or chair to car), accomplish mobility (walk with or without gait aids or operate a wheelchair), speak, hear, see, and think have an impact on the ability to live independently. Disability occurs when these and other skills of independent living are impaired. These functional skills must be assessed to identify the most appropriate rehabilitation intervention. For example, consider a patient with recent hemiparesis and aphasia. The neurologist evaluates the patient to determine cause (cerebral thrombosis, hemorrhage, embolism, or tumor), proper acute management, and prevention of progression of the impairment (hemiparesis and aphasia). The physiatrist evaluates the patient not only to identify strategies for impairment reduction (muscle reeducation and strengthening) but also to decipher maneuvers that minimize the disability (inability to dress, bathe, or ambulate) that has resulted from the impairment.

One soon realizes that the rehabilitation evaluation is not limited to a specific organ system. Instead, a truly comprehensive quality to the assessment emerges. In that the goal of rehabilitation is to maximize an individual's mental, social, vocational, and physical usefulness, the influence of the individual's impairment on work, play, family life, and sexuality must also be assessed and appropriate strategies identified.

Following is an outline of a clinical evaluation applicable to rehabilitation. In its complete form it should be useful for the comprehensive assessment of a patient admitted to a rehabilitation unit. For patients evaluated as outpatients or in consultation with a nonrehabilitation physician, parts of it may be used.

OUTLINE OF CLINICAL EVALUATION

History

Chief complaint
History of present illness, including medications and dosages
Functional abilities (Table 2–1)

TABLE 2–1 Assessment of Functional Abilities

Function	*Independent*	*Independent With Aids*	*Needs Some Assistance*	*Totally Dependent*
Feeding				
Dressing				
Hygiene				
Toileting				
Bed activities				
Transfers				
Mobility/ wheelchair				
Mobility/gait				
Driving				

Review of Systems

Constitution: fever, chills, sweats, fatigue, weight change
HEENT
- Head: headaches
- Eyes: scotoma, pain, dryness
- Ears: earache, drainage
- Nose: epistaxis, drainage, congestion
- Throat and mouth: teeth, gums, tongue, eating, sores, masses, voice

Respiratory: cough, sputum, hemoptysis, wheezing, dyspnea, pleuritic chest pain
Cardiovascular: chest pain, dyspnea, orthopnea, paroxysmal nocturnal dyspnea, palpitations, claudication, murmur, exercise tolerance
Gastrointestinal: pain, nausea, vomiting, stool consistency, blood from mouth or rectum, jaundice, change in bowel habits
Genitourinary: dysuria, pyuria, hematuria, retention, incontinence, sensation, stones, urinary tract infection
- Females: menses and bleeding, pain, pregnancies, miscarriages, live births, menopause
- Males: erection, ejaculation, progeny, pain

Neurologic
- Cranial nerves
  - I: altered smell
  - II, III, IV, VI: diplopia, blurring, field cuts, glasses
  - V: weakness of masticating muscles
  - VII: facial weakness, dysarthria, loss of taste
  - VIII: deafness, imbalance, dizziness, tinnitus
- Motor: weakness, tremors, clumsiness
- Gait: stability, falls, endurance
- Sensory: loss or change, pain
- Cognitive, perceptual: changes in memory or thinking
- Personality: changes

Muscles: pain, weakness, hypertrophy, atrophy
Skeleton: fracture, deformity
Joints: stiffness, limited motion, pain, swelling

Past Medical History

Allergies
Blood transfusions and reactions
Childhood illness
Surgical procedures
Hospitalizations not involving surgical procedures
Injuries
Immunizations: include Pneumovax and flu vaccines
Illnesses: diabetes, hypertension, pneumonia, coronary artery disease, hepatitis, bronchitis, chronic obstructive pulmonary disease, scarlet fever, rheumatic fever, cancer
Travel

Family History

Family members and their health
History of hereditary disease, hypertension, cancer, diabetes, heart disease

Patient Profile

- Social history
  - Habits
    - Diet: for secondary prevention of risk factors
    - Drugs, alcohol, smoking
  - Family: members, others at home, marital status
  - Architectural accessibility of home
  - Vocational history
  - Avocational interests
- Psychologic history
  - Previous life-style
  - Past and current responses to stress

Physical Examination

- Vital signs: blood pressure, pulse, temperature, respiration
- Skin and lymphatics
- HEENT
  - Head: signs of trauma, surgical wounds
  - Eyes: nystagmus, conjunctivae, sclerae, funduscopic examination
  - Ears: otoscopic examination
  - Nose: inspection
  - Throat and mouth: inspection and palpation, gums and teeth, swallowing
- Neck: quality of jugular and carotid pulsations, bruits, nodes, thyroid
- Chest: structure, respiratory rhythm, clubbing, inspection, palpation, percussion, auscultation, diaphragm
- Cardiovascular: heart sounds, peripheral pulses (grading)
- Abdomen: bowel sounds, tenderness, organomegaly, masses
- Genitourinary: flank tenderness, external genitalia, pelvic examination
- Rectal: sphincter tone, masses, prostate, stool
- Neurologic
  - Mental status
    - Level of consciousness: coma, stupor, somnolence, confusion, reaction to verbal, visual, tactile, and painful stimuli
    - Intellect: orientation, calculation, retention, recent and past memory, general information, similarities, abstractions
    - Personality: description of cooperation, behavior and affect
    - Thought: fears, preoccupations, insight, fixed ideas, delusions, illusions, hallucinations
    - Complex sensory functions: agnosias, body scheme, concepts of time, space, configuration
    - Performance of complex acts: apraxia, perseveration

Language: listening (single- and multiple-step commands), reading, speaking, writing
Speech: respiration, phonation, articulation, resonance, prosody
Handedness
Handwriting sample
Cranial nerves
I: smell
II: visual acuity and fields
III, IV, VI: pupillary responses, extraocular muscles, nystagmus
V: masseter, pterygoids
VII: corneal reflex, facial muscles
VIII: hearing (watch), Weber, Rinne, Romberg tests
IX, X, XI: sternocleidomastoid, taste, gag
XII: tongue
Reflexes
Muscle stretch reflexes: jaw (nerve V), biceps (C5–C6), brachioradialis (C5–C6), triceps (C6–C8), quadriceps (L2–L4), internal hamstring (L4–L5, S1–S2), external hamstring (L5, S1–S2), gastrocnemius-soleus (L5, S1–S2)
Superficial reflexes: corneal (nerves V–VIII), gag (nerves IX–X), epigastric (T6–T9), hypogastric (T11–L1), cremaster (L1–L2), anal (S3–S5), bulbocavernosus (S2–S4)
Pathologic reflexes: Babinski, Chaddock
Sensation
Test extremities, thorax, abdomen, genitalia, perineum
Superficial touch and pain, deep pain, position sense, vibration, stereognosis, temperature (hot and cold), extinction to bilateral confrontation
Coordination/rapid alternating movements
Sitting and standing balance
Rapid alternating movements
Finger-nose-finger test
Heel-toe test
Musculoskeletal
Inspection: atrophy, swelling, skin changes
Palpation: swelling, spasm, tenderness
Range of motion
Passive
Active
Joint stability: tests, subluxations, dislocations
Manual muscle testing (see below)
Gait (see below)

Manual muscle testing

Manual muscle testing is helpful for ascertaining the degree and extent of muscle weakness. Grading muscle strength involves assigning a specific value (by adjective or number) to the strength of muscles (Table 2–2). Manu-

TABLE 2–2 Systems Used to Grade Muscle Strength

		Grading System[3]					
Strength	*Criteria*	*Mayo Clinic PM & R* (number)*	*Mayo Clinic Neuro* (number)*	*Kendall (%)*	*National Foundation for Infant Paralysis (%)*	*Wright and Lovett (word & letter)*	*Aids to Investigation of Peripheral Nerve Injury (number)*
Normal	Muscle has the ability to move the body part through the available arc of motion and hold against gravity and maximal resistance	0	0	90%–100%	100%	Normal N	5
Good	Muscle moves the part through the available arc of motion against gravity but accepts less than maximal resistance	1	−1	70%–90%	75%	Good G	4
Fair	Muscle moves the part through the available arc of motion against gravity but cannot accept any additional resistance	2	−2	40%–60%	50%	Fair F	3
Poor	Muscle can complete the arc of motion but only with elimination of the effects of gravity	3	−3	10%–30%	25%	Poor P	2
Trace	A feeble visible or palpable contraction of muscle (or prominence of a tendon) without production of motion	3+†	−3, −4	5%		Trace T	1
Total paralysis	No contraction of muscle	4	−4	0%	0%	Zero 0	0

* Neuro, neurology; PM & R, physical medicine and rehabilitation.
† In the Mayo Clinic PM & R system (following the numerical value): + = weaker than designated grade; − = stronger than designated grade.

al muscle testing is of benefit clinically for diagnosing neuromuscular diseases, designing effective therapy programs, evaluating the need for assistive devices, and following the course of a disease and its response to treatment (through periodic reevaluations); it can also be of benefit for determining subsequent physical, medical, and surgical management of neuromuscular diseases. Various factors influence manual muscle testing, including the presence or absence of pain, fatigue, age and sex of a patient, upper motor neuron disorders, communication problems, conversion reactions, other psychologic factors (for example, low motivation or fear), and the expectations of the examiner.

When manual muscle testing is performed,[3] joint motion should be assessed, preferably with the patient moving the part actively through the available range of motion. Evaluation of the presence of co-contraction and substitution patterns is important. Positioning should be checked. The muscle should be tested in an antigravity position, and stabilization proximal to the segment tested should be ensured. The examiner applies resistance proximal to the next distal joint and in the direction opposite to the movement produced by the muscle contraction. Assessment of posture as a clue to muscle weakness, as well as ambulation patterns, is recommended. Also, strong antigravity muscles such as the dorsiflexors and plantar flexors of the ankle should be evaluated by heel and toe gait, respectively.

Gait

Numerous factors cause deviations in the normal pattern of walking, including (1) restriction of joint motion (including contractures), (2) pain with movement or weight-bearing, (3) muscle weakness, (4) changes in sensation, (5) lack of coordinated movement, and (6) amputations or other changes in soft-tissue status. Careful observation of the patient during standing and walking with identification of deviations is a valuable component of the physical evaluation process.

DIAGNOSES

A logical listing of a patient's diagnoses based on the history and physical examination summarizes the clinical findings. Both medical and rehabilitation diagnoses are stated, along with a succinct comment on the prognosis and the expected duration of treatment. It is increasingly important to document the diagnoses in order of rehabilitation significance because third-party payers

(Medicare, workmen's compensation, and private insurance carriers) review them to determine payment based on the appropriateness of admission.

GOALS

Rehabilitation goals should continue to be refined at patient care conferences; however, at the time of the initial evaluation, general statements are made relating to short- and long-term goals. Plans for impairment reduction and improvement in functional status are clearly stated, as is the expected placement after dismissal. Medical goals are determined, including diagnostic studies and medications needed and problems requiring close scrutiny.

COMMENT

The requirements of a clinical evaluation can vary from evaluation of a specific joint to a comprehensive examination for admission to a rehabilitation unit. The detail needed and the time available will guide the examiner in determining the items to be selected for the clinical evaluation.

Presenting the results of the history and physical examination to an experienced clinician can help the medical student develop skills for problem identification and problem solving.

Clearly, the clinical evaluation remains a most important skill for the medical student to develop. Learning this skill never really ends.

REFERENCES

1. Mayo Clinic and Mayo Foundation. Clinical examinations in neurology. 5th ed. Philadelphia: WB Saunders, 1981.
2. Kottke FJ, Stillwell GK, Lehmann JF. Krusen's handbook of physical medicine and rehabilitation. 3rd ed. Philadelphia: WB Saunders, 1982.
3. Kendall FP, McCreary EK. Muscles testing and function. 3rd ed. Baltimore, Maryland: Williams & Wilkins, 1983.

3 PSYCHOLOGIC ASPECTS OF DISABILITY

James F. Malec, Ph.D.

This chapter briefly reviews the psychologic aspects of rehabilitation. Specific psychologic problem areas are discussed, followed by a brief summary of standardized assessment and treatment techniques.

PSYCHOLOGIC SEQUELAE

Psychosis

Persistent psychosis (disorganized thinking and behavior typically accompanied by hallucinations or delusions) is rare after the onset of disability. Persistent psychosis, if present, is most likely associated with severe premorbid personality disorder (for example, schizophrenia or schizotypal or borderline personality) or with brain injury. Even among brain-injured patients, psychotic episodes occur in only a small minority and are usually short lived.

Transient, acute psychotic episodes may also occur among patients whose disability or treatment imposes long periods of sensory deprivation. Some patients with burns or spinal cord injuries must lie in a fixed position with little change in visual or auditory stimulation on a specially designed mattress that reduces tactile irritation (for example, a water bed, mud bed, or bead bed). These patients may experience a loss of reality contact in reaction to such sensory deprivation, as may patients who are deprived of sensation because of impaired peripheral vision, hearing, or touch.

Depression

Criteria for a major depressive episode and for dysthymia (neurotic depression), as defined by the American Psychiatric Association's *Diagnostic and Statistical Manual of Mental Disorders* (DSM-III), Third Edition,[1] are outlined in Table 3–1. Depression is more common than psychosis after the onset of disability, but it occurs in only a minority of cases. Fullerton et al.[2] found that 10% of patients with spinal cord injuries suffered a major depressive episode and 20% had a minor depression or a mixed affective disorder. Patterson and Foliart[3] reported that 18% to 25% of patients with multiple sclerosis experienced depression. Robinson et al.[4] reported that 27% of patients with stroke experienced major depression and 20%, minor depression. Estimates of the incidence of depression after traumatic brain injury are not available. Clinical experience suggests that limited self-awareness and self-control pose more frequent problems than depression for patients with traumatic brain injury.

Geisler et al.[5] reported that about 1.5% of their sample of patients died by suicide after spinal cord injury. This relatively small percentage was nonetheless almost 3 times that in the general population. Although *active* suicide attempts or completions are easily identified, disabled or chronically ill persons may also invite *passive* suicide through noncompliance with medical recommendations. Other authors[6] estimate that 12% of deaths after spinal cord injury are due to active suicide and that as many as 46% of deaths may result from self-neglect.

It is important to recognize that the incidence of depression after disability varies with social and environmental factors affecting the patient. For instance, the Mayo Clinic experience is that depression is not nearly as frequent in patients with stroke from rural areas and small towns who return to stable family and social networks as in the urban population studied by Robinson et al.[4]

Patients with certain central nervous system lesions causing pseudobulbar palsy may show a type of emotional uncontrol termed *pathologic laughing or crying* in the absence of significant depression. This disorder sometimes occurs in patients with stroke or multiple sclerosis. The patient may respond with laughter or tears without any subjective sense of strong emotion. In severe cases, even the production of speech may trigger a pathologic laughing or crying response. The neurologic mechanism responsible is poorly understood, but it is believed to be associated with anterior cerebral lesions possibly involving the basal ganglia.

Anxiety

Fears of specific things or situations (phobias) are uncommon after a disabling event, but they may occur, particularly in reaction to a traumatic experience. A person severely injured in a car accident, for instance, may experience debilitating anxiety when trying to enter a car. A patient who has fallen several times may begin to experience interfering anxiety during ambulation training.

Some patients become so anxious to do well in rehabilitation therapy that a high level of emotional arousal interferes with learning and performance. Performance anxiety may also result from fear of failure in specific performance situations.

TABLE 3–1 Diagnostic Criteria (DSM-III) for Major Depressive Episode, Dysthymic Disorder, and Adjustment Disorder

Diagnostic criteria for Major Depressive Episode

A. Dysphoric mood or loss of interest or pleasure in all or almost all usual activities and pastimes. The dysphoric mood is characterized by symptoms such as the following: depressed, sad, blue, hopeless, low, down in the dumps, irritable. The mood disturbance must be prominent and relatively persistent, but not necessarily the most dominant symptom, and does not include momentary shifts from one dysphoric mood to another dysphoric mood, e.g., anxiety to depression to anger, such as are seen in states of acute psychotic turmoil. (For children under six, dysphoric mood may have to be inferred from a persistently sad facial expression.)

B. At least four of the following symptoms have each been present nearly every day for a period of at least two weeks (in children under six, at least three of the first four).

(1) poor appetite or significant weight loss (when not dieting) or increased appetite or significant weight gain (in children under six, consider failure to make expected weight gains)
(2) insomnia or hypersomnia
(3) psychomotor agitation or retardation (but not merely subjective feelings of restlessness or being slowed down)(in children under six, hypoactivity)
(4) loss of interest or pleasure in usual activities, or decrease in sexual drive not limited to a period when delusional or hallucinating (in children under six, signs of apathy)
(5) loss of energy; fatigue
(6) feelings of worthlessness, self-reproach, or excessive or inappropriate guilt (either may be delusional)
(7) complaints or evidence of diminished ability to think or concentrate, such as slowed thinking, or indecisiveness not associated with marked loosening of associations or incoherence
(8) recurrent thoughts of death, suicidal ideation, wishes to be dead, or suicide attempt

C. Neither of the following dominate the clinical picture when an affective syndrome (i.e., criteria A and B above) is not present, that is, before it developed or after it has remitted:
(1) preoccupation with a mood-incongruent delusion or hallucination (see definition below)
(2) bizarre behavior

D. Not superimposed on either Schizophrenia, Schizophreniform Disorder, or a Paranoid Disorder.

E. Not due to any Organic Mental Disorder or Uncomplicated Bereavement.

Diagnostic criteria for Dysthymic Disorder

A. During the past two years (or one year for children and adolescents) the individual has been bothered most or all of the time by symptoms characteristic of the depressive syndrome but that are not of sufficient severity and duration to meet the criteria for a major depressive episode (although a major depressive episode may be superimposed on Dysthymic Disorder).

From American Psychiatric Association.[1] By permission.

B. The manifestations of the depressive syndrome may be relatively persistent or separated by periods of normal mood lasting a few days to a few weeks, but no more than a few months at a time.

C. During the depressive periods there is either prominent depressed mood (e.g., sad, blue, down in the dumps, low) or marked loss of interest or pleasure in all, or almost all, usual activities and pastimes.

D. During the depressive periods at least three of the following symptoms are present:

(1) insomnia or hypersomnia
(2) low energy level or chronic tiredness
(3) feelings of inadequacy, loss of self-esteem, or self-deprecation
(4) decreased effectiveness or productivity at school, work, or home
(5) decreased attention, concentration, or ability to think clearly
(6) social withdrawal
(7) loss of interest in or enjoyment of pleasurable activities
(8) irritability or excessive anger (in children, expressed toward parents or caretakers)
(9) inability to respond with apparent pleasure to praise or rewards
(10) less active or talkative than usual, or feels slowed down or restless
(11) pessimistic attitude toward the future, brooding about past events, or feeling sorry for self
(12) tearfulness or crying
(13) recurrent thoughts of death or suicide

E. Absence of psychotic features, such as delusions, hallucinations, or incoherence, or loosening of associations.

F. If the disturbance is superimposed on a preexisting mental disorder, such as Obsessive Compulsive Disorder or Alcohol Dependence, the depressed mood, by virtue of its intensity or effect on functioning, can be clearly distinguished from the individual's usual mood.

Diagnostic criteria for Adjustment Disorder

A. A maladaptive reaction to an identifiable psychosocial stressor, that occurs within three months of the onset of the stressor.

B. The maladaptive nature of the reaction is indicated by either of the following:

(1) impairment in social or occupational functioning
(2) symptoms that are in excess of a normal and expectable reaction to the stressor

C. The disturbance is not merely one instance of a pattern of overreaction to stress or an exacerbation of one of the mental disorders previously described.

D. It is assumed that the disturbance will eventually remit after the stressor ceases or, if the stressor persists, when a new level of adaptation is achieved.

E. The disturbance does not meet the criteria for any of the specific disorders listed previously or for Uncomplicated Bereavement.

Adjustment Reaction

A broad generalization is that about a third of patients experience depression or other severe psychologic disorders after the onset of disability, a third adjust to disability without any emotional or behavioral disturbance requiring professional attention, and a third experience mild adjustment problems. These mild affective disorders often fit the DSM-III category of adjustment disorder (Table 3–1). An adjustment disorder may be characterized primarily by depressive mood, anxiety, or inappropriate behavior.

Many adjustment problems and stressors affect the disabled patient. People often find self-worth and a means for dealing with stress in their activities. Disability may limit work, hobbies, and social and recreational activities and thus result in diminished self-esteem, boredom, or frustration. At the same time, the patient is prevented from engaging in activities that may have formerly provided a distraction from or a method of addressing such stress. Patients may need considerable time and support to discover new, rewarding activities.

Communication problems, sexual problems, and other disabilities that interfere with interpersonal relationships and intimacy can result in particularly severe stress. Disability and disfigurement can also produce self-consciousness and concerns about body image, more so for persons whose self-worth was based on physical beauty, strength, or skill.

Grief Reactions

Other mild affective or behavioral problems after becoming disabled do not clearly fit the DSM-III scheme. Some patients, for instance, seem to experience genuine grief for a lost body part, physical function, or activity. The grief does not seem inappropriate in degree and usually resolves if the patient is allowed a period of grieving.

A grief reaction is not a universal phenomenon after the onset of disability. At one point in the study of the psychology of rehabilitation, it was vogue to believe that, after becoming disabled, all persons went through a period of grief or through predictable stages of adjustment similar to those Kübler-Ross[7] identified as stages of adjustment to terminal illness (that is, denial, anger, depression, bargaining, and acceptance). Contemporary research, however, has failed to identify any predictable course or series of stages of emotional adjustment to disability.[6]

Denial

After brain injury, some patients are unable to recognize their illness (anosognosia) or to recognize an impaired body part (autotopagnosia). Such extreme denial rarely occurs on a purely psychologic basis, that is, as a defense against negative feelings associated with illness or disability. When extreme denial does occur without brain injury, it raises a strong suspicion of premorbid personality disturbance.

Alternatively, many patients tend to minimize the permanence or consequences of their disabilities. Most contemporary clinicians believe this form of mild "denial" can be an effective means for emotional coping, particularly during the acute period after the onset of disability, and becomes problematic only if it interferes with participation in the rehabilitation process. At a time when medical and rehabilitation staff are often themselves uncertain about the ultimate degree of recovery that can be expected, the patient who does not have the background knowledge to appreciate the subtleties of medical prognosis often hopes for the best. Just as it may be appropriate for medical staff to advise patients of the possibility of a less-than-hoped-for outcome at this time, patients may appropriately be more optimistic. Their optimism allows them to find the energy to manage negative feelings, to learn more about their conditions, and to participate fully in the rehabilitation process.

Cognitive Impairment

In addition to nonrecognition of disability, brain-injured patients may show an array of impaired cognitive abilities that interfere with social functioning, such as poor concentration, language disturbance, visuoperceptual disturbance, confusion, poor judgment, impulsiveness, and limited self-awareness and social awareness, including sexual inappropriateness. Cognitive impairment may interfere with coping abilities and may be associated with episodes of extreme distress.

Substance Abuse

Among drivers requiring emergency hospital treatment after a nonfatal automobile accident, 25% to 35% are intoxicated (that is, they have a blood alcohol level of 0.10% or more).[8] In a prospective study, Rimel[9] reported that ethanol was present in the bloodstream of 72% of 1,330 patients with central nervous system trauma and that 55% of these patients had a blood alcohol level of more than 0.10%. This relatively high percentage indicates the need for evaluation for substance abuse disorders among this patient group.

For the evaluation of substance abuse disorders, a distinction can be made between patients who are substance dependent or have a pattern of abuse and those who are not alcoholics but were intoxicated at the time of an injury. Substance-dependent or substance-abusing patients typically show a pattern of regular, problematic use that interferes with occupational or social functioning. They often have a family history of substance dependency. Such patients are appropriately treated in traditional programs with an Alcoholics Anonymous philosophy that emphasizes total abstinence.

Nonalcoholics are not physically or psychologically dependent on alcohol. Their use of ethanol does not significantly interfere with work or social adjustment. In fact, an episode of irresponsible use leading to injury in these persons is often associated with a work or social function. The nonalcoholics who are intoxicated at the time of injury often resist traditional treatment because—with some justification—they do not see themselves as "alcoholic" or "hooked" and are unwilling to commit themselves to lifelong sobriety. A behavioral treatment program emphasizing moderation and responsible use may be most appropriate for these patients. It must be emphasized, however, that differentiating the chemically dependent or substance-abusing patient who denies and minimizes the extent of use from the nonalcoholic with a history of intoxication is very difficult.

Personality

The DSM-III has made a valuable distinction between acute psychologic disorders (Axis I) such as depression or psychosis and more long-standing personality disorders (Axis II) evidenced in maladaptive coping and interpersonal styles. A thorough discussion of personality theory is beyond the scope of this chapter. However, an assessment by a psychologist or psychiatrist of personality style and of possible premorbid maladaptive personality tendencies can be invaluable for planning a rehabilitation program that maximally elicits the patient's cooperation and reduces interpersonal friction between patient and staff.

The possibility of a relationship between specific personality traits and specific disabilities is controversial. Shontz[10] presented the argument that personality traits are not associated with specific disabling illnesses or events. Rohe and Athelstan[11] and Malec[12] presented evidence that identifiable personality traits predispose patients to severe traumatic injury and must be considered in rehabilitation planning.

The person who is most likely to sustain a severe traumatic injury, such as a spinal cord injury, is likely to be an activity-oriented, risk-taking person who learns best by doing rather than through study and introspection. This type of person, whose traits resemble Eysenck's[13] description of extroversion, typically prefers occupations in which tangible effects are produced by physical labor. Because of their risk-taking behavior, persons with this sort of personality may rebel against the cautious, conservative restrictions of inpatient rehabilitation but eventually are more likely to adjust successfully to disability than persons who are less willing to try new things.[14] Frictions may develop between the more extroverted patient and staff, who often value introspection, conceptual thinking, caution, and careful planning. Such frictions can be avoided if rehabilitation planning is activity oriented and incorporates some planned "risks" that allow patients to test themselves. Often employed as a mechanic, plumber, welder, or carpenter, for example, patients with this type of personality often find great difficulty in shifting vocational interests to less physically demanding occupations such as accounting or computer programming. Vocational counseling thus requires creativity in discovering occupations in which the more extroverted patient's limited physical abilities can still be used to produce a tangible (and marketable) product or service.

Family Reactions

Close family members may also experience significant affective or adjustment disorders after the onset of disability in a loved one. Spouses often find they must exchange responsibilities; for instance, a wife may become the primary wage earner and her disabled husband assume the role of homemaker and primary caregiver for the children. Such role reversals may result in loss of self-esteem, guilt, sexual problems, and affective distress for one or both partners.

Family members often find that a loved one who has sustained brain damage shows subtle—or not so subtle—changes in personality. Unlike when a loved one is lost in death, however, society offers no avenue for the family's grief. On the contrary, the family is expected to be overjoyed that the loved one has not died and to maintain love and responsibility for that person despite personality changes. Lezak[15] offered an excellent discussion of problems facing families after brain injury of a family member.

ASSESSMENT

As a supplement to the clinical interview, practitioners in clinical psychology and neuropsychology have developed methods for standardized assessment of various factors of psychologic functioning, including mood, acute psychopathology, personality, intelligence and cognitive functioning, interpersonal relationships, and vocational interests and aptitudes. Standardized assessment means that such procedures are conducted in a standard, invariable manner. Typically, results are then interpreted with reference to a normative group, usually a sample of persons whose age and sex are similar to those of the patient and who exhibit normal functioning. Selection, administration, and interpretation of standardized assessment instruments are technical enterprises for which qualified clinical psychologists have specialized training.

TREATMENT

Antidepressant medication is often of benefit to patients who meet criteria for a biologically based depression. Pathologic laughing or crying may be reduced with antidepressant medication given at doses lower than those typically recommended for treating depression, probably because of the dopamine agonistic, not the antidepressant, properties of the medication.[16] Levodopa has also been reported to decrease pathologic laughing or crying.[17]

Beck et al.[18] described an alternative treatment approach in which depressed patients are guided to rethink ideas that maintain depression, such as overgeneralized assumptions (for example, "no one cares about me" or "I can't do anything right") or selectively negative perceptions (for example, "I'm not making any progress in ambulation training" when the patient is making good progress in all other areas). Contemporary psychologic treatment involves increasingly sophisticated procedures and thus is best offered by or in consultation with a qualified psychiatrist or clinical psychologist. The most effective treatment for depression is often a combination of antidepressant medication and Beck's cognitive-behavioral approach. Medication reduces dysphoria and improves the energy level during the initial stages, and therapy teaches improved self-control and the interpersonal skills needed to maintain adjustment.

Cognitive-behavioral therapy can also help people learn to make decisions, reassess life-styles, think constructively, and plan activities in order to resolve an adjustment disorder. Yet another approach that has been found to reduce dysphoria is systematically increasing pleasant and valued activities.[19] Active involvement in a comprehensive rehabilitation program offers many patients the opportunity to participate in various activities that they enjoy and value.

Resolution of grief requires a somewhat different approach involving the acknowledgment and experience of feelings related to loss in association with psychologic support.

Changing maladaptive personality traits may be accomplished in long-term psychodynamic psychotherapy, but it is usually an unrealistic goal for the relatively short period of inpatient physical rehabilitation. During inpatient rehabilitation, patients are typically focused not on psychologic but on physical change. Behavioral programs (in which desired behaviors are consistently rewarded and undesirable behaviors are not rewarded), behavioral contracts, or simple limit setting offers rehabilitation staff the avenues for restricting the expression of maladaptive personality tendencies and for increasing compliance with medical and rehabilitation treatment. To obtain cooperation from patients with less flexible and adaptable personalities, the rehabilitation staff must also adapt. In consultation with the staff psychologist, the rehabilitation team may attempt to elicit the patient's participation by accommodating their expectations and their own style of interpersonal interaction to those of the patient.

REFERENCES

1. American Psychiatric Association diagnostic and statistical manual of mental disorders. 3rd ed. Washington DC: American Psychiatric Association, 1980.
2. Fullerton DT, Harvey RF, Klein MH, Howell T. Psychiatric disorders in patients with spinal cord injuries. Arch Gen Psychiatry 1981; 38:1369–1371.
3. Patterson MB, Foliart R. Multiple sclerosis: understanding the psychologic implications. Gen Hosp Psychiatry 1985; 7:234–238.
4. Robinson RG, Starr LB, Kubos KL, Price TR. A two-year longitudinal study of post-stroke mood disorders: findings during the initial evaluation. Stroke 1983; 14:736–741.
5. Geisler WO, Jousse AT, Wynne-Jones M, Breithaupt D. Survival in traumatic spinal cord injury. Paraplegia 1983; 21:364–373.
6. Trieschmann RB. Spinal cord injuries: psychological, social and vocational adjustment. New York: Pergamon Press, 1980.
7. Kübler-Ross E. On death and dying. New York: Macmillan, 1969.
8. Lowenfels AB, Miller TT. Alcohol and trauma. Ann Emerg Med 1984; 13:1056–1060.
9. Rimel RW. A prospective study of patients with central nervous system trauma. J Neurosurg Nurs 1981; 13:132–141.
10. Shontz FC. Physical disability and personality: theory and recent research. In: Marinelli RP, Dell Orto AE, eds. The psychological and social impact of physical disability. New York: Springer-Verlag, 1977:105–129.
11. Rohe DE, Athelstan GT. Vocational interests of persons with spinal cord injury. J Counsel Psychol 1982; 29:283–291.
12. Malec J. Personality factors associated with severe traumatic disability. Rehabil Psychol 1985; 30:165–172.
13. Eysenck HJ. Dimensions of personality. London: Routledge & Paul, 1947.
14. Athelstan GT, Crewe NM. Psychological adjustment to spinal cord injury as related to manner of onset of disability. Rehabil Counsel Bull 1979; 22:311–319.
15. Lezak MD. Living with the characterologically altered brain injured patient. J Clin Psychiatry 1978; 39:592–598.
16. Schiffer RB, Herndon RM, Rudick RA. Treatment of pathologic laughing and weeping with amitriptyline. N Engl J Med 1985; 312:1480–1482.
17. Udaka F, Yamao S, Nagata H, Nakamura S, Kameyama M. Pathologic laughing and crying treated with levodopa. Arch Neurol 1984; 41:1095–1096.
18. Beck AT, Rush AJ, Shaw BF, Emery G. Cognitive therapy of depression. New York: Guilford Press, 1979.
19. Lewinsohn PM, Hoberman HM. Depression. In: Bellack AS, Hersen M, Kazdin AE, eds. International handbook of behavior modification and therapy. New York: Plenum Press, 1982:397–431.

4 SEXUALITY AND DISABILITY

Daniel E. Rohe, Ph.D.

Concern about the sexual functioning of persons with disabilities began in earnest in the late 1960s in the United States. This concern was an outgrowth of various social forces operating at the time, such as the human rights movement, alternative lifestyles, and increased societal willingness to examine sexual attitudes. During the early 1970s, an experiential learning program entitled Sexual Attitude Restructuring (SAR) was devised through the Glide Urban Center, an agency of the United Methodist Church, and implemented to help professionals examine their sexual beliefs and values. These programs helped raise consciousness about the topic of sexuality, and soon SAR workshops were devised for persons with physical disabilities.

The rehabilitation literature blossomed with articles expounding the importance of sexuality issues, commonly encountered sexuality concerns, and how to provide counseling.[1-3] The heightened interest in this area led to publication of the journal *Sexuality and Disability*.[4] Interest became so intense that rehabilitation professionals were found to actually overestimate the importance of sexual function for recently disabled persons.[5] Addressing the sexuality concerns of disabled patients has now become a well-established and accepted part of comprehensive rehabilitation services.

The goal of this chapter is to provide a succinct overview of how sexuality is affected by the presence of a physical disability. The sexual response cycle and common sexual dysfunctions in nonphysically disabled persons are summarized, and the conceptual distinctions among sex drive, sex acts, and sexuality are delineated. Disabilities are classified according to their effect on sexual function, and associated interfering medical conditions are explained. The sexuality concerns of persons with spinal cord injury, a disability affecting multiple areas of sexual functioning, are discussed. The topic of sexual counseling is also addressed.

SEXUAL RESPONSE CYCLE AND COMMON DYSFUNCTIONS

Understanding sexuality in physically disabled patients presumes a working knowledge of the sexual response cycle and common sexual difficulties encountered in nonphysically disabled persons. The work of Masters and Johnson demonstrated that male and female responses are similar and can be divided into four phases: excitement, plateau, orgasm, and resolution. The excitement phase occurs when psychologic or physical stimuli result in increased muscle tension, blood pressure, and heart rate. It is accompanied by penile erection or vaginal lubrication. During the plateau phase, maximal vasocongestion of the sexual organs occurs with additional increases in heart rate and blood pressure. Orgasm involves rhythmic contractions of the penis in men and the vagina in women and the perineal muscles in both sexes. The resolution phase involves return to the body's normal resting state.

Common male sexual difficulties include premature ejaculation, impotence, and retarded ejaculation. Common female sexual difficulties include preorgasmia, secondary orgasmia, dyspareunia, sexual aversion, and vaginismus. Various publications [6-8] have detailed descriptions of the sexual dysfunctions. Not infrequently, professionals fail to understand that persons with physical disabilities are subject to the same sexual dysfunctions as nondisabled persons. The treatment approaches are frequently similar, if not identical.

SEX DRIVE, SEX ACTS, AND SEXUALITY

A proper understanding of human sexuality requires careful differentiation among sex drive, sex acts, and sexuality.[9] Sex drive is a primary drive similar to others such as hunger, thirst, and avoidance of pain. These drives are innate and involve complex interrelationships among bodily receptors, hormone levels, and autonomic and central nervous system functions. Because the sex drive does not have immediate consequences for survival, other drives usually take precedence. For example, if a person is experiencing pain, the probability of the sex drive being expressed is greatly diminished. In a physically disabled person, should he or she be struggling with anxiety, pain, malaise, or fatigue, interference with the sex drive may result.

Sex acts are behaviors that result in pleasurable sensations through contact with one's own or another person's body. Contact is most frequently made with the erogenous zones or genitals, which are maximally responsive to such stimulation. Yet, it is important to understand that many other areas of the body may provide pleasurable sensations. This fact is especially important for physically disabled persons, who may have reduced or absent sensation in certain areas of the body. The various human behaviors that result in pleasurable sensations are exceedingly diverse.[10] Sexual intercourse is but one of an infinite number of sex acts.

Sexuality can be defined as the expression of one's sex drive, through learned sex acts, within the context of the sexual identity of the person. Sexuality is more than sexual organs or sexual behaviors. Berkman et al.[11] described sexuality as a dynamic process grounded in developmental learning experiences and having three components. These components are the individual's self-concept, relationships with others, and specific repertoire of sexual behaviors. Sexuality is frequently confused with intimacy because physical closeness is often equated with psychologic closeness. Intimacy is a special state of mutual understanding, trust, and acceptance. Intimacy may or may not involve the satisfaction of a sex drive through sex behaviors. Although physical disability may interfere with sex drive and sex behaviors, the ongoing basic human need and capacity for intimacy remain.

SEXUAL DYSFUNCTION IN DISABLED PERSONS

Sexual dysfunction in disabled persons can be categorized according to four causes. First, those constantly under the stress of pain, fatigue, or malaise may have decreased sexual activity due to a reduction in sex drive. A second cause of sexual dysfunction is limited learning opportunities involving sexual behaviors or the lack of social skills necessary for initiation and maintenance of relationships. Third, sexual dysfunction may arise because of bodily changes that directly interfere with the ability to either receive sexual pleasure or engage in previously learned sex acts. Examples include spinal cord injury, stroke, arthritis, and multiple sclerosis. Fourth, major changes in self-image, self-esteem, and body image may result in sexual dysfunction. These changes are especially likely with the sudden onset of disability.

For all of the above-mentioned conditions, the ultimate goal of the helping professional is to increase comfort with changes in sexual function and encourage a willingness to experiment with alternative methods of expressing one's sexuality. Persons with the fewest inhibiting attitudes and greatest willingness to use alternative methods have the most potential to achieve a satisfactory sexual life-style.

TYPES OF DISABILITY ACCORDING TO THEIR IMPACT ON SEXUAL FUNCTION

Cole and Cole[12] suggested that severe disabilities can be grouped into four types with respect to their impact on sexual function. Type I disabilities are nonprogressive and occur at birth or before puberty. Examples include congenital loss of sight or hearing, spina bifida, and mental retardation. Persons with these disabilities often fail to encounter the social learning opportunities associated with adolescent sexual development. This occurs for various reasons, including overprotective parents and societal ambivalence about sexuality training for developmentally disabled persons. The naive belief, associated with this group to an even greater degree than for nondisabled persons, is that sexuality education will be interpreted as an endorsement and thus increase the frequency of sexual behavior.

Type II disabilities also begin before puberty but are progressive. Examples include cystic fibrosis, muscular dystrophy, diabetes mellitus, and juvenile rheumatoid arthritis. Persons with these disabilities find it difficult to establish a stable body image and constantly face the uncertainty of further physical deterioration. As in the case of persons with type I disabilities, these persons frequently miss important socializing opportunities of a psychosexual nature.

Type III disabilities occur after adolescence and are nonprogressive. These stable, late-onset disabilities include spinal cord injury (discussed below), amputation, and burns. Affected persons have gone through the socializing experiences connected with adolescence and often have engaged in various sexual behaviors. They have developed the interpersonal skills required to initiate and maintain intimate social relationships, particularly of a sexual nature. After injury, their task is to adapt already developed skills in order to maximize the likelihood of a fulfilling sexual life-style.

Type IV disabilities include progressive degenerative diseases and are usually found in older adults. These disabilities include arthritis, multiple sclerosis,[13] heart disease, stroke, cancer, and chronic renal disease. Affected patients usually have a long history of intimate relationships. They face the problem of coping with either a discrete event or slow deterioration that may impair their intellectual and physical ability to communicate sexually. Others face negligible impairments but may harbor fear of further losses should they engage in strenuous physical activity. These fears coupled with the necessity of frequent medical interventions often result in marked changes in sexual behavior.

SEXUAL CONCERNS OF PERSONS WITH SPINAL CORD INJURY

Spinal cord injury is a disability with widespread impact in all areas of sexual functioning. Currently, approximately 250,000 persons in the United States have a spinal cord injury. About four-fifths of these persons are male, and most are in their early twenties at the time of injury. Hohmann[14] provided data suggesting that male patients with spinal cord injury may have some reduction in sex drive, possibly due to disruption of the autonomic nervous system. Many of his subjects reported reduced sexual interest and fewer sexual feelings. The author concluded that the quality of the relationship with the partner becomes a critical issue in maintaining sexual activity after injury.

The sexual behaviors of male and female patients with spinal cord injury are often significantly altered by the disability.[15-17] Male patients have two types of potential erections after injury: psychogenic and reflexogenic. Psychogenic erections result primarily from mental stimulation and occur in approximately 30% of male patients with lower motor neuron lesions; they are absent in those with complete upper motor neuron lesions. Although these patients may emit sperm, few have an actual ejaculation. Reflexogenic erections result when an external stimulus is applied to the genitals or pelvic area. These erections occur in 90% of male patients with upper motor neuron lesions. Ejaculation in these patients is also rare. Those unable to achieve a usable erection have the option of obtaining a penile prosthesis; these have proved useful, but their reliability remains a concern.[18,19]

All male patients with a complete spinal cord injury usually become infertile because of reduced sperm motility and viability soon after injury. Women with spinal cord injury remain fertile; menstruation usually resumes 2 to 3 months after injury. Both sexes report the loss of orgasm as experienced before injury. Some describe the presence of a "phantom orgasm"; this consists of a buildup of muscle tension accompanied by pleasurable sensations in body areas that are still innervated followed by a feeling of relaxation. Sexual behaviors of persons with spinal cord injury are usually altered because of limitations in body movements. If the partner who incurs the injury was previously the most active, significant changes in roles may be needed. Sexual positions may have to be changed and new methods of stimulating the partner used.[15]

The effect of spinal cord injury on a person's sexuality and the resulting social and economic changes place tremendous stress on any already established relationship. Studies examining marriage among persons with spinal cord injury are confounded by several factors, including the amount of time since the onset of disability. Several studies of male veterans suggest that divorce rates are not significantly different from those of nondisabled persons.[20,21] A recent study of a civilian sample, however, showed that persons with spinal cord injury have fewer marriages and more divorces than the general population.[22] Divorce was more likely if the person with spinal cord injury was young, female, black, childless, previously divorced, or more dependent in self-care activities. Data from another nonveteran sample suggested that persons who married after injury were happier and more satisfied than those married before injury.[23]

SEXUAL COUNSELING: PLISSIT MODEL

All physicians, physiatrists in particular, are in a central position to detect and provide help to patients with sexually related concerns. Studies have shown that persons who have sexually related difficulties typically turn to either their physician or their pastor. Until the relatively recent introduction of sexual medicine into the curriculum of medical schools, few physicians had any specific training to deal with these concerns.

Effectiveness with sexual concerns requires that physicians have a thorough understanding of their own sexual values, a knowledge of sexual function and dysfunction, and the interpersonal skills to establish rapport and obtain a sexual history. Wiens and Brazman[24] stated that taking a sexual history produces a therapeutic effect by giving the patient permission to be sexual, filling knowledge gaps, and providing reality-based feedback. Estimates are that as many as half of all sexual concerns can be ameliorated through the provision of information alone. Physicians are often ambivalent when asking about sexuality concerns. Annon and Robinson[6] described a simple yet useful model to help guide interventions for sexual concerns primarily related to response difficulties connected with orgasm, arousal, or desire. The system is the PLISSIT model or, more accurately, the P–LI–SS–IT model. The letters refer to three levels of brief therapy—*p*ermission, *l*imited *i*nformation, and *s*pecific *s*uggestions— and a fourth level of *i*ntensive *t*herapy.

The first and most basic level of intervention is permission. Often, disabled individuals seek a knowledgeable person in a position of authority to listen to their sexual concerns, reassure them that they are not unique or unusual, and, in most instances, provide permission to continue doing what they have been doing. This level of intervention may provide reassurance and affirm the individual as a sexual being. Permission is most appropriate when directed toward a patient's thoughts, fantasies, feelings, and sexual acts. Permission should be limited to activities that do not carry the risk of being dangerous or illegal.

Limited information entails provision of specific information relevant to a sexual concern. This level of intervention seeks to remove sexual myths that may be the basis of much anxiety and fear. Such myths might include issues such as genital size, masturbation, sexual frequency, and sexual performance. Disabled persons might need information about alternative methods of giving and receiving sexual pleasure, changes in sexual response secondary to disease or medications, and fertility. The focus of this intervention is on information directly relevant to the client's concerns.

The final level of brief therapy involves providing specific suggestions. The first step in this process is to obtain a limited history about the sexual problem. This history would include items such as a description of the problem, information about problem onset and course, the client's concept of cause and maintenance of the problem, past treatment outcome, and current expectations and goals of treatment. Once this history is obtained, specific interventions are provided that have proved helpful and usually reliable for ameliorating a particular problem. Descriptions of these interventions are available in standard texts of sexual therapy. These interventions are usually simple, have a behavioral focus, and emphasize the necessity to engage in practice sessions alone or with a partner at home.

Intensive therapy is usually initiated for sexual problems other than those related to sexual response, such as sexual identity problems.[25] Because few persons require intensive therapy, physicians are less likely to encounter them. This level of intervention involves obtaining a comprehensive developmental history of the patient or partner or both. The goal is to define a person's sexual identity, behaviors, and fantasies thoroughly. Therapeutic intervention in such cases is usually lengthy, involves multiple areas of sexual functioning, and is usually done by a therapist having extensive training and appropriate credentials.

In summary, the PLISSIT model provides a method for conceptualizing appropriate levels of intervention for the physician. Given the likelihood that persons will expect their physician to be knowledgeable about sexual function, the physician must have appropriate self-knowledge and factual knowledge to guide the patient appropriately. All physicians working with physically disabled patients can achieve the skills needed for the first two levels of therapy—permission and limited information. Some may have further training and develop the skills needed to intervene at the third level—specific suggestions. Problems requiring intensive therapy require referral to appropriate sources.

REFERENCES

1. Eisenberg MG, Rustad LC. Sex education and counseling program on a spinal cord injury service. Arch Phys Med Rehabil 1976; 57:135–140.
2. Robinault IP. Sex, society, and the disabled: a developmental inquiry into roles, reactions, and responsibilities. Hagerstown, Maryland: Harper & Row, 1978.
3. Romano MD, Lassiter RE. Sexual counseling with the spinal-cord injured. Arch Phys Med Rehabil 1972; 53:568–572.
4. Daniels SM, Nowinski J. Sexuality and disability. New York: Human Sciences Press, 1978.
5. Hanson RW, Franklin MR. Sexual loss in relation to other functional losses for spinal cord injured males. Arch Phys Med Rehabil 1976; 57:291–293.
6. Annon JS, Robinson CH. Treatment of common male and female sexual concerns. In: Ferguson JM, Taylor CB, eds. The comprehensive handbook of behavioral medicine. Vol 1. New York: SP Medical & Scientific Books, 1980:273–296.
7. Godow AG. Human sexuality. St. Louis: CV Mosby, 1982.
8. Leiblum SR, Pervin LA, eds. Principles and practice of sex therapy. New York: Guilford Press, 1980.

9. Griffith ER, Trieschmann RB, Hohmann GW, Cole TM, Tobis JS, Cummings V. Sexual dysfunctions associated with physical disabilities. Arch Phys Med Rehabil 1975; 56:8–13.
10. Ford CS, Beach FA. Patterns of sexual behavior. New York: Harper & Brothers, 1951.
11. Berkman AH, Weissman R, Frielich MH. Sexual adjustment of spinal cord injured veterans living in the community. Arch Phys Med Rehabil 1978; 59:29–33.
12. Cole TM, Cole SS. Sexual adjustment to chronic disease and disability. In: Stolov WC, Clowers MR, eds. Handbook of severe disability. Washington DC: United States Department of Education, Government Printing Office, 1981:279–288.
13. Barrett M. Sexuality and multiple sclerosis. New York: National Multiple Sclerosis Society, 1982.
14. Hohmann GW. Some effects of spinal cord lesions on experienced emotional feelings. Psychophysiology 1966; 3:143–156.
15. Mooney TO, Cole TM, Chilgren RA. Sexual options for paraplegics and quadraplegics. Boston: Little, Brown & Company, 1975.
16. Narum GD, Rodolfa ER. Sex therapy for the spinal cord injured client: suggestions for professionals. Prof Psychol Res Pract 1984; 15:775–784.
17. Trieschmann RB. Spinal cord injuries: psychological, social and vocational adjustment. New York: Pergamon Press, 1980.
18. Beutler LE, Scott FB, Karacan I, Baer PE, Rogers RR Jr, Morris J. Women's satisfaction with partners' penile implant: inflatable vs noninflatable prosthesis. Urology 1984; 24:552–558.
19. Fallon B, Rosenberg S, Culp DA. Long-term followup in patients with an inflatable penile prosthesis. J Urol 1984; 132:270–271.
20. Comarr AE. Marriage and divorce among patients with spinal cord injury I. J Indian Med Prof 1962; 9:4353–4359.
21. El Ghatit AZ, Hanson RW. Marriage and divorce after spinal cord injury. Arch Phys Med Rehabil 1976; 57:470–472.
22. DeVivo MJ, Fine PR. Spinal cord injury: its short-term impact on marital status. Arch Phys Med Rehabil 1985; 66:501–504.
23. Hoch Z. Sex therapy and marital counseling for the disabled. Arch Phys Med Rehabil 1977; 58:413–415.
24. Wiens A, Brazman R. A rationale and method for the sexual history in family practice. J Fam Pract 1977; 5:213–215.
25. Annon JS. Behavior treatment of sexual problems: brief therapy. Hagerstown, Maryland: Harper & Row, 1976.

5 EXAMINATION OF JOINTS

John L. Merritt, M.D., F.A.C.P.
Mehrsheed Sinaki, M.D.

A prerequisite for the examination of any part or system of the human body is a thorough understanding of that part's anatomy and function for correct examination, recording, and interpretation. This chapter is not a review of joint anatomy or function because excellent texts on these subjects are already available; instead, this chapter is intended to present principles of joint examination that will assist the examiner in obtaining and interpreting the results.

An incomplete and inaccurate examination can result from the imposing number of human joints and the prodigious extent of joint landmarks, functions, and signs. All these factors may provide a setting for random and careless joint evaluation. The best guard against such is to develop a "routine" or system, whether the evaluation is of 1, 10, or 174 joints.

METHODICAL EXAMINATION

Adherence to a methodical evaluation is essential when a thorough examination of joints is needed.[1] Whether one begins with the upper extremities and then proceeds to the trunk and then the lower extremities or the reverse can often be determined by personal choice, patient position, or convenience, but variation in the order of examination should only rarely be the case. Deviations from one's established routine invite oversights and errors. The following sequence is suggested. With the patient standing, the lower back should be examined first, including the sacrum, coccyx, and sacroiliac and lumbar spine. The thoracic spine should be examined next; the patient will need to lie down to complete this part of the evaluation. Then the patient sits on the edge of the examination table or bed. The neck, skull, and temporomandibular joints are examined. The upper extremities are next approached, proceeding from proximal to distal joints. Finally, the lower extremities are examined, also from proximal to distal. Whether examining the back, neck, or upper or lower extremities, each joint pair should be symmetrically evaluated, first the right side and then the left (the "right first rule")—with one exception, which is described below. Measurements are recorded similarly: right/left (for example, knees [passive]: 5° to 110°/15° to 75°).

MOTION

Joint motion should be determined before the joints are palpated.[2,3] Range of motion should include first active motion, then active assisted or passive motion. When the range is abnormal, goniometry (for peripheral joints) or skin distraction measurements (for the spine) should be added.[4,5] Motions that cause pain and painful arcs of motion should be noted and recorded. After active and passive motions have been recorded, resistance to active motion (this may also serve as an evaluation of muscle strength) and any pain caused by isometric contractions are noted.[6] Although strength assessment includes appraisal of active, against-gravity movements, strength determination concludes with isometric resistance.

In patients with suspected or known arthritis, bursitis, or tendinitis, it is essential for the examiner to position himself or herself so as not to be overcome and not to allow movement during testing of resistance to motion.[7-9] Isometric resistance is usually tolerated, but painful isotonic movements are unwarranted and uncomfortable and may interfere with the remainder of the examination. Every effort should be made to ensure as little discomfort as possible.[1] If the examination is unnecessarily painful, patient trust and confidence in the examiner are undermined and assessment of relaxed, passive motions becomes impossible. This mistrust may even spill over into poor compliance to treatment recommendations and thus sabotage the very purpose of the joint examination.

In this light, whenever joint pain is reported to be asymmetric, relaxed passive examination of *the least painful side* should be performed first in order to enhance trust between patient and examiner and to allow the patient a better understanding of what motion or activity is to be attempted. This is the single exception to the "right first rule." A simple explanation to the patient before each step as to what is to be performed and what is to be examined aids the patient and examiner. Pain, muscle spasm, and splinting are thus minimized. When active assisted or passive movements are to be performed, a gentle, careful grip that supports the painful joint and avoids other tender areas is essential.

LIMITATION OF MOTION

When evaluating joint motion, one is, of course, already formulating a differential diagnosis. During this time, keep in mind that the causes of limitation of joint motion generally fall into one of four categories.[10]

The first cause of limitation of joint motion is contractures. Contractures may be caused by the shortening of collagen fibers in muscle, tendon, ligaments, or, most frequently, the joint capsule itself. Capsular contractures (adhesive capsulitis) are a common consequence of infrequent or incomplete ranging of joints and often of surgical procedures, trauma, arthritis, tendinitis, bursitis, or neuromuscular disorders. Ligamentous contractures have similar broad causes but are more significant in the neck and back than in peripheral joints. Tendon and muscle contractures are often considered congruous, but careful studies have shown that these contractures are predominately intramuscular and that associated tendons themselves are not frequently contracted.

Motion limited by contractures has a special "feel" when the joint is passively moved.[6,8] This has been called a soft "end-feel" and is a slow gradual resilience at the end of an arc of passive motion. This is in contrast to the hard "end-feel" or "block" at the end of an arc of motion described below.

The second cause is capsular distention.[10] Joint capsules allow full arcs of joint motion only because of the existence of large, lax capsular redundancies (Fig. 5–1). These capsular redundancies may restrict motion not only when they are contracted (for example, adhesive capsulitis) but also when they are distended by fluid or synovial proliferation. This is the primary cause of loss of motion in inflammatory arthritis and after trauma. The capsular redundancies are already tense, and further movement of the joint is thus limited by the already taut, interlaced capsular collagen fibers. Further movement will thus only cause pain or tears of the joint capsule fibers.

The third cause is intra-articular loose bodies, which may limit joint motion by mechanically impinging on joint surfaces. Torn menisci, synovial plicae, loose cartilaginous fragments, and villonodular synovitis are some examples of intra-articular loose bodies.

The fourth cause is cartilaginous incongruity. Degenerative or inflammatory erosion of joint surface cartilage is the frequent cause. The resulting lack of a smooth surface for joint approximation may result in a sudden barrier to motion. Both intra-articular loose bodies and cartilaginous incongruity usually have a hard "end-feel"—the joint comes to an abrupt halt and does not move as further slow, gentle, unidirectional pressure is applied.[6]

Limitation of joint motion may, of course, and frequently does, result from combinations of these four causes. For example, traumatic hemarthrosis may restrict motion by capsular distention, but a torn meniscus may also be present. As the hemarthrosis resolves

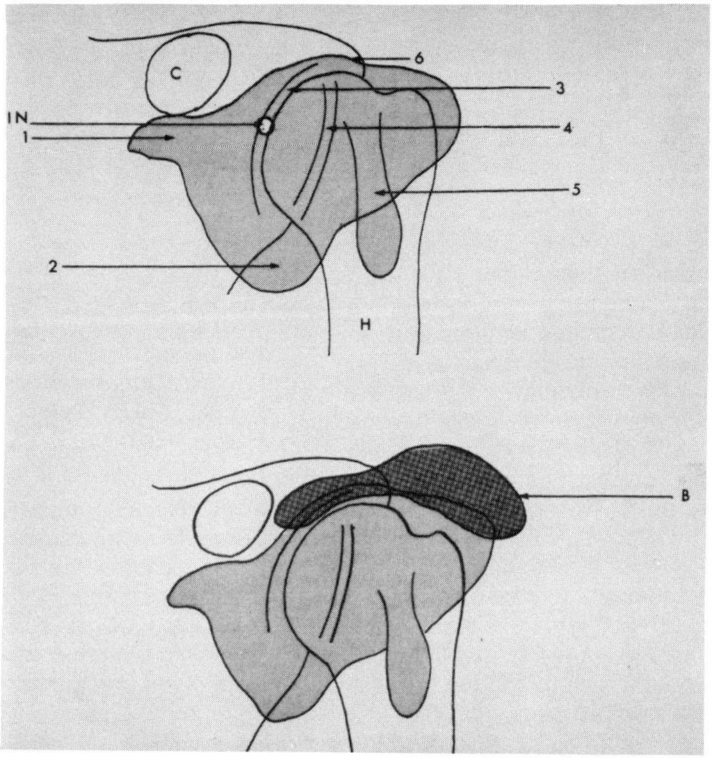

Figure 5–1 Arthrograms. Shaded area on shoulder joint depicts normal arthrogram. C, Coracoid process; H, humerus; IN, anterior site of injection into glenohumeral joint. (1) Subscapular bursa that normally communicates directly with shoulder joint and thus fills in normal arthrogram. As dye injection distends capsule, it hangs as dependent pouch under joint 2. (3) Superior medial surface of humerus. (4) Line of lesser density caused by underlying glenoid labrum. (5) Synovial lining that is pouch accompanying biceps tendon sheath in intertubercular groove a distance of some 2 inches. (6) Subacromial bursa and rotator cuff. Rotator cuff tear will permit dye to extend into subacromial bursa, superior to smooth line above humeral head, above and "around corner" of greater tuberosity, B. (From Cailliet R. Shoulder pain. Philadelphia: FA Davis, 1966:61. By permission.)

but motion continues to be restricted by cast, splint, pain, or inactivity, the joint capsule may contract as the joint fluid is absorbed.[10] An adhesive capsulitis may be the consequence.[9] Degenerative joint disease may limit motion by joint surface incongruity, but associated degenerative meniscal fragments may further limit motion. Pain and inactivity may concomitantly contribute to a superimposed joint capsule contracture. However, because the treatment strategies for each of the four categories of limitation of motion are divergent, understanding the contribution of each will promote a more logical and efficacious therapeutic plan. The physical examination of the joint is essential for development of such a therapeutic plan.

PALPATION

Palpation should be performed only after active, passive, and resistive joint motions have been assessed. Palpation should include joint margins, synovium, bursae, and accessible tendons. Palpation includes an appraisal of swelling, tenderness, stability, crepitation, deformities, and "joint play."[1,8]

The synovium is the soft tissue of the joint proper. Normal synovium is not palpable because it is only a few cells in thickness. A swollen synovial membrane has a "boggy" feel, somewhat like the feel of modeling clay or fresh dough.[1,7] An inflammatory arthritis is synonymous with synovitis. Synovitis is readily palpated. Therefore, learning to "feel" synovial thickening is a fundamental skill for the diagnosis of arthritis. A thickened, inflamed synovial membrane is readily palpable to the experienced examiner in all extremity joints from the elbow and knee distally. Practice is required to appreciate swollen, proliferative synovium, but this skill is not difficult to achieve with practice and frequent comparison with normal joints.

Synovial fluid is present in a normal joint in such minute quantities that it, like normal synovium, also is not palpable.[1] Palpation of fluid in a joint is abnormal and usually associated with synovitis. Joint fluid (effusion) may be obvious by visual or palpatory inspection. Fluid may be further identified by applying pressure over the joint and observing a readily reducible bulge at the margins of the joint.

Crepitations are grating vibrations that may be palpated or sometimes heard during motion. They result from cartilaginous roughening from degenerative or, less frequently, inflammatory processes. Inflammatory or degenerative changes in tendons and associated structures, however, may also produce crepitations. Of less significance is joint "snapping" due to tendon and ligament slipping over bony surfaces during motion. The stability of the supporting ligamentous structures should next be determined by passive joint manipulation. Specific techniques are available for each joint. Deformities of bony architecture, contractures, and articular subluxations should be noted and recorded.

"JOINT PLAY"

In addition to testing ligamentous stability by specific relaxed passive joint manipulation techniques, minor joint motions should also be estimated. A typical joint has major and minor motions.[5,6,8] Major motions may include flexion, extension, adduction, abduction, or rotation.[5] All joints also have minor motion, called "joint play."[8] This small motion is a passive gliding motion perpendicular to and along the axis of the articulating bones (Fig. 5–2). Restrictions of joint play motions are associated with tight joint capsules and intra-articular obstructions.[6] These minor joint motion restrictions, restrictions of joint play, are the basis for spinal and peripheral joint mobilization and manipulation techniques.[8]

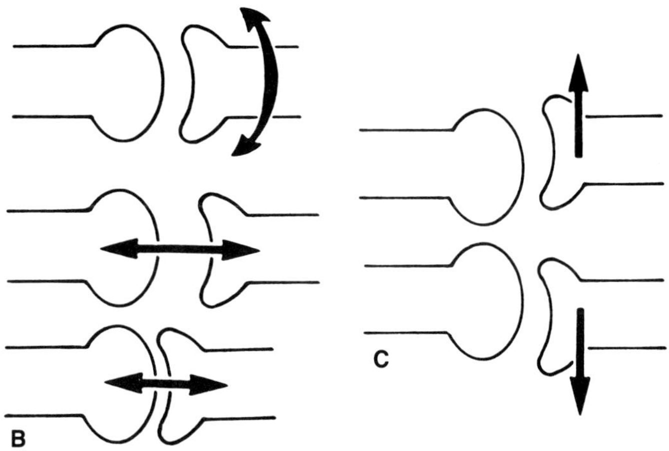

Figure 5–2 Joint play. *A*, Major motions: flexion, extension, and rotation. *B*, Longitudinal minor motion. *C*, Transitional, gliding, minor motion.

THE RECORDING CHART

Collection of a large amount of data can lead to a record that is unwieldy and difficult to review.[2,3] However, a permanent record of all joint examinations is essential for prescribing and monitoring treatment. A convenient and useful charting system, the STL system, has been in use at the Mayo Clinic for many years (Fig. 5–3).[1] "S" indicates synovitis (objective and palpable synovial swelling or synovial effusion), "T" denotes joint tenderness, and "L" designates limitation of motion. "S," "T," and "L" can all be graded from 1 to 4: grade 1 is the slightest detectable involvement, grades 2 and 3 are moderate to severe abnormalities, and grade 4 is the most severe (rarely used) grade. Motions of the shoulder, elbow, wrist, fingers, knee, and ankle are often recorded more precisely by goniometry, when abnormal. Incomplete finger flexion can also be recorded in centimeters of flexion lag from the end of the nail bed to the transverse palmar crease. Thoracic and lumbar motions are best recorded with a motion diagram, onto which one can record grades of motion (0 to 4) and color in the arcs that are painful.[6] Traditional goniometry of thoracolumbar spine motion is an inaccurate and worthless effort. The skin distraction

Name ______________________________ Date ______________________

Joint	Right (Rt.) S	T	L	Comments	Left (Lt.) S	T	L	Comments
T-M	0	0	0		0	0	0	
S-C	0	0	0		0	0	0	
M-S	0	0	0					
A-C	0	0	0		0	0	0	
Sh	0	2		Abd. 60° (or grade 1+) Ext. rot. 60° (or grade 1+) Int. rot. 60° (or grade 1+)	0	0	0	
Elb	0	0	0		0	0	0	
Wr	1+	1−		Dorsiflexion 35° (or grade 2)	0	0	0	
MCP	0	0	0	Fist 100% (MCP, PIP, DIP) MCP_2	1	1−	0	Fist 100% (MCP, PIP, DIP)
PIP	0	0	0	PIP_2	1+	0	0	
DIP	0	0	0		0	0	0	
Hip	0	0	0		0	0	0	
Kn	1	1		Ext. 15° (or grade 1) Flex. 115° (or grade 1)	0	0	0	
Ank	0	0	0		0	0	0	
S-T	0	0	0		0	0	0	
MTP	0	0	0	MTP_2	1	1	0	
PIP	0	0	0		0	0	0	
DIP	0	0	0		0	0	0	

Spine

	T	L
Cervical		
Atlas (vertebrae 1 & 2)	T_0	L_0
Vertebrae 3–7	T_0	L_0
Thoracic		
Costochondral	T_0	L_0
Chest expansion	12.5 cm	
Lumbar	T_0	L_0
Lumbosacral	T_0	L_0
Sacroiliac	T_0	
Coccyx	T_0	

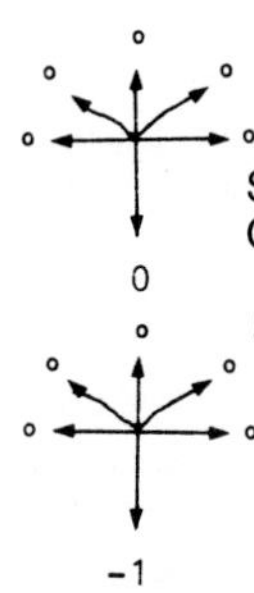

Spine flexion: C7-S1 = 8.5 cm

Schober = 5.0 cm

Posture_Mild upper thoracic rounding

Gait_Normal

Examiner ______________________

Figure 5–3 Example of chart used to record results of joint examination. Joints: T-M, temporomandibular; S-C, sternoclavicular; M-S, manubriosternal; A-C, acromioclavicular; Sh, shoulder; Elb, elbow; Wr, wrist; MCP, metacarpophalangeal; PIP, proximal interphalangeal; DIP, distal interphalangeal; Kn, knee; Ank, ankle; S-T, subtalar; MTP, metatarsophalangeal. Finding: S, swelling; T, tenderness; L, limitation of motion. (From Polley and Hunder.[1] By permission of the publisher.)

methods of Martin[1] (C7–S1 distraction during flexion) and of Schober (Fig. 5–4) and the inclinometer method of Loebl (Fig. 5–5) (lumbar spine) are the most convenient and reproducible objective clinical measurements of spine motion.[4]

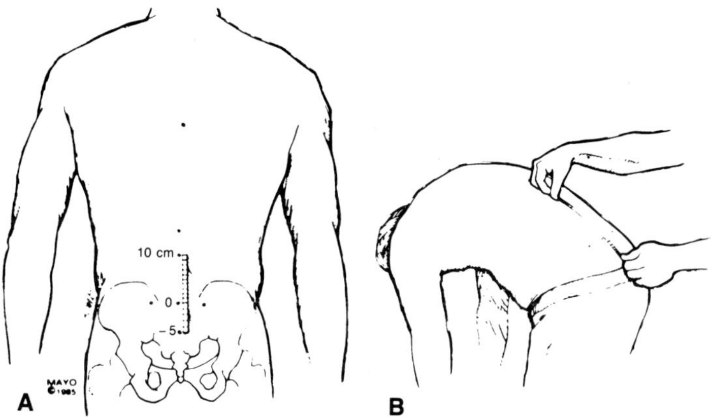

Figure 5–4 Modified Schober flexion test. *A*, With subject standing erect but relaxed, top of sacrum ("0") is identified by spinal intersection of horizontal line joining dimples of Venus (denoted by small circular marks to left and right of zero), and points 10 cm above and 5 cm below are marked. *B*, Subject bends forward maximally, and distance between the upper and lower marks is measured in centimeters. This value minus 15 is amount of lumbar flexion. (From Merritt et al.[4] By permission of Mayo Foundation.)

TENDINITIS AND BURSITIS

The most common joint symptom is pain. Most joint pain is not from arthritis but from tendinitis and bursitis. Because the prognoses and therapies for arthritis, bursitis, and tendinitis are different, distinguishing these disorders is important. A regard to some simple observations, however, can help to differentiate them.[6] Pain is produced by active and passive motions in all planes in the presence of significant synovitis. In contrast, tendinitis produces pain primarily with active and resistive motions but not with, or as intensely with, passive motion, and then only in planes where the tendon or its associated muscle is placed under tension. Pain

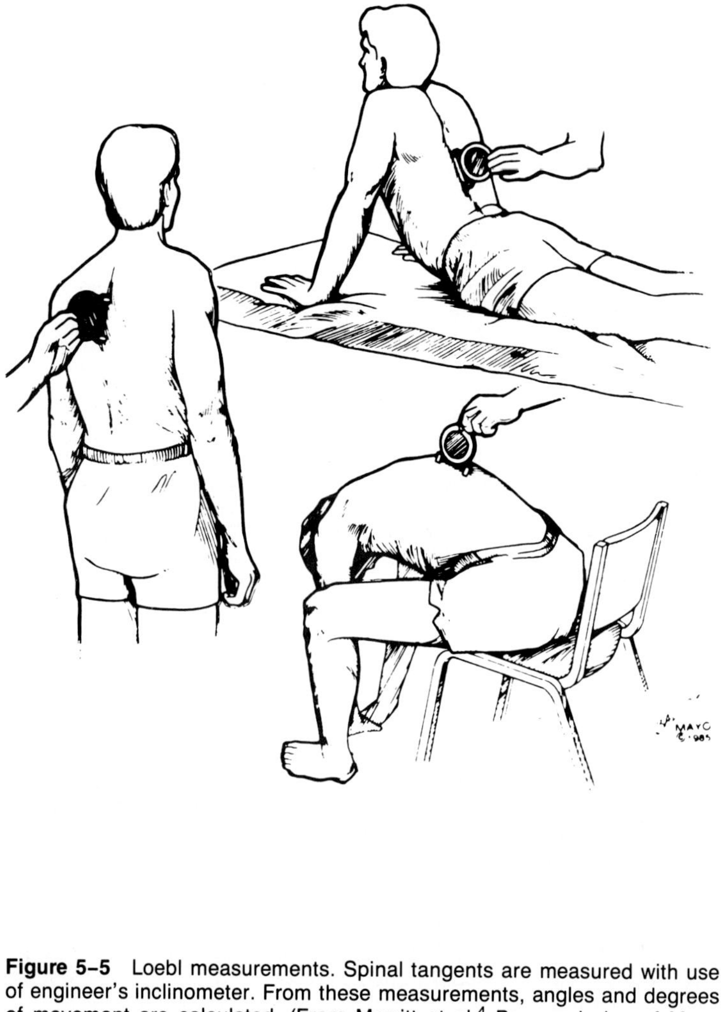

Figure 5–5 Loebl measurements. Spinal tangents are measured with use of engineer's inclinometer. From these measurements, angles and degrees of movement are calculated. (From Merritt et al.[4] By permission of Mayo Foundation.)

can be elicited by isometric resistance in tendinitis (Fig. 5–6). Bursitis is associated with painful arcs of active and passive motion but not with isometric resistance. Thus, if one observes active and then passive movements and finally isometric resistance to that motion, the differentiation is clearer. Confirmation can then be established by direct palpation.

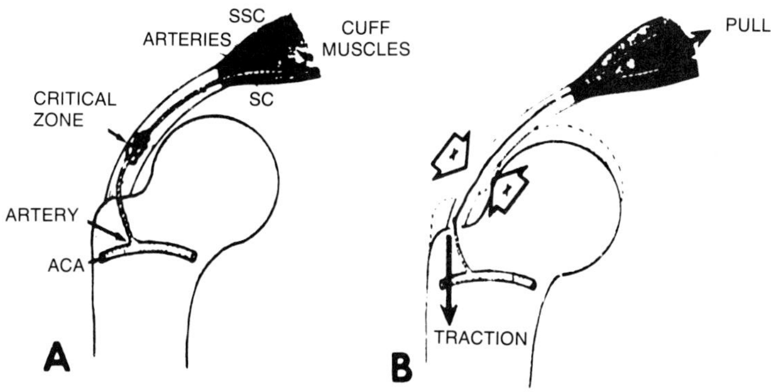

Figure 5–6 Blood circulation. *A*, Circulation to rotator cuff. Arterial branch from anterior circumflex artery (ACA) enters from bone. Suprascapular (SSC) and subscapular (SC) branches merge to enter from muscle. Critical zone of tendon is anastomosis that is patent when arm is supported and inactive. *B*, Traction on cuff from dependent arm or from pull of contracting cuff muscle elongates tendon and renders critical zone (arrows) relatively ischemic. (From Cailliet.[9] By permission of the publisher.)

As an example, if one noted shoulder and arm pain with active shoulder abduction but not with passive abduction or active flexion, supraspinatus tendinitis would be suspected.[6] Shoulder arthritis and subacromial bursitis (both are causes of shoulder pain during active abduction) would be less likely diagnoses. Further confirmation of the diagnosis of supraspinatus tendinitis could (and should) be made by isometrically resisting abduction while the arm is in an abducted and internally rotated position. Finally, palpation of the supraspinatus tendon is performed with the shoulder in internal rotation, adduction, and extension. Subacromial bursitis would produce pain on active and passive abduction but not with isometric resistance to abduction and not with active or passive shoulder flexion.

Lateral epicondylitis ("tennis elbow," common extensor tendinitis) should, likewise, be established not only by direct palpation but also by reproduction of pain during active and resisted wrist extension and supination. Medial epicondylitis ("golfer's elbow") should similarly be confirmed by resisted wrist pronation and flexion.

SHOULDER IMPINGEMENT SYNDROME

The impingement syndrome is a common shoulder syndrome that results from the unique characteristics of the rotator cuff muscle groups.[9] The supraspinatus muscle is a major shoulder abductor, but it also, during active contraction, pulls the head of the humerus inferiorly into the inferior portion of the glenoid. This active muscular contraction may, however, be disrupted in conditions of cuff degeneration, rupture, or tears. When this mechanism fails to pull the head downward and the humerus is rotated, the greater tuberosity impinges on the acromion, trapping the intervening supraspinatus tendon and subacromial bursa (Fig. 5–7). Repeated impingement results in trauma and further inflammatory changes in these structures, which in turn result in edema and swelling in these structures, which further increase impingement with less abduction.

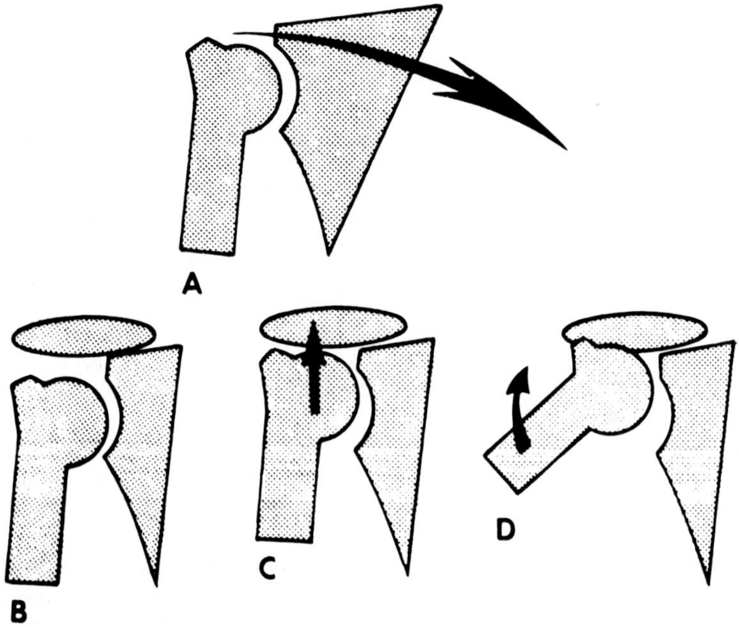

Figure 5–7 Impingement syndrome. *A*, Supraspinatus muscle and tendon abduct and set head of humerus inferiorly into glenoid. *B*, Normal, relaxed relationship. *C*, Defective rotator cuff results in superior gliding of humerus in glenoid. *D*, Impingement of greater tuberosity on inferior surface of acromion.

PRINCIPLES OF GONIOMETRY

The method of measuring and recording joint motion as presented here is based on the principles of the neutral zero method described by Cave and Roberts in 1936.[11] In this method, all motions of the joint are measured from a defined zero starting position. Thus, the degrees of motion of the joint are added in the direction of the joint motion from this position. The extended "anatomic position" of an extremity is, therefore, accepted as 0° rather than 180°.

GENERAL PRINCIPLES OF MEASUREMENT OF RANGE OF MOTION OF JOINTS

The instrument used is called a goniometer (Fig. 5–8). It consists of two rigid shafts that intersect at a hinged joint.[5] The protractor is fixed to the shafts so that motion can be read directly from the scale in degrees. The axis of the goniometer should coincide with the appropriate axis of motion in the joint being measured. This point can be determined by moving the joint through the range of motion and visually estimating the site of rotation. The shaft of the goniometer should be aligned parallel to the long axis of limb segments that are associated with the joint being measured. One of these segments must be stabilized for an accurate reading of the actual joint motion. The "starting position" in Figures 5–9 through 5–27 is defined as the point at which the movable segment is at 0°.[12] With minor exceptions, this is also the anatomic position. If the subject has a limitation of motion that prevents assuming the starting position, this is recorded as the number of degrees from zero. (Example: Normal flexion of the elbow is expressed as 150°. In the case of a flexion contracture, the reading might be 15° to 150°. If the subject has excessive mobility beyond the starting position, this reading is expressed as a negative value from the zero position. This is frequent in the elbow and the knee and is sometimes termed "hyperextension.") The "measurement" is defined as the reading on the scale that reflects the maximal amount of motion available in a joint in a given plane of orientation. Two types of substitution that must be avoided in measurement are (1) deviation from the plane of motion and (2) movement of the limb segment designated as the baseline. When recording data, the motion should be indicated as passive or active.

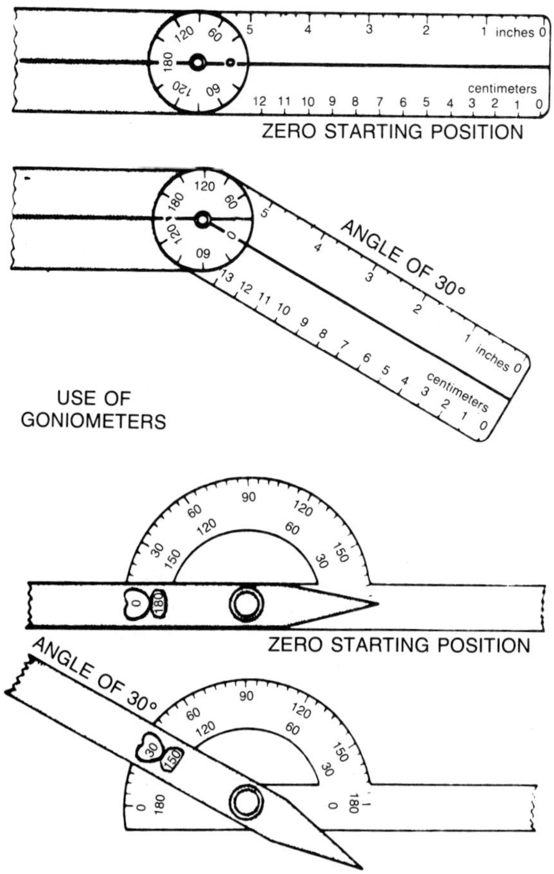

Figure 5–8 After the landmarks of a joint are defined, the goniometer is used to measure motion. (From Measuring and recording of joint motion.[12] By permission of the publisher.)

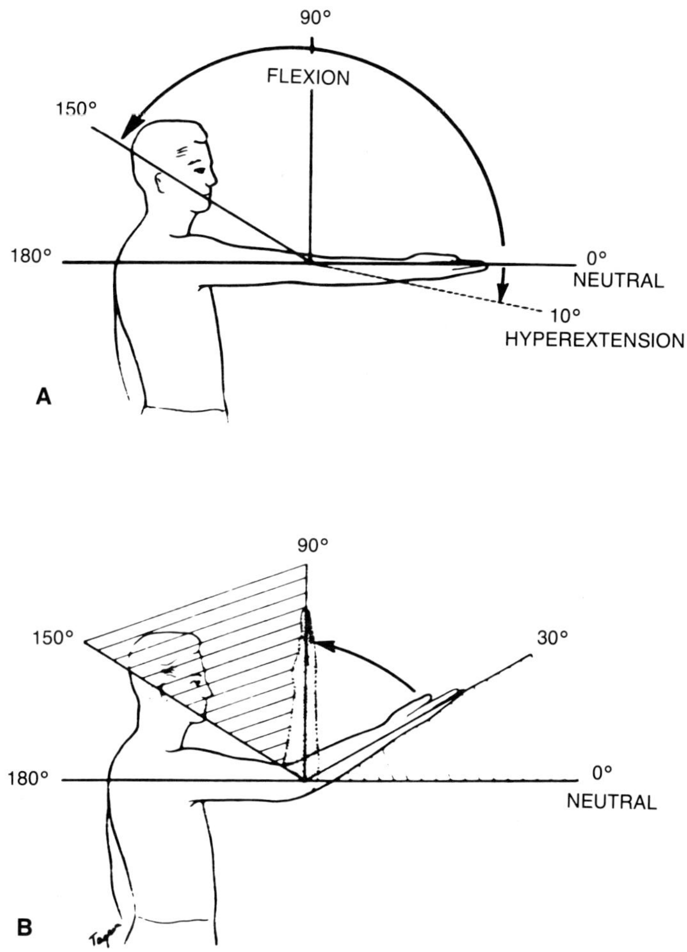

Figure 5–9 Elbow. *A*, Flexion and hyperextension. *B*, Limited motion. Unshaded area is range of limited motion. (From Measuring and recording of joint motion.[12] By permission of the publisher.)

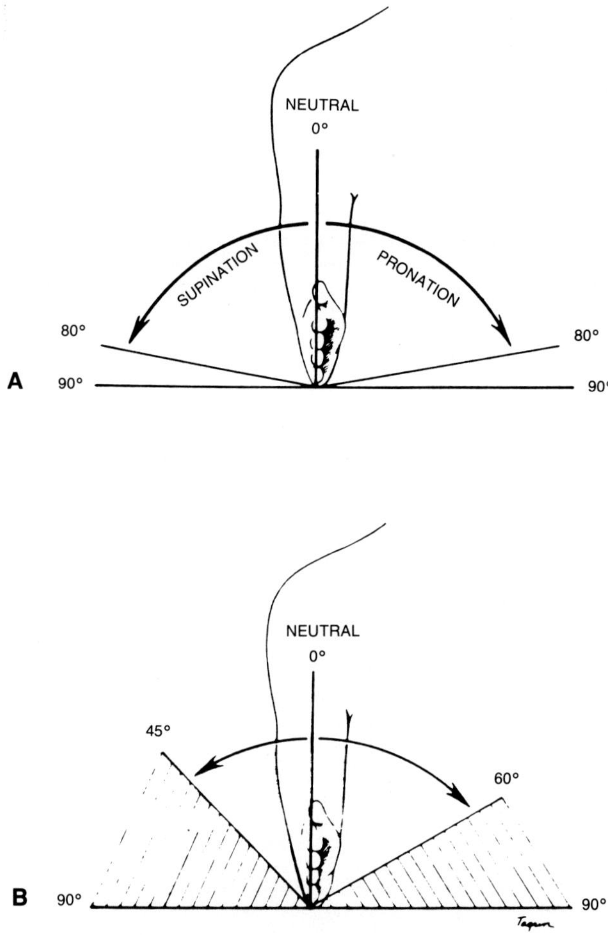

Figure 5–10 Forearm. *A*, Pronation and supination. *B*, Limited motion. Unshaded area is range of limited motion. (From Measuring and recording of joint motion.[12] By permission of the publisher.)

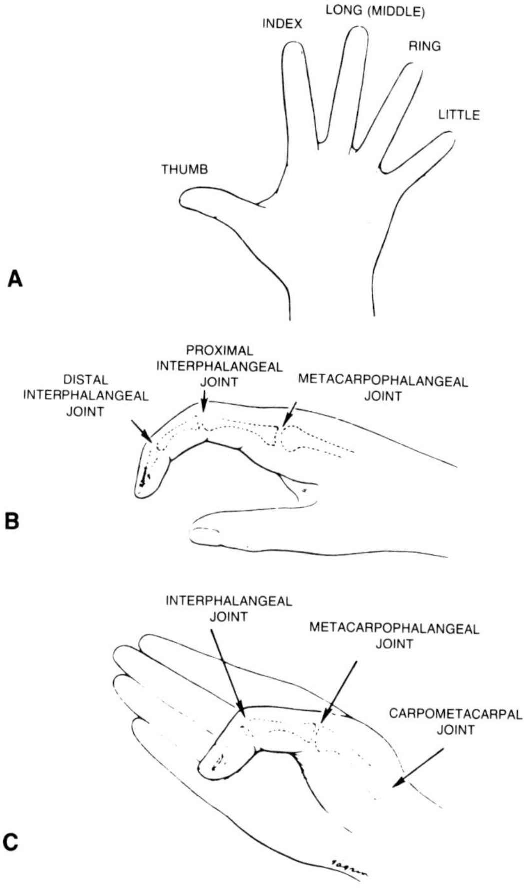

Figure 5–11 Hand. *A*, Nomenclature for fingers. *B*, Joints of fingers. *C*, Joints of thumb. (From Measuring and recording of joint motion.[12] By permission of the publisher.)

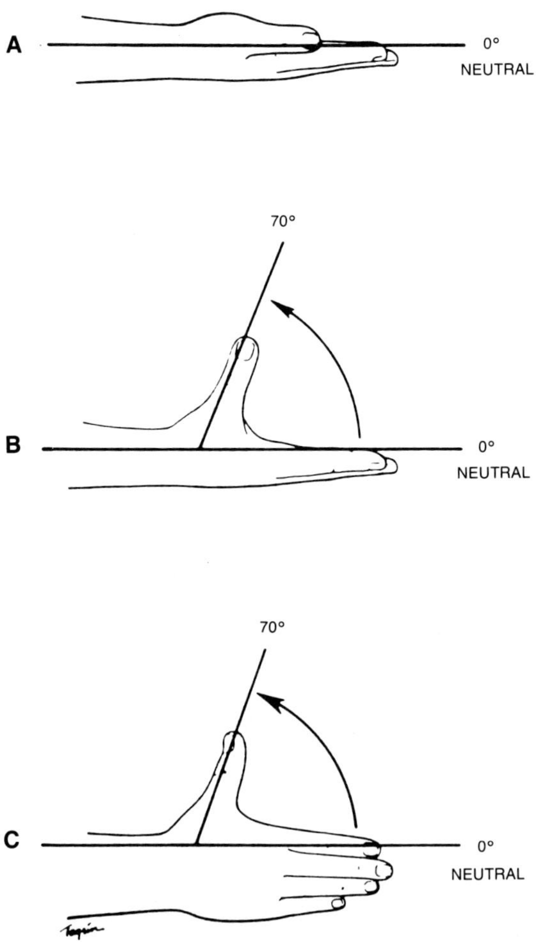

Figure 5–12 Thumb, abduction. *A*, Zero starting position. *B*, Abduction at right angle to plane of palm. *C*, Abduction parallel to plane of palm (abduction-extension). (From Measuring and recording of joint motion.[12] By permission of the publisher.)

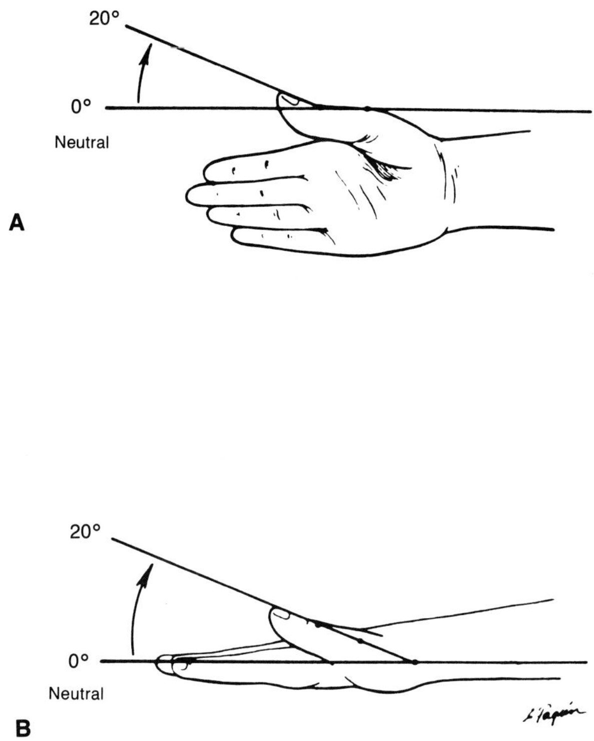

Figure 5–13 Thumb, hyperextension and extension. *A*, Hyperextension of distal interphalangeal joint. *B*, Extension of carpometacarpal joint. (From Measuring and recording of joint motion.[12] By permission of the publisher.)

A

B

C

D

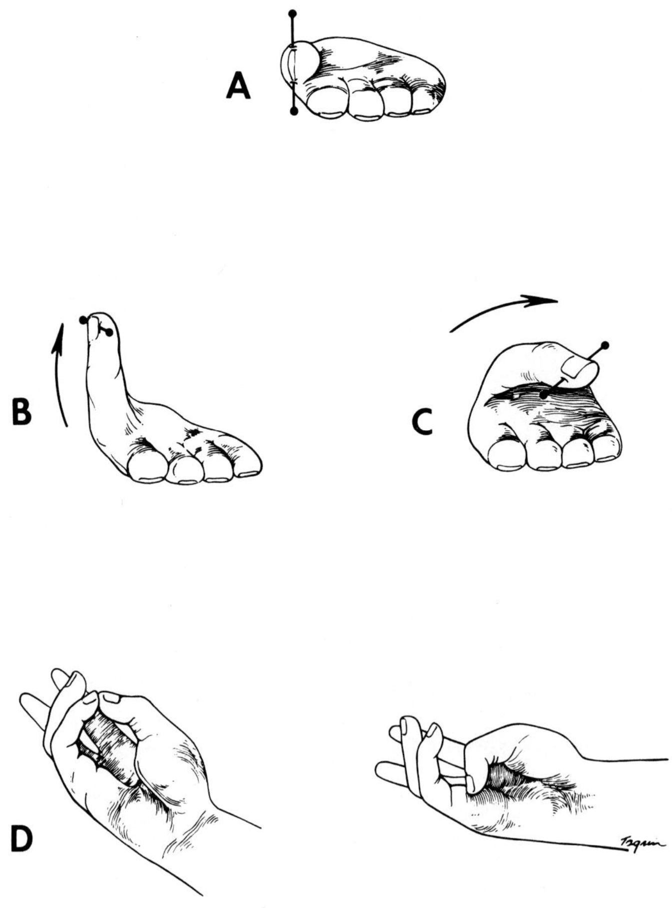

Figure 5–14 Thumb, opposition. *A*, Zero starting position. *B*, Abduction. *C*, Rotation. *D*, Flexion, two methods: tip, or pulp, of thumb touches tip of fifth finger (left) or tip of thumb touches base of fifth finger (right). (From Measuring and recording of joint motion.[12] By permission of the publisher.)

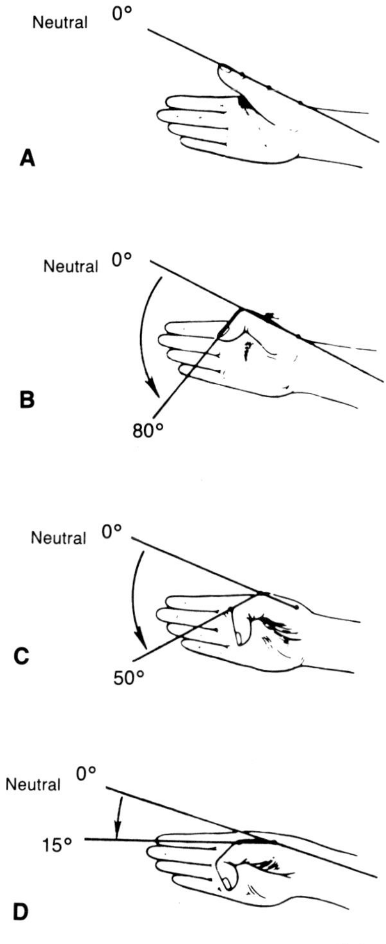

Figure 5–15 Thumb, flexion. *A*, Zero starting position. *B*, Flexion of distal interphalangeal joint. *C*, Flexion of metacarpophalangeal joint. *D*, Flexion of carpometacarpal joint. (From Measuring and recording of joint motion.[12] By permission of the publisher.)

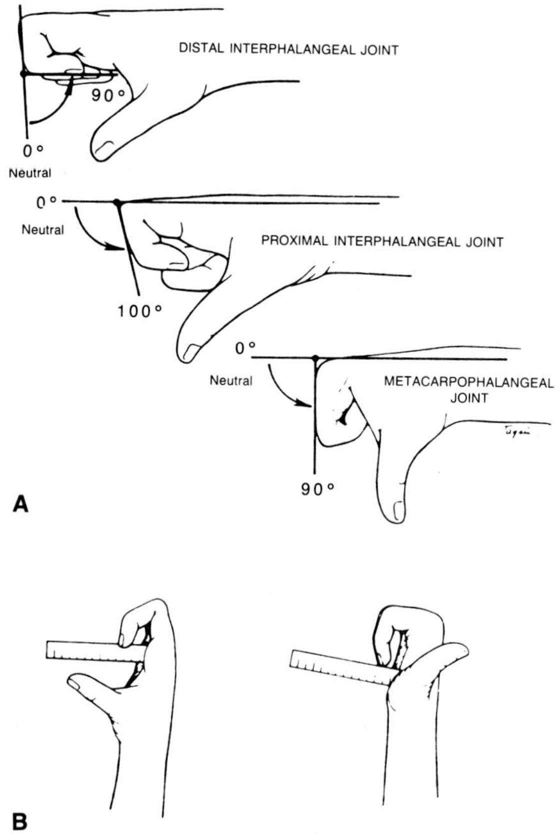

Figure 5–16 Fingers, flexion. Zero starting position: extended fingers parallel to each other, in line with plane of dorsum of hand and wrist. *A*, Flexion of joints of fingers. *B*, Composite motion of flexion, estimated with a ruler as distance from tip of finger to (1) distal palmar crease (left) and (2) proximal palmar crease (right). (From Measuring and recording of joint motion.[12] By permission of the publisher.)

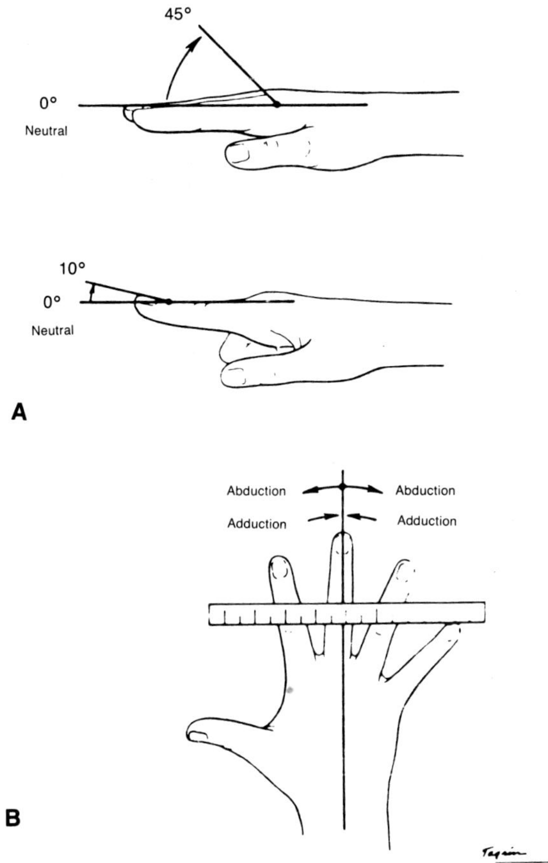

Figure 5–17 Fingers, extension. *A*, Extension of metacarpophalangeal joint (top) and hyperextension of distal interphalangeal joint (bottom). *B*, Abduction and adduction (finger spread). (From Measuring and recording of joint motion.[12] By permission of the publisher.)

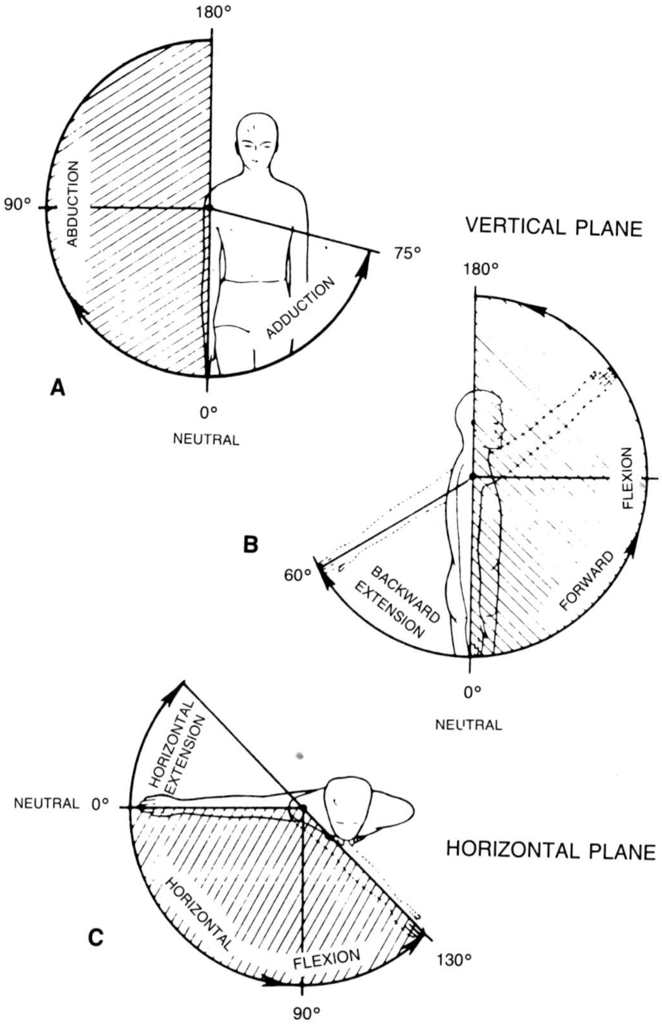

Figure 5–18 Shoulder. Zero starting position: patient standing erect, arm at side of body. *A* and *B*, Vertical or upward motion: abduction and adduction (*A*) and forward flexion and backward extension (*B*). *C*, Horizontal motion: flexion and extension. (From Measuring and recording of joint motion.[12] By permission of the publisher.)

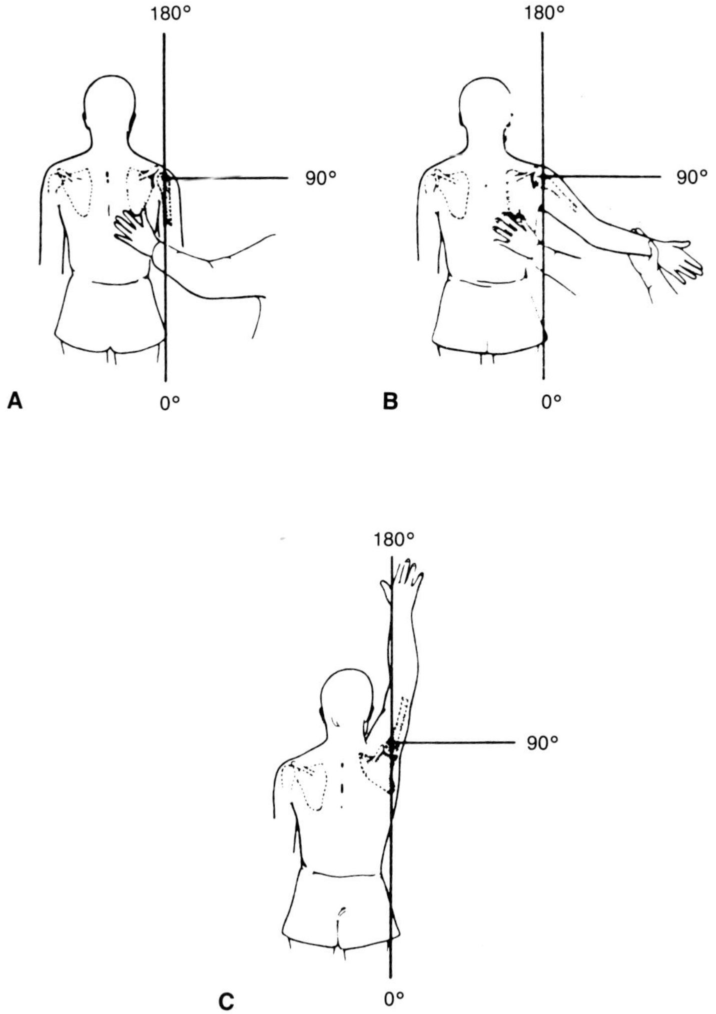

Figure 5–19 Shoulder, glenohumeral motion. *A*, Neutral starting position. *B*, Range of true glenohumeral motion, estimated by examiner fixing scapula with one hand and passively elevating arm with other hand. *C*, "Combined" glenohumeral and scapulothoracic motion. (From Measuring and recording of joint motion.[12] By permission of the publisher.)

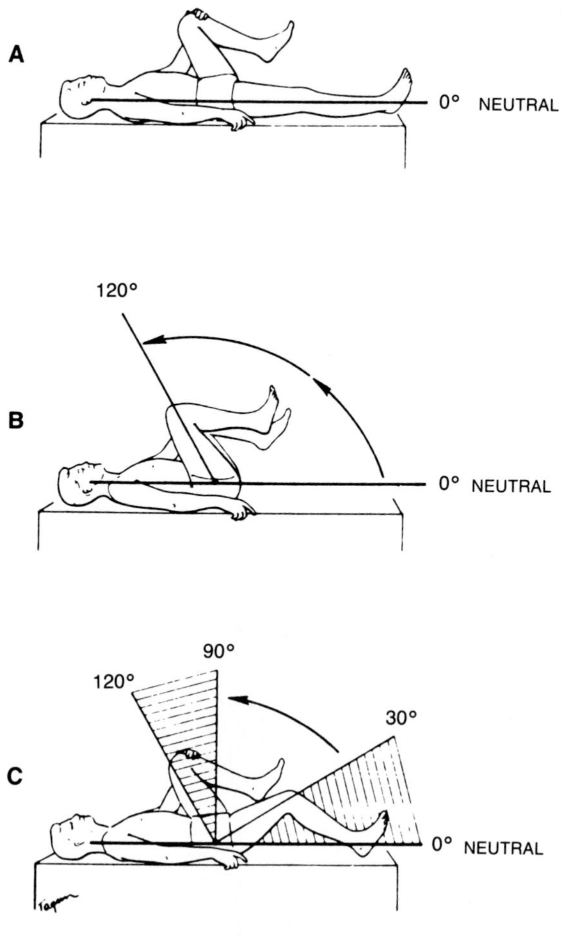

Figure 5–20 Hip, flexion. *A*, Zero starting position for right hip. *B*, Flexion. Examiner should place one hand on iliac crest to note point at which pelvis begins to rotate. *C*, Limited motion in flexion. Unshaded area is range of limited motion. (From Measuring and recording of joint motion.[12] By permission of the publisher.)

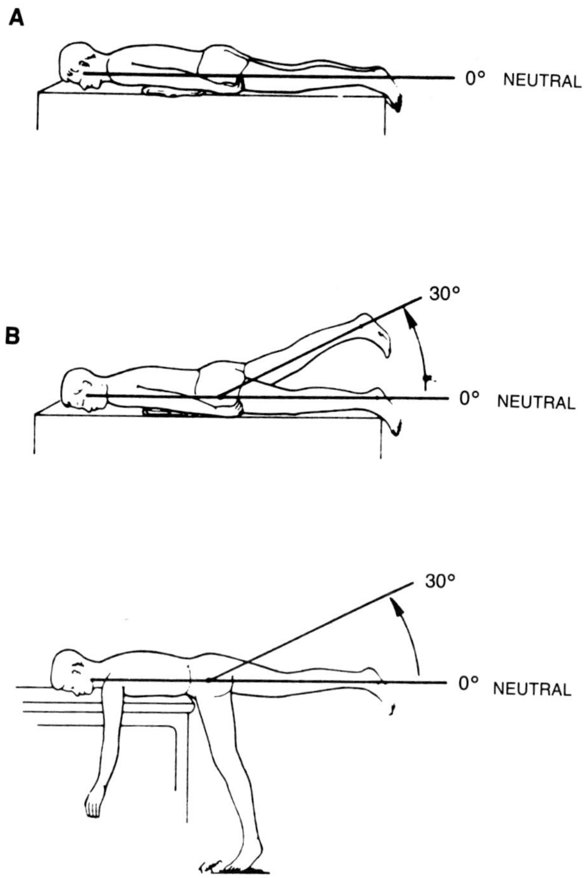

Figure 5–21 Hip, extension. *A*, Zero starting position. *B*, Extension. Two methods are used: (1) with patient face down and a small pillow under abdomen, leg is extended with knee straight or flexed (top) and (2) with opposite extremity placed over end of examining table, hip is extended (more accurate method) (bottom). (From Measuring and recording of joint motion.[12] By permission of the publisher.)

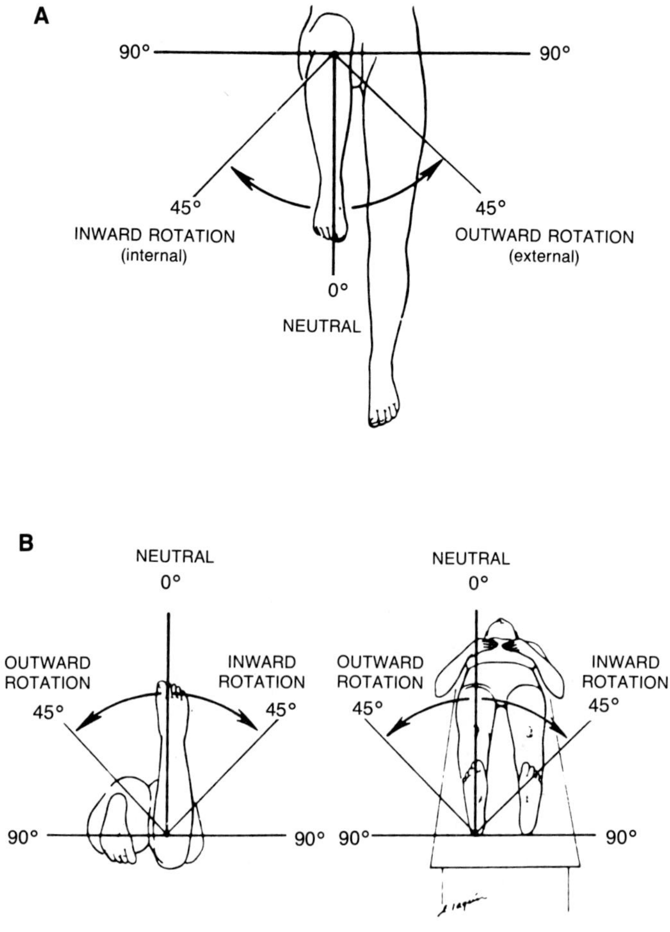

Figure 5–22 Hip, rotation. *A*, Rotation in flexion. Zero starting position: patient supine, hip and knee flexed 90° each, thigh perpendicular to transverse line across anterior-superior spines of pelvis. *B*, Rotation in extension. Two methods of measurement: (1) patient prone, knee flexed 90° and perpendicular to transverse line across anterior-superior spines of pelvis (left) and (2) patient supine. (From Measuring and recording of joint motion.[12] By permission of the publisher.)

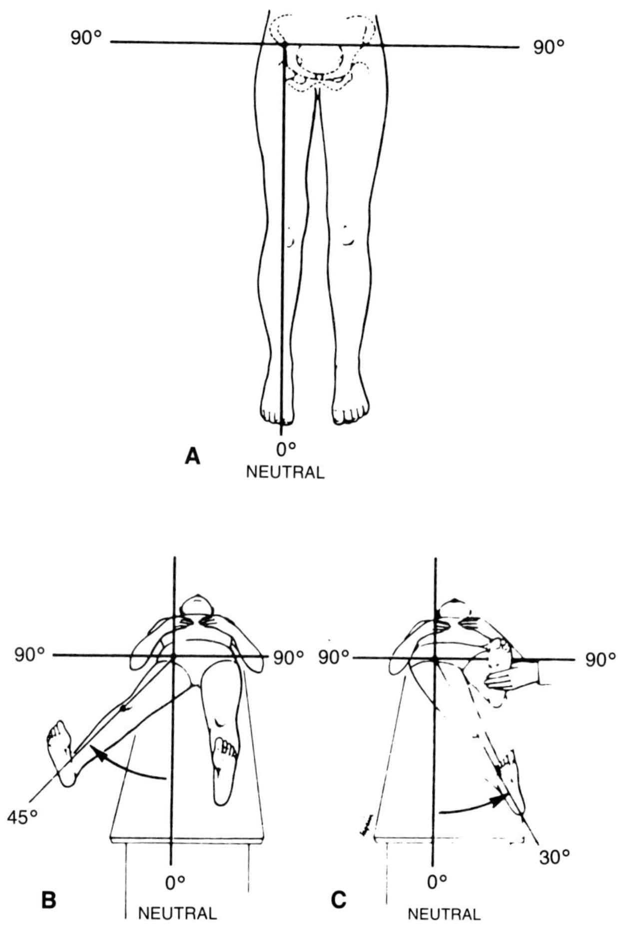

Figure 5–23 Hip, abduction and adduction. *A*, Zero starting position: patient supine, legs extended at right angles to transverse line across anterior-superior spines of pelvis. *B*, Abduction. *C*, Adduction. Examiner should elevate opposite extremity a few degrees, to allow leg to pass under it. (From Measuring and recording of joint motion.[12] By permission of the publisher.)

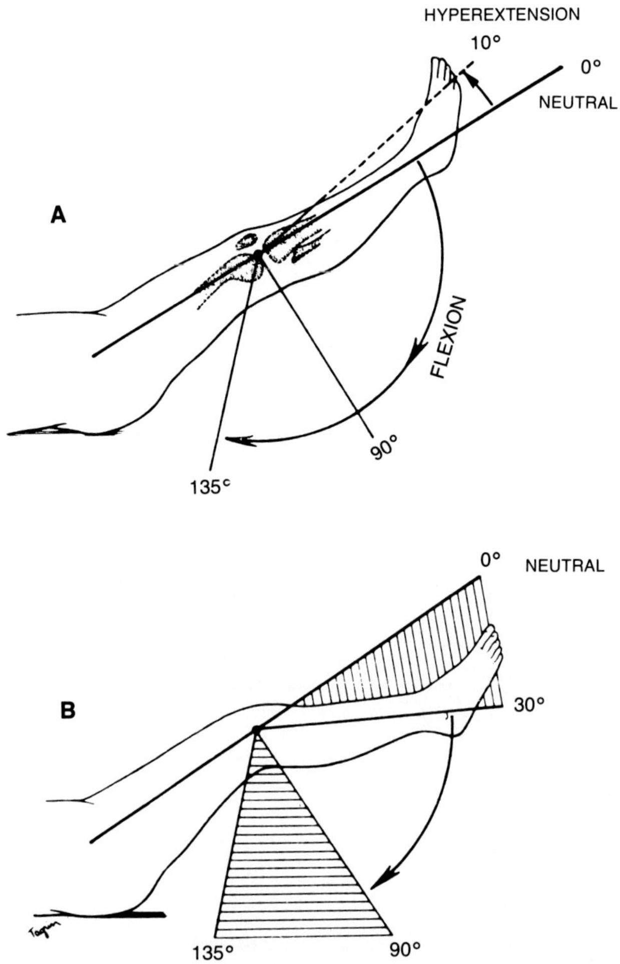

Figure 5-24 Knee. Zero starting position: extended straight knee with patient supine or prone. *A*, Flexion and hyperextension. *B*, Limited motion. Unshaded area is range of limited motion. (From Measuring and recording of joint motion.[12] By permission of the publisher.)

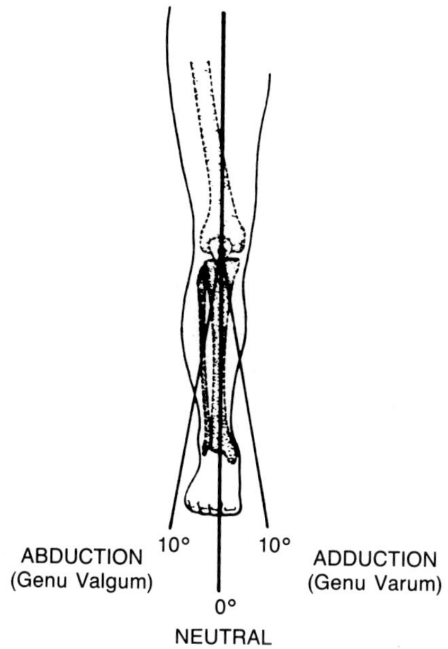

Figure 5–25 Knee, abduction and adduction—best measured in degrees and compared with opposite or normal knee. (From Measuring and recording of joint motion.[12] By permission of the publisher.)

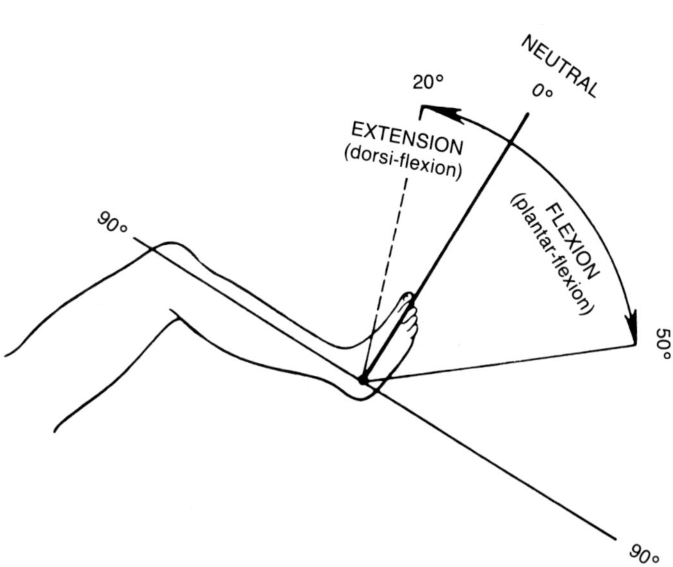

Figure 5–26 Ankle. Zero starting position: leg at right angles to thigh, foot at right angle to leg. Extension and flexion—best measured in degrees from right-angle neutral position and compared with opposite ankle. (From Measuring and recording of joint motion.[12] By permission of the publisher.)

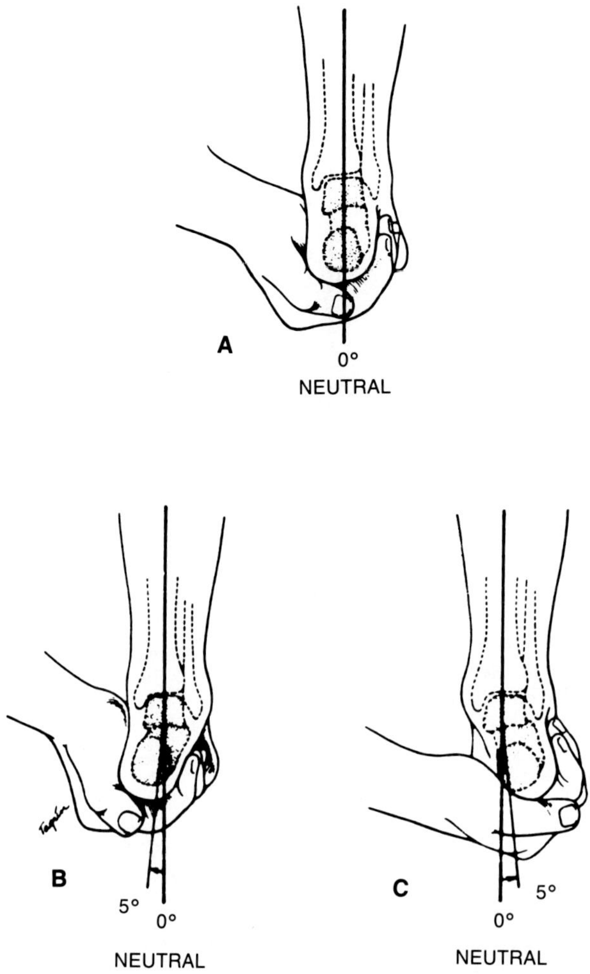

Figure 5–27 Hind part of foot (passive motion). *A*, Zero starting position: heel aligned with midline of tibia. *B*, Inversion. *C*, Eversion. (From Measuring and recording of joint motion.[12] By permission of the publisher.)

BONY LANDMARKS

The following are fixed bony landmarks or guides for alignment of the goniometer for accurate measurements.[1]

Surface Anatomy

Scapula:
- Spine
- Acromial process
- Axillary and vertebral borders
- Inferior angle

Clavicle:
- Sternal (convex) or acromial (concave) extremity
- Suprasternal notch or jugular notch

Humerus:
- Greater tubercle
- Lesser tubercle
- Bicipital groove
- Lateral epicondyle
- Medial epicondyle

Ulna:
- Olecranon process
- Head of ulna
- Styloid process
- Medial border

Radius:
- Lateral surface
- Styloid process

Carpal bones

Metacarpal bones

Phalanges:
- Distal and proximal extremity
- Medial and lateral borders

Pelvis:
- Crest of the ilium
- Anterosuperior iliac spine
- Posterosuperior iliac spine
- Iliac tuberosity
- Pubic symphyses

Femur:
- Greater trochanter
- Adductor tubercle
- Lateral epicondyle
- Medial epicondyle

Tibia:
  Medial condyle
  Lateral condyle
  Tibial tuberosity
  Anterior border
  Medial surface
  Medial malleolus

Fibula:
  Styloid process
  Head
  Lateral malleolus

Tarsals

Metatarsals

Phalanges

Spine:
  Spinous processes (C–2 to L–5)
  Sacrum
  Coccyx

REFERENCES

1. Polley HF, Hunder GG. Rheumatologic interviewing and physical examination of the joints. Philadelphia: WB Saunders, 1978.
2. Hoppenfeld S. Physical examination of the spine and extremities. New York: Appleton-Century-Crofts, 1976.
3. Kapandji IA. The physiology of the joints: annotated diagrams of the mechanics of the human joints (translated by L.H. Honoré). 2nd ed. Vols 1–3. Edinburgh: E & S Livingstone, 1970.
4. Merritt JL, McLean TJ, Erickson RP, Offord KP. Measurement of trunk flexibility in normal subjects: reproducibility of three clinical methods. Mayo Clin Proc 1986; 61:192–197.
5. Kottke FJ, Stillwell GK, Lehmann JF, eds. Krusen's handbook of physical medicine and rehabilitation. 3rd ed. Philadelphia: WB Saunders, 1982.
6. Cyriax JH. Textbook of orthopaedic medicine. 7th ed. Vols 1 and 2. London: Baillière Tindall, 1978.
7. Ehrlich GE, ed. Rehabilitation management of rheumatic conditions. Baltimore: Williams & Wilkins, 1980.
8. Saunders HD. Evaluation, treatment and prevention of musculoskeletal disorders. Minneapolis: Viking Press, 1985.
9. Cailliet R. Soft tissue pain and disability. Philadelphia: FA Davis, 1977.
10. Medical knowledge self-assessment program in physical medicine and rehabilitation syllabus. Philadelphia: American Academy of Physical Medicine and Rehabilitation, 1977.
11. Cave EF, Roberts SM. A method for measuring and recording joint function. J Bone Joint Surg 1936; 18:455–465.
12. Measuring and recording of joint motion. Chicago: American Academy of Orthopaedic Surgeons, 1963.

6 THERAPEUTIC HEAT AND COLD

G. Keith Stillwell, M.D., Ph.D.

The therapeutic uses of heat and cold are based on their physiologic effects. There are no absolute indications for their application, and there are almost no absolute contraindications. The indications for the prescription of heat or cold are covered briefly here.[1]

LOCAL HEATING

Physiologic Effects

These effects are demonstrated in Figure 6–1. The mechanism underlying the analgesia is probably the same as that involved with other types of cutaneous stimulation, such as massage, transcutaneous electrical nerve stimulation, or local cooling. The role of the axon reflex is questionable. Its absence might allow denervated skin to be more easily burned, but the evidence on this point is conflicting. The local removal of heat by increased blood flow is vital for the prevention of excessive heating. A patient whose vasculature cannot respond adequately is more easily burned.

Aside from sedation, the systemic effects of local heating (Fig. 6–1) essentially involve thermoregulatory responses, and their magnitude will be influenced by the ambient temperature and humidity. Measures should be taken so that patients who fall asleep during treatment are not harmed by falls and that elderly or debilitated patients do not exceed their cardiorespiratory reserves. An infant with inadequate thermoregulatory control should be treated cautiously with heat, if at all.

In patients with impaired sensation for heat or pain in the area being heated, adjusting the intensity of the heat appropriately will be difficult. The difference between the dosages for adequate heating and burning is small.

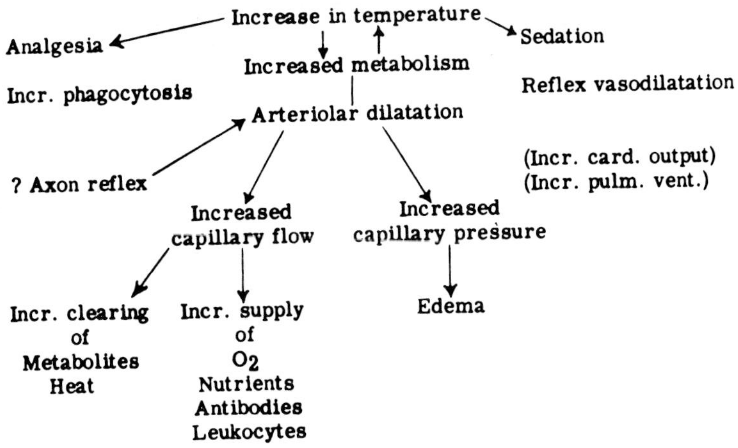

Figure 6–1 Physiologic effects of local heating: local effects that probably are not directly attributable to an increase in local metabolic rate (left) and systemic effects (right). (From Stillwell GK. The use of physical medicine in office practice with particular emphasis on the aftercare of fractures. J Iowa Med Soc 1963; 53:12–18. By permission of the Society.)

Indications

Local heating is indicated for analgesia, to increase cutaneous blood flow, to accelerate the suppurative process, and for sedation.

Contraindications

Impaired cutaneous blood flow, impaired sensation, and noninflammatory edema are contraindications for the use of local heating. It should also be avoided in very young, elderly, or debilitated patients.

Methods

Conductive. In this type the source of heat is in contact with the surface to be heated. The amount of heat transferred is proportionate to the temperature difference, the area of contact, and the duration of contact. Examples of conductive heating are a hot water bottle and an electric heating pad. With heating pads, the temperature of the heat source is maintained, and patients lying on them are sometimes burned. The part being heated can be elevated but the skin cannot be observed. Conductive heating is not suitable for open wounds.

Convective. With convective heating the source of heat is in contact with the skin but it is in motion. Examples of this type are the whirlpool bath and various hot-air devices. The part being heated can be observed during treatment, but in the whirlpool bath it cannot be elevated. This type is frequently used for open wounds.

Conversion. For conversive heating a form of energy is delivered to the tissues and converted to heat. The most simple is radiant or infrared heat. The part being treated can be observed during heating and can be elevated. Shortwave diathermy uses electromagnetic radiation in the short-wave radio frequencies, and microwave diathermy uses higher frequencies. With either of these methods the dose entering the patient cannot be measured directly; thus, the presence of heat and pain sensibility is essential. These forms cannot be used in the presence of significant pieces of embedded metal. Ultrasound therapy uses inaudibly high sound frequencies, can be measured more precisely, and can be used in the presence of embedded metal.

LOCAL COOLING

Physiologic Effects

The effects of cooling are largely the opposite of those of heating. The reduction in local blood flow decreases the convective transfer of heat by the blood; thus, cold is sometimes said to be "more penetrating" than heat. Cooling of peripheral nerves is associated with a reduction in their conduction velocities. Blocking of nerve conduction can be achieved. In humans, the order of loss of function is light touch and cold, motor power, vasoconstriction, and, last, pain and gross pressure. Spasticity may be reduced. Muscle viscosity can be increased so that a moderately weak muscle may become clinically weaker. Rare individuals are hypersensitive to cold, developing wheals, facial flushing, and syncope even from immersion of one hand in water at 8°C for 6 minutes; such persons may need to be rescued if they attempt to swim in cold water.

Indications

The indications for local cooling are to reduce extravasation of blood and fluid into the tissues after trauma, for analgesia, to reduce spasticity, and to preserve the viability of parts that are temporarily ischemic.

Contraindications

Hypersensitivity to cold, Raynaud's phenomenon, and previous frostbite are contraindications to local cooling.

Methods

Conductive. Cold packs, wet or dry, are used. If the cold pack has been in the freezer compartment of a refrigerator, it must not be placed in direct contact with the skin. Immersion in an unstirred cold water bath can be used, or the area can be massaged with ice.

Convective. Cold air or cold water may be used with forced circulation.

Evaporation. Spraying with ethyl chloride has been used.

REFERENCE

1. Lehmann JF, de Lateur BJ. Diathermy and superficial heat and cold therapy. In: Kottke FJ, Stillwell GK, Lehmann JF, eds. Krusen's handbook of physical medicine and rehabilitation. 3rd ed. Philadelphia: WB Saunders, 1982:275–350.

7 THERAPEUTIC ELECTRICITY

Gudni Thorsteinsson, M.D.

Within the field of physical medicine and rehabilitation, electricity is used for activating muscles and controlling pain. The use of electricity for stimulating specific organs (for example, the heart or urinary bladder) is not discussed in this chapter.

MUSCLE ACTIVATION

Electricity is used to activate muscle through either its nerve supply (innervation intact) or the muscle itself when the nerve supply has been interrupted (denervated muscles).

The amount of electricity (voltage or amperage) needed to stimulate a nerve is much less than that needed to stimulate a muscle directly, and it is also less painful to stimulate a nerve. The effectiveness of electrical stimulation is a function of the rate (frequency) and duration of the stimulus and the magnitude of its change. The minimal duration of an effective stimulus for a nerve is about 0.03 msec and that for a muscle, 1 msec.

Nerve Supply Intact

The indications for electrical stimulation include (1) phrenic nerve stimulation (for example, cases of spinal cord injury above the C–4 segment), (2) electrophysiologic orthosis (for example, in cases of cerebrovascular accidents with loss of central motor control), (3) spasticity control (for example, in cases of multiple sclerosis, spinal cord injury, or stroke), (4) treatment of scoliosis, (5) neuromuscular reeducation and sensory-motor retraining, (6) fecal incontinence, (7) urinary incontinence, and (8) electroejaculations.

This type of stimulation is used to activate muscles that have lost control from the higher central nervous system but the nerve supply from the spinal cord is intact. For example, phrenic nerve stimulation for respiration is used in cases of spinal cord injury higher than the C–4 level; the diaphragm still has its nerve supply through the phrenic nerve originating below the spinal cord lesion. The same type of electrical stimulation is applied in functional electrical orthosis. The stimulation of muscle with an intact nerve supply may also be used for muscle reeducation. For example, this type is used in cases of disuse atrophy of muscle after trauma, orthopedic procedures, tendon transfers, and tendon repairs. The objective of stimulation is to facilitate and restore mobility, strength, control, endurance, speed, and precision.

The mode of application depends on the condition being treated. The electrode may be implanted, as in the case of phrenic nerve stimulation and some of the electrophysiologic orthoses, or surface electrodes can be used. The intensity, frequency, and duration depend on the condition being treated and differ from one patient to another. They are determined by the function or results one is trying to obtain. For example, rhythmic contractions can be used to obtain different types of function such as breathing, walking, or changes in muscle tones for spasticity control. Surface electrical stimulation of the paraspinal muscles on the apex site of the curve is used to treat scoliosis of 20° to 40° (Cubb); 77% of curves improve or are maintained when treated to bone maturity.[1]

Denervated Muscle

Denervated muscle can be stimulated by the bipolar method. One electrode is applied over the muscle origin, and the second electrode is at the distal musculotendinous junction. Another method that can be used is the monopolar method, which stimulates the motor points of the muscles. Electrical stimulation retards denervation atrophy. Its effectiveness in such cases depends on the duration, frequency, and intensity used, the electrode placement, and the duration and number of treatment sessions. The therapeutic stimulation should be both isometric and isotonic to obtain maximal results. A rest period of more than 10 minutes is optimal between stimulations.

ANALGESIA

The physiologic basis for the use of electrical stimulation to control pain is the modulation (change) of pain sensation. This occurs at the spinal cord level (dorsal horn) or diencephalon (thalamus). Innocuous stimulation is activated by the use of electrical stimulation, and, at the same time, modulation is achieved by closing the pain gate or overbalancing the scales of modulation in disfavor to the pain. Also, electrical stimulation activates some brainstem reticular nuclei, which activates descending pain control fibers. One type of electrical stimulation also activates the endorphin system, which favors pain control.

Various types of electrical stimulation are used for pain control. One of these is high-frequency transcutaneous electrical nerve stimulation (hi-TENS or traditional TENS). This term is a misnomer because the frequency is less than 200 Hz, but it is used to distinguish it from low-frequency TENS of 1 to 2 Hz. Low-frequency TENS (low-frequency, high-intensity TENS or acupuncture-like TENS) is another type of electrical stimulation used for pain control. High-voltage galvanic stimulation (high-voltage, high-peak current [HVHPC] or Microdyne stimulation) and interferential therapy (medium frequency; 4,000 Hz) are electrical stimulations that have been used recently.

Basically, two types of modulation are being achieved. One activates the thick myelinated fibers and causes modulation at the spinal cord, brainstem, and thalamus levels, and the other, which is not as comfortable, involves endorphin activation. Electrical stimulation can be used to control chronic and acute pain. Originally, it was mainly used for chronic pain, but its use for acute pain has gained popularity because the more penetrating stimulation (HVHPC and interferential therapy) also seems to reduce edema, which is so often associated with acute pain that occurs with trauma or postoperatively. Electrical stimulation should not be used with a cardiac pacemaker when it might affect it.

Electrical stimulation has especially been used for neurogenic pain located in the periphery (for example, chronic painful peripheral neuropathy). It has also been used with reasonable results for chronic myofascial pain syndromes, low back pain syndromes, cancer pain, and arthritis. It has not proved successful for controlling central pain.

To control acute pain, electrical stimulation has been used postoperatively and has decreased atelectasis after thoracic operation and decreased ileus associated with abdominal operation. Its application has been shown to decrease the use of narcotics and allowed earlier ambulation when used after orthopedic operation.

Thorough evaluation of patients before prescribing electrical stimulation is important because other conditions such as depression may be present and may need special attention. Electrical stimulation is rarely prescribed alone but is combined with other physical therapy measures, such as exercises and training for relaxation, conditioning, and proper posture.

The efficacy of electrical stimulation is usually partial relief (25% to 90%), although complete relief is not uncommon, especially when the stimulation is first introduced. There is a definite placebo effect, but it is not different from that associated with other therapies used to control pain. A definite decline in efficacy occurs over time when treating chronic pain.

The stimulation is applied either over a nerve innervating the area or over the area of pain. Most often the stimulation is used two to three times per day, but sometimes it is used continuously or under certain circumstances when pain is increased, such as while working.[2,3]

REFERENCES

1. Herbert MA. The treatment of scoliosis using electrical stimulation of muscle. IEEE Eng Med Biol Mag, September, 1983; 43–49.
2. Thorsteinsson G. Electrical stimulation for analgesia. In: Stillwell GK, ed. Therapeutic electricity and ultraviolet radiation. 3rd ed. Baltimore: Williams & Wilkins, 1983:109–123.
3. Jacobs SR, Jaweed MM, Herbison GJ, Stillwell GK. Electrical stimulation of muscle. In: Stillwell GK, ed. Therapeutic electricity and ultraviolet radiation. 3rd ed. Baltimore: Williams & Wilkins, 1983:124–173.

8 AMBULATORY AIDS

David L. Nash, M.D.

Practitioners in the field of physical medicine and rehabilitation encounter a wide range of people with physical impairments, many of whom are having some difficulty with ambulation. These gait difficulties may be temporary or permanent. Sometimes a permanent impairment shows improvement with time, such as in a person who has suffered a cerebrovascular accident. In some other conditions the gait impairment will progressively worsen, such as in a person with a progressive neuromuscular disease. This chapter addresses the various conditions that may be associated with gait difficulties and the characteristics of an antalgic gait. Evaluating a patient's needs, the type of gait aid to meet these needs, and the various types of crutch gaits are also discussed, as is applying these principles to write a physical therapy prescription for a gait impairment.

CONDITIONS ASSOCIATED WITH GAIT IMPAIRMENTS

Conditions associated with gait impairments can be classified in many ways. I prefer to divide them into three categories. The first condition is pain, possibly with some additional structural lesion in the lower extremity. The second includes conditions that are usually not painful but are associated with impaired balance, coordination, or strength. The third condition is amputation, which is discussed in Chapter 9.

Pain With or Without a Structural Lesion

The most commonly encountered patients with temporary needs for a gait aid have pain. Both in emergency rooms and in outpatient clinics, patients present daily with sprains or strains of ligaments or tendons, contusions, lacerations, torn knee cartilage, or tendon or nerve injury. These injuries need proper rest and protection, which can be provided with a gait aid to relieve weight-bearing stresses.

Fracture or Operative Intervention. Fractures or surgical intervention in the lower extremity may be associated with the types of traumatic lesions mentioned above. However, many lower extremity operations are not related to trauma, such as correction of a congenital deformity or treatment of an acquired disease such as osteoarthritis of the hip with a total joint arthroplasty or a focal atherosclerotic obstruction with vascular bypass. These conditions also usually require a gait aid for protection during healing and to minimize pain from excessive weight bearing.

Inflammatory Diseases. Other conditions requiring protection from painful weight bearing are associated with inflammatory processes. Lower extremity joints may be affected with a systemic connective tissue disease such as rheumatoid arthritis, a crystal-induced arthropathy such as gout, or infection such as septic arthritis. Osteoarthritis can certainly have a painful inflammatory appearance too. Painful inflammatory processes of other soft tissues, such as cellulitis, myositis, or thrombophlebitis, can also warrant the use of a gait aid during the acute phases. Again, the primary goal of a gait aid in these conditions is to facilitate ambulation while protecting painful healing tissue from the stress of weight bearing.

Impaired Balance and Coordination

In this group of disorders, pain is usually not a feature, but unsteadiness of gait places the patient at risk for falls and injuries.

Spasticity secondary to an upper motor neuron injury is most commonly encountered in patients after stroke resulting in hemiplegia, spinal cord injury resulting in quadriparesis or paraparesis, or traumatic brain injury. Spastic cerebral palsy, a perinatally acquired brain injury, certainly fits into this category. The excessive tone and central motor lesion cause difficulties in voluntarily activating and inhibiting muscle groups and result in stiff, jerky styles of gait. Patients with hemiplegia often need to swing their stiff, straight leg out to the side to keep from catching a toe. This type of gait abnormality is referred to as circumduction.

Weakness can result from any number of diseases affecting the motor units. There are many myopathies described that include the muscular dystrophies. The lower motor neuron can be affected in several ways also, for example, by an inflammatory process such as Guillain-Barré syndrome or by inherited idiopathic or acquired peripheral neuropathies, such as occurs with Charcot-Marie-Tooth disease, diabetes, folic acid or vitamin B_{12} deficiency, or environmental toxin exposure. Amyotrophic lateral sclerosis is typified by progressive painless weakness. Also, weakness can be associated with a prolonged illness and bed rest resulting in marked deconditioning.

Ataxias, disorders of muscular coordination, can be divided into two types. The first is based on impaired cerebellar function that limits, on a central processing basis, the brain's capacity to coordinate muscle activation. Foot placement appears haphazard or drunken and lurching with a wide base. The other type is based on sensory deficits limiting peripheral feedback from the limbs regarding their position in space. Affected patients may have a more noticeable slapping of their feet and become significantly more impaired in the dark because compensatory visual cues are decreased.

Rigidity most commonly occurs in the gaits of patients with Parkinson's disease who have an extrapyramidal disorder resulting in a gait disturbance characterized by short, shuffling steps, no arm swing, flexed posture, and sometimes difficulty initiating the first step. Their gait may also have a peculiar acceleration referred to as festination.

A combination of the features mentioned above may also be present in some diseases with weakness, upper and lower motor neuron deficits, cerebellar dysfunction, and sensory loss. The most common disease that can include all of these features is multiple sclerosis.

THE ANTALGIC GAIT

The characteristic gait resulting from weight-bearing pain in one of the lower extremities has several distinguishing features (Table 8–1). The foot is placed flat rather than with the typical heel strike in order to reduce the jarring of impact. Push off may also be avoided to eliminate the associated transmission of forces. The duration of time with weight on the painful leg is shortened relative to the time on the other leg, which results in a shortened swing phase and a prolonged stance phase on the normal side. The normally smooth cadence and rhythm are disrupted. The center of gravity is typically shifted to the painful side, especially with hip disease, to decrease forces at the joint that would be normally increased because of the mechanical properties of the lever arm.

TABLE 8–1 Characteristics of an Antalgic Gait

No heal strike
No push off
Reduced stance phase on painful leg
Shortened swing phase of normal leg
Prolonged stance phase on normal leg
Abnormal cadence and rhythm
Center of gravity shifts to painful side during weight bearing

When a person stands on one leg with the body weight centered over the pelvis, the pelvis acts as a lever arm and the femoral head in the acetabulum acts as a fulcrum. The hip abductors have to increase the forces at the fulcrum further by contracting to counterbalance the body weight and hold the pelvis level. Shifting one's weight to the painful side reduces these forces.

SELECTION OF ASSISTIVE DEVICES

Evaluation of Assets and Impairment of Patient

Before a gait aid can be prescribed, the patient must be evaluated to determine his or her strengths and limitations and any potential complicating factors. The strength and condition of the upper extremities need to be assessed, particularly the shoulder adductors, elbow extensors, and grip strength. Pain or deformity such as in rheumatoid arthritis must be taken into consideration. The strength and condition of the "good leg" are also important to evaluate. Pain or weakness on the less involved side, circulation problems such as claudication, and possibly fragile, vulnerable skin on the weight-bearing surface of the foot affect the choice of gait aids and techniques.

Also pertinent to the assessment is a past history of falls and whether the patient is taking anticoagulants that might warrant extra precautions against falls. A history of cardiac problems, syncope, angina, or orthostatic hypotension should be noted, as should significant pulmonary impairments with marked shortness of breath or general debilitation from prolonged illness and bed rest. The hemoglobin or hematocrit value is also worth noting, especially if the patient has recently undergone an operation.

Ambulatory Aids

The three basic categories of aids are canes, crutches, and walkers (Fig. 8–1).

Canes. A cane is used for conditions with the least degree of gait impairment. It is always used in the hand opposite the impaired leg. In normal gait, the opposing arm and leg swing together in a reciprocal fashion. Using the cane in the hand opposite to the affected limb allows one to simulate this normal gait pattern, and it functionally provides significant weight-bearing relief when used in this manner. A cane is of proper length if, when placed with the tip 6 inches lateral to the forefoot, the elbow is flexed 30°. The cane is used in patients with mild pain or slight instability. After a cemented total hip replacement, one usually advances from crutches to a cane when pain is largely resolved

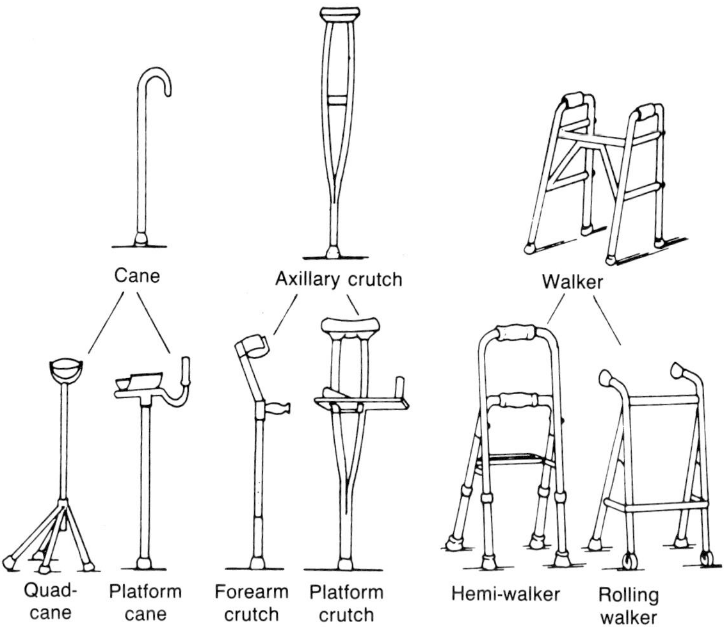

Figure 8–1 Three basic types of ambulatory aids—canes, crutches, and walkers—and some common modifications.

and strength and stability have improved significantly. A cane might be used in cases of femoral trochanteric bursitis to decrease the tension of the hip abductor on the trochanter. Hemiplegia is another common condition for which a cane is used. A quadripod cane (Fig. 8–2) is commonly used by hemiplegic patients to broaden the base of support for additional stability.

Crutches. Crutches, in contrast to canes, are most commonly used bilaterally for greater weight-bearing relief. The fitting of crutches is similar to that of a cane; when the hand is resting on the grip and the tip is 6 to 8 inches lateral to the forefoot, the elbow should be flexed 30°. In addition, there should be room for approximately two fingers between the axillary pad and the axilla. Axillary crutches are probably the most commonly used gait aid to protect against painful weight bearing on a lower extremity after injury or operation. Crutches may also be used in cases of mild to moderate ataxia or weakness related to a neuromuscular condition. When crutches are expected to be used for a long duration, light-weight aluminum ones are sometimes preferred to the less expensive wooden ones. Also, in patients with chronic conditions who have good shoulder strength, forearm (Lofstrand) crutches may be more convenient because they are shorter and made of aluminum and allow for limited use of the hands while standing.

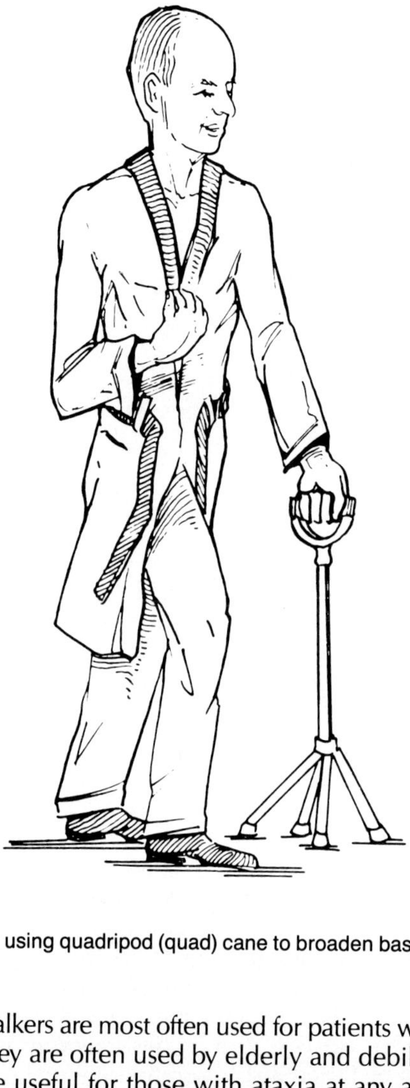

Figure 8–2 Patient using quadripod (quad) cane to broaden base of stability.

Walkers. Walkers are most often used for patients with moderate instability. They are often used by elderly and debilitated persons, but they are useful for those with ataxia at any age and, in particular, young children with spastic cerebral palsy who are learning to walk. The walker may also be preferred for some persons who are physically capable of using crutches but do not have the motor planning ability required for some crutch gaits.

Several modifications and special features may benefit certain persons. A rolling walker with wheels on the front is beneficial to those with moderately severe ataxia because it eliminates the relatively unstable and unsupported phase of gait that occurs when the walker is lifted up to be advanced. With the wheels, a steady, continuous forward force on the walker keeps it advancing.

The addition of sandbags or ankle weights to the walker may be required to provide additional stability for persons with severe ataxia. Patients who have Parkinson's disease with retropulsive instability may also benefit from these modifications.

For patients with rheumatoid arthritis who have severe involvement of the wrists and hands, platform attachments are available both for axillary crutches and walkers (Fig. 8–3). These attachments distribute the weight-bearing pressure across the forearm and decrease the stress to the hands and wrists. The swivel walker that can be advanced one side at a time or the rolling-type walker function best for patients using platform attachments on a walker.

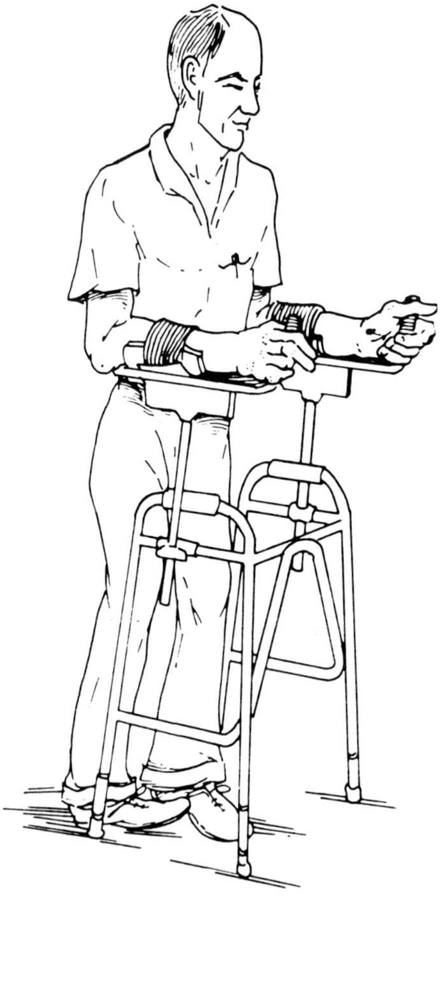

Figure 8–3 Patient using walker with platform attachment.

CRUTCH GAITS

Gaits for Disorders Involving One Leg

The most common crutch gait prescribed and used is called the 3-point gait. In this gait, the two crutches and the involved leg move together as a unit while the "good leg" supports the body weight by itself. When ordering 3-point crutch gait, one also needs to specify the weight-bearing restrictions. For nonweight bearing, the goal is to maintain the normal reciprocal gait pattern with no weight-bearing forces on the affected limb. Touch-only weight bearing has been arbitrarily set at 10 to 30 lb of weight bearing. Some orthopedic surgeons prefer this gait early after total joint arthroplasty. Partial weight bearing allows for up to 40 to 80 lb of weight bearing. When the actual amount of weight is not critical, weight bearing as tolerated is often ordered. It should be noted that it is difficult to reproduce a precise amount of weight bearing consistently. Therefore, these amounts are only approximate and not a precise standard.

The swing gait can be used for one affected lower extremity but it is often discouraged because it does not simulate normal reciprocal motion of the lower extremities. The crutches are advanced together, then the legs are advanced together as a unit. Young patients often prefer this gait because it is conducive to greater speed. The primary indication for its use, however, is for paraplegic patients with long leg braces.

Gaits for Two Affected Limbs

The 4-point (or 4-count) gait is characterized by moving one crutch or limb at a time and always having three points remaining in contact with the floor at any one time. An example of the sequence would be left crutch, right foot, right crutch, left foot. For most people this is a tediously slow gait, but it is tolerated in conditions such as rheumatoid arthritis, with which joints in both legs need protection from weight bearing. Also, some patients with moderately severe ataxia benefit from this gait pattern with its added stability. After starting with the 4-point gait, patients often advance to the quicker 2-point gait, in which one crutch and the opposite foot move together in a more natural reciprocal fashion. This gait is faster than the 4-point gait and has a more natural rhythm, but only one crutch and one leg are in contact with the floor at any one time.

The "walk to" gait is most commonly used with the walker but can be used with crutches. The patient first advances the crutches or walker as a unit and then steps up one foot at a time to the position of the gait aid. This pattern is commonly used by elderly persons who have very limited mobility.

For safety and comfort, axillary and grip pads are standard on most axillary crutches. Also, crutches usually have large rubber tips to prevent slipping. As part of gait training, it is important to instruct patients in the proper technique to be used when encountering curbs or steps or carpeting. For unsteady patients, a safety belt around the waist that the therapist can hold to prevent a sudden fall is the best precaution.

PRESCRIPTION FOR AMBULATORY AIDS

Prescriptions for aids for a gait impairment (Table 8–2) always need to be individualized and may include orders for exercises (including range of motion, stretching, strengthening, pregait training, balance, coordination, transfers, and gait reeducation) and occupational therapy for additional assistance with training and devices for activities of daily living.

TABLE 8–2 Sample Prescriptions for Ambulatory Aids

Clinical Problem	*Prescription*
Painful soft tissue injury, leg	3-Point axillary crutch gait, nonweight bearing. Instructions for safety on curbs, carpet, and stairs
Rheumatoid arthritis, acute flair or severe chronic deformity with weakness or pain	4-Point platform axillary crutches; advance to 2-point as tolerated or Platform walker with swivel or rolling mechanism
Multiple sclerosis with marked ataxic gait	"Walk to" or through gait with rolling, weighted walker

9 PROSTHESES AND ORTHOSES

Rolland P. Erickson, M.D.
Malcolm C. McPhee, M.D.

DEFINITIONS

Prosthesis

A prosthesis is an artificial substitute for a missing body part. Although this definition may relate to absent ears, breasts, or dentition, the following discussion pertains only to those devices that are designed to replace a partially or completely absent limb.

Orthosis

An orthosis is a device that, when in contact with the body, improves function. In the greatest sense, this definition could encompass wheelchairs, feeding and grooming aids that improve one's ability to accomplish activities of daily living, crutches, and walkers. However, the following discussion is limited to devices that improve limb function.

INDICATIONS FOR PROSTHESES OR ORTHOSES

Amputation

"Major amputation" is generally defined as proximal to and including complete amputation of the hand or foot. In the United States alone, about 43,000 major amputations are performed every year. The yearly incidence is thus nearly 0.3 amputation per 1,000 persons; the prevalence is about 1 amputation per 250 persons.

Disease. Although etiologic reports vary by region and country, the most common reason for amputation is disease. Peripheral vascular disease manifested as atherosclerosis, thromboangiitis, and diabetes mellitus accounts for 58% to 93% of all amputations and is, as expected, most frequent in elderly populations. The lower extremity is affected most often.

Trauma. Trauma is the second most frequent reason for amputation and is responsible for 29% to 33% of all cases. Like other traumatic conditions, amputations most often affect young adults and certain occupational groups and are most frequent during wartime. Approximately a third involve the upper extremity.

Tumor. Accounting for approximately 5% of the indications for amputation, tumor as an etiologic agent peaks twice. The higher peak occurs during adolescence and is due to osteosarcoma and chondrosarcoma, and a less significant peak occurs during late middle age. Certain medical centers with comprehensive cancer treatment programs have a much greater proportion of amputations due to cancer.

Congenital Limb (Skeletal) Deficiency. In about 5% of persons with absent limbs, the condition has been present since birth. It is more than semantically incorrect to consider such limb loss as a "congenital amputation." Congenital limb deficiencies can be transverse or longitudinal. A transverse deficiency is the absence of all skeletal parts distal to the deficiency along a transverse axis and results in limb loss similar to that of most acquired amputations. Conversely, a longitudinal deficiency extends parallel to the long axis of the limb; an example is absence of the radius, radial carpal bones, and one or more radially situated digit rays. The medical and prosthetic management of transverse deficiencies often parallels that of acquired amputations. However, special surgical, prosthetic, and orthotic interventions are frequently required for the management of longitudinal deficiencies.

In contradistinction to acquired amputations, congenital limb deficiences occur more frequently in the upper extremity; a transverse deficiency below the elbow is the single most frequent deficiency.

Paralysis

Paralysis as an indication for use of an orthosis cannot be classified as simply as amputations. A myriad of neurogenic lesions involving a single or diffuse portion of the central or peripheral nervous system and also myopathic processes can impact an individual to a degree that orthotic intervention may be required. However, common conditions often requiring one or more orthoses include cerebrovascular accidents with hemiplegia, spinal cord injuries, head injuries, traumatic and entrapment mononeuropathies, Guillain-Barré syndrome, peripheral neuropathies, poliomyelitis, and congenital maladies.

Skeletal Instability

A multitude of conditions with skeletal instability also may benefit from orthotic intervention. Ligamentous injuries to weight-bearing joints, monoarthropathies and polyarthropathies with or without inflammation, and fractures of long bones often require one or more orthotic devices to augment or maintain stability. Conditions resulting in painful extremities, although often unassociated with skeletal instability, are included in the discussion.

BIOMECHANICAL PRINCIPLES

Lower Extremity

The human gait cycle (Fig. 9–1) is often addressed using relatively standard terminology. Stance phase is the portion of the gait

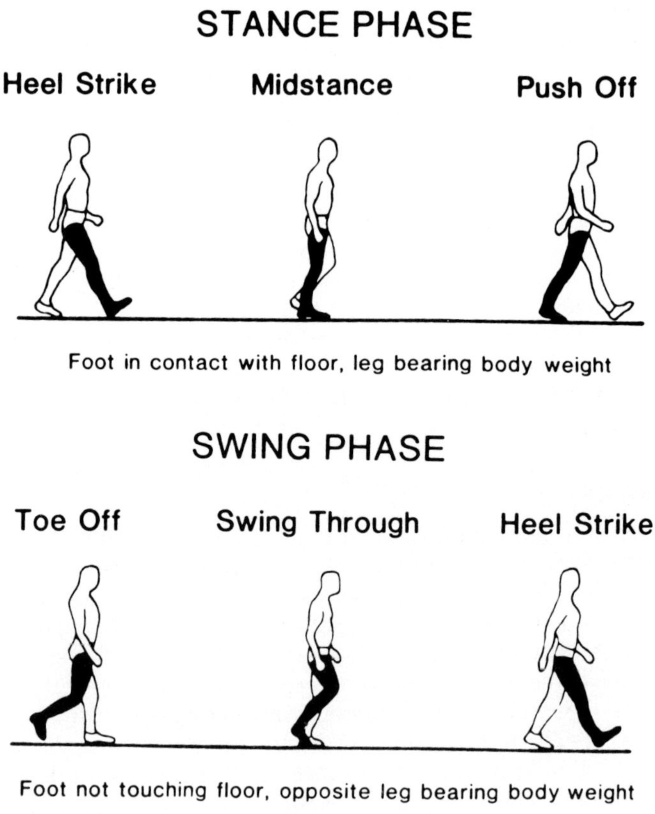

Figure 9–1 Analysis of a single forward step. (From Anderson MH, Bechtol CO, Sollars RE. Clinical prosthetics for physicians and therapists: a handbook of clinical practices related to artificial limbs. Springfield, Illinois: Charles C Thomas, 1959:169. By permission of the publisher.)

cycle in which the reference limb is in contact with the floor; it is initiated when the heel first contacts the floor (heel strike). It progresses through full foot-floor contact (midstance) and culminates with heel lift (push off). Swing phase is the portion of the gait cycle in which the reference limb does not contact the floor. It begins with loss of foot-floor contact (toe off), progresses through unencumbered forward movement (swing through), and ends with heel strike.

We walk the way we do, given our anatomic limitations, because it is the most energy-efficient way to transport ourselves physically from one place to another. At first analysis, ambulation may seem to be an easy and automatic activity. Yet, with closer analysis, human gait becomes exceedingly complex.

The body's center of gravity has been calculated to be just anterior to the second sacral vertebra. The energy costs of ambulation would be minimized if we could transport that center of gravity forward in a straight line without vertical or lateral displacement. In that we do not have wheels, this is impossible. Instead, we move ourselves forward by alternating movements of two stick levers (legs), a decidedly inefficient activity because we are constantly raising, lowering, and laterally displacing our center of gravity as it is moved forward. To damp these displacements, our extrapyramidal system uses a complex repertoire of arm, pelvic, hip, knee, ankle, and foot movements and forces constantly practiced and improved on since our first steps as a toddler. Any condition that causes a deviation from our normal gait pattern results in an increased cost of ambulation.

Compared with an able-bodied walker, the average person with a below-knee amputation ambulates with a 41% increase in energy expenditure, and one with an above-knee amputation experiences an 89% increase. In hemiplegics, ambulation consumes 63% more calories.

As energy expenditure rises, the ability for ambulation declines and disability occurs. When coupled with environmental barriers (stairs, lengthy hallways, or rough ground), the disability becomes a handicap.

Clearly, it is prudent to design, fabricate, and assess the usefulness of all lower extremity prosthetic and orthotic devices for their ability to approximate normal gait.

Upper Extremity

Just as ambulation depends on normal lower extremity function, our ability to accomplish the activities of daily living depends on normal upper extremity function. Through complex and coordinated force and movement patterns of the trunk, shoulder, elbow, wrist, and hand, we have the dexterity to thread a needle as well as the strength to lift heavy weights. Any significant disruption in these patterns yields deficits in our ability to feed, dress, groom, toilet, write, work, or recreate.

Upper extremity prosthetic and orthotic devices must be developed and assessed for their ability to approximate normal upper extremity function.

Prosthetic and Orthotic Materials

Materials suitable for prosthetic and orthotic devices have certain desirable characteristics. The material should be lightweight because the intact parts of the impaired limb must not only have the strength to accomplish the activity but also be able to move the device that will perform or assist in the performance of the activity. Newer thermoplastic and metal alloy developments are continually applied to device fabrication to minimize weight. The material should be resistant to fatigue to assist in the repetitious activities of living. The material should be smooth and inert to minimize skin trauma and irritation. For externally powered devices, desirable factors include small size, constant and long-lasting power, and an intimate interface between skin and machine. Every effort should be made to manufacture low-maintenance components. Few prosthetic and orthotic devices accomplish all these goals.

PROSTHETIC PRINCIPLES

Lower Extremity Components

Foot and Ankle. The human foot and ankle absorb decelerating forces during heel strike, provide a stable base of support during midstance, and, in concert with the triceps surae, furnish a rigid lever arm to propel the body up and forward during the later stages of stance phase. Designed to mimic these activities, the standard foot and ankle mechanism for most prostheses is currently the solid ankle-cushion heel. A compressible heel cushions heel strike, and the lack of an articulated ankle provides the lever arm to propel the body forward at the end of stance phase (Fig. 9–2).

Below-Knee Amputation Sockets. A socket is the portion of the prosthesis that incorporates the residual limb. The most frequent design used in below-knee sockets is the patellar-tendon-bearing socket (Fig. 9–3). In that the standard below-knee amputation stump is bony with many pressure-intolerant areas, the patellar-tendon-bearing socket is designed to allow the lion's share of weight bearing at the patellar tendon, just distal to the patella. Edema and skin problems are minimized if the socket is skillfully molded to provide total contact with the stump. Even then, a fabric sock usually separates the stump from direct contact with the prosthesis. The prosthesis is prevented from falling off the stump during swing phase by suspending it either by molding the sides of the prosthesis snugly above the femoral condyles or through a fastening-tape (Velcro) strap. For situations in which the patellar tendon cannot tolerate the weight bearing, or when the knee joint

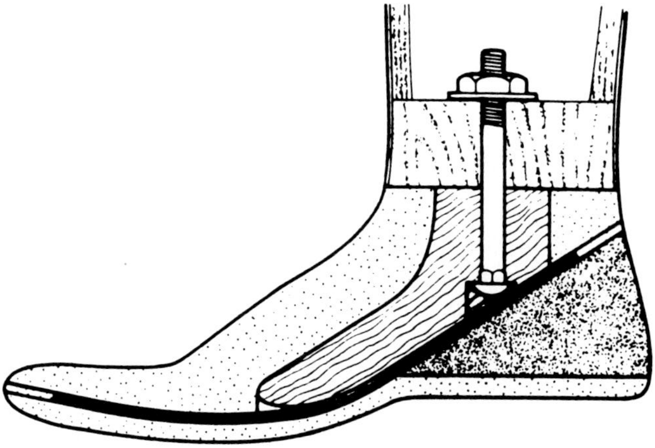

Figure 9–2 Solid ankle-cushion heel. (From Levy SW. Skin problems of the amputee. St. Louis, Missouri: Warren H. Green, 1983:82. By permission of the publisher.)

is painful or unstable, significant weight may be redistributed to more proximal tissues via a thigh lacer attached to the prosthesis through lateral and medial knee joints.

Knee Units. Prostheses for amputations above the knee require a mechanical knee. The constant friction unit is the most basic type. It consists of a simple bolted articulation in which constant friction can be applied to resist free swing at the knee. Additional security against unexpected knee flexion during stance phase can be provided by the safety knee. When weight is placed on the limb, a friction brake provides resistance against buckling into flexion.

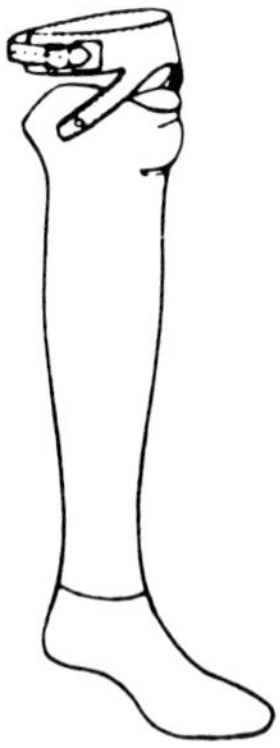

Figure 9–3 Below-knee prosthesis with patellar-tendon-bearing socket. (From Hosmer-Dorrance, Campbell, California. By permission.)

Additional stability against knee flexion during stance phase is provided in virtually all knee units by situating the articulation posteriorly. If the wearer is agile and ambulates at multiple speeds, hydraulic mechanisms are often used to provide variable resistance during swing phase.

Above-Knee Amputation Sockets. The standard above-knee amputation socket is the quadrilateral type (Fig. 9–4). It molds the soft tissues of the stump such that the ischial tuberosity is maintained on a horizontal shelf on the posterior aspect of the socket. Consequently, much of the weight bearing occurs at this point, and the distal pressure-intolerant areas of the stump are thus relieved of significant weight-bearing tasks. Unlike the patellar-tendon-bearing socket, the quadrilateral socket is often used without an intervening sock, and thereby an intimate fit provides suction during swing phase to maintain suspension of the prosthesis on the stump. Modifications to the basic design include the use of a fabric sock and suspensory belt for persons who have difficulty accomplishing the vigorous donning efforts. Recently, flexible thermoplastics have been used in the fabrication of the socket to accommodate dynamic changes of muscle size and stump shape during gait. Another innovation is a socket redesigned to incorporate greater hip adduction, which thereby stretches the hip abductors for more efficiency.

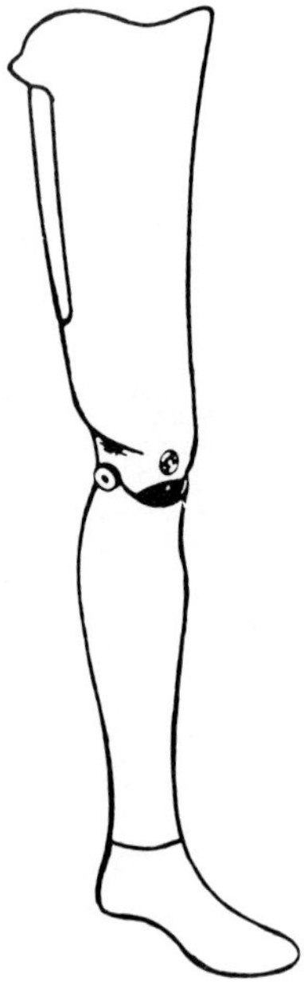

Figure 9–4 Standard above-knee prosthesis. (From Hosmer-Dorrance, Campbell, California. By permission.)

Hip Disarticulation and Hemipelvectomy Prostheses. Although energy inefficient, the Canadian design is used by many people with hip disarticulation and hemipelvectomy (Fig. 9–5). The knee and hip articulations are placed so that simple downward weight bearing stabilizes the joints against buckling. The socket is large and encompasses much of the remaining pelvic soft tissues. Suspension is maintained through a belt that passes above the opposite iliac crest.

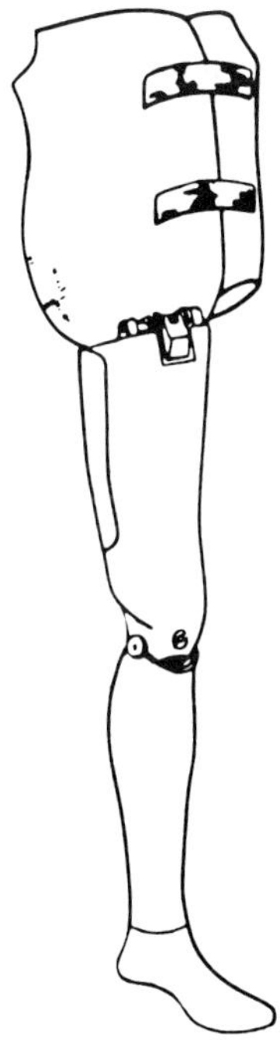

Figure 9–5 Hip disarticulation and hemipelvectomy prosthesis. (From Hosmer-Dorrance, Campbell, California. By permission.)

Upper Extremity Components

Terminal Devices. In an effort to approximate normal prehension, maintain visual monitoring of manual tasks, and accomplish acceptable cosmesis, many prosthetic hooks and hands have been developed. The terminal device used by many persons with upper extremity amputations is a curved and split hook in which sturdy rubber bands maintain the closed position. It is opened by traction on a cable powered by intact proximal muscles on either side or both sides. Similar mechanisms operate many mechanical hands. Mechanisms to use the cable for closing instead of opening the hook or hand are also available. In recent years, battery-operated hooks and hands have been developed that are controlled by electromyographic signals from proximal muscles.

Wrist Units. Mechanical wrist units are used to allow operation of the terminal device close to the body and in various degrees of supination and pronation.

Below-Elbow Amputation Sockets. Below-elbow amputation sockets use a double wall to provide both cosmetically acceptable exterior contours and total socket-stump contact. Suspension is provided by either snug capture of the epicondyles or a harnessing system suspended from the involved and uninvolved shoulders (Fig. 9–6).

Elbow Units. For above-elbow amputations, a prosthetic elbow unit is required. This unit must be able to be positioned and maintained in various angles. Both of these operations are usually accomplished through cable systems similar to the one that operates the terminal device. Expensive and complex externally powered systems have also been designed to perform these actions.

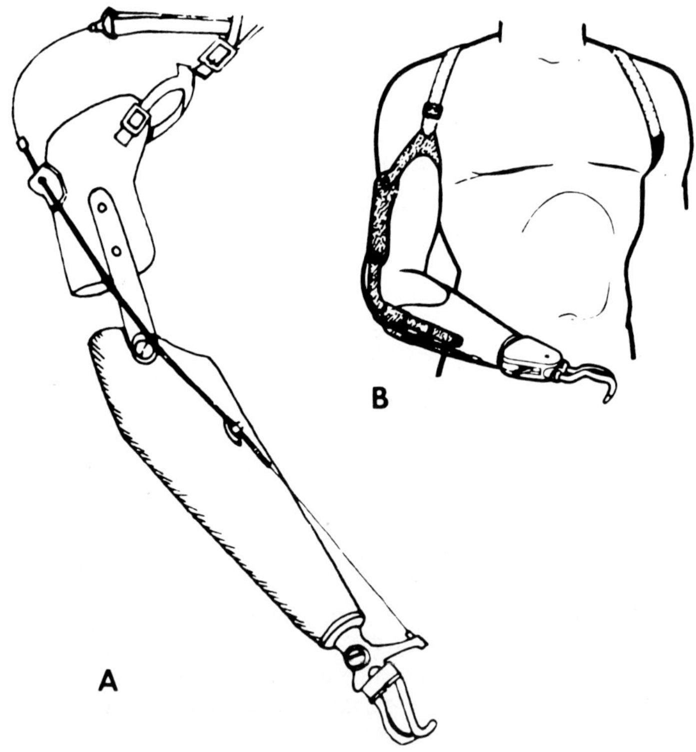

Figure 9–6 *A* and *B*, Below-elbow prostheses. (*A*, From Below and above elbow harness and control system, Evanston, Illinois: Northwestern University Prosthetic-Orthotic Center, 1966. *B*, From Pursley RJ. Harness patterns for upper-extremity prostheses. In: American Academy of Orthopaedic Surgeons. Orthopaedic appliances atlas. Vol. 2. Artificial limbs. Ann Arbor, Michigan: JW Edwards, 1960:105–128. By permission of the Academy.)

Above-Elbow Amputation Sockets. As with below-elbow amputation sockets, above-elbow amputation sockets are usually double walled, and suspension is provided through a harnessing system (Fig. 9–7).

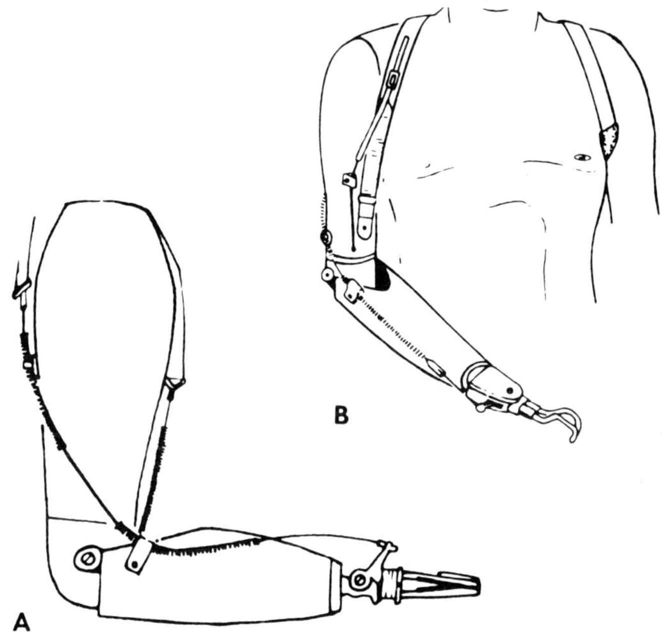

Figure 9–7 *A* and *B*, Above-elbow prostheses. (*A*, From Below and above elbow harness and control system, Evanston, Illinois: Northwestern University Prosthetic-Orthotic Center, 1966. *B*, From Pursley RJ. Harness patterns for upper-extremity prostheses. In: American Academy of Orthopaedic Surgeons. Orthopaedic appliances atlas. Vol. 2. Artificial limbs. Ann Arbor, Michigan: JW Edwards, 1960:105–128. By permission of the Academy.)

Shoulder Disarticulation and Forequarter Prostheses. Although functional shoulder disarticulation and forequarter prostheses are available, the lack of proximal muscles for cable operation on the involved side and the complexity of actions required for the prosthesis to be functional generally negate effective use. Frequently, affected persons opt for a cosmetic shoulder cap or an endoskeletal system passively positioned by the opposite hand.

Exoskeletal and Endoskeletal Prosthetic Systems. Most prostheses are fabricated with an exoskeleton of laminated plastic. To improve cosmesis and minimize weight, endoskeletal component systems have been devised with carefully molded soft surfaces that appear similar to the contralateral limb.

ORTHOTIC PRINCIPLES

Lower Extremity Devices

Ankle-Foot Orthoses. With instability about the ankle, a stable base of support is never achieved during stance phase. With paralytic conditions, not only is stance unstable but footdrop leads to catching of the toe during swing phase. If the triceps surae is involved, no push off is provided.

The conventional (double-upright) orthosis is the prototype ankle-foot orthosis (see Fig. 11–7). A steel stirrup attaches the device to the sole of the shoe. Mechanical ankle joints situated on both the medial and the lateral aspects of the ankle at approximately the height of the anatomic ankle joint connect the stirrup to two metal uprights that pass proximally along the calf. The proximal ends of the uprights are attached to a cuff surrounding the calf. The mechanical ankle joints can be locked or stopped at various angles or fitted with springs that provide resistance to either ankle dorsiflexion or plantar flexion.

With the conventional ankle-foot orthosis, footdrop can be prevented with a stop that prevents plantar flexion during swing phase. Push off is simulated through use of a dorsiflexion stop. With conditions of gross ankle instability, the ankle joints can be rendered immobile. If weight-bearing relief is required, a patellar-tendon-bearing piece is added to redistribute the weight proximally.

With the development of sturdy and resilient thermoplastics, in-shoe ankle-foot orthoses have been designed to incorporate many of the characteristics of the double-bar upright type and yet be lighter weight and provide greater cosmesis (see Fig. 17–1).

Common conditions amenable to the use of an ankle-foot orthosis include hemiparesis, multiple sclerosis, head injury, lumbar radiculopathies, and peroneal neuropathies.

Knee-Ankle-Foot Orthoses. When paralysis or instability occurs at both the knee and the ankle, support must be extended to the proximal thigh, and the knee must be crossed with joints that can be locked. If weight-bearing relief is required at the knee or the ankle, forces can be redistributed even more proximally, incorporating the ischial tuberosity and soft tissues of the proximal thigh.

Upper Extremity Devices

Although upper extremity orthoses vary considerably in design and purpose, there are two basic types. Static orthoses provide structural stability through immobilization to prevent contractures and support joints and muscles weakened by disease or injury. A single joint or several joints may be immobilized with a single device. A burned hand is often immobilized by a static hand orthosis to prevent contractures during healing. A static (resting) wrist-hand orthosis is often used to immobilize and protect joints inflamed by rheumatoid arthritis (see Fig. 25–1). The shoulder can be maintained in abduction for several weeks after a rotator cuff repair to protect the healing tissues.

Functional orthoses improve function through the use of joints, levers, pulleys, and external power sources. The power sources include rubber bands, springs, batteries, and cartridges of compressed gas. Peripheral nerve lesions can be made less disabling by using power sources to simulate the lost motor function. A wrist-hand orthosis that assists wrist and metacarpophalangeal extension through springs or rubber bands may provide added function to a person with radial nerve palsy (see Fig. 25–2). An elbow with posttraumatic instability may be stabilized with a hinged splint. External power may be added to assist elbow flexion or place dynamic stretch to an accompanying flexion contracture.

REHABILITATION

Provision of a prosthesis or an orthosis does not constitute rehabilitation. Rehabilitation is the medical and educational process by which a person, disabled by disease or injury, regains independence in all spheres of life.

Comprehensive rehabilitation is an interdisciplinary team process in which health-care professionals bring together special expertise to maximize a patient's independence.

Because of the large influx of amputees into the health-care system at the end of World War II, Army and Veteran's Administration physicians soon recognized that management of these patients was inadequate and rife with inefficiencies, duplicated services, and patient misconceptions. The team concept was developed and has since succeeded in improved care.

Team Members

Physician. The physician provides the team leadership, directs the amputee clinic, provides the prosthetic prescription, and manages the medical issues. Although most often a physiatrist, the physician may be an orthopedist, a vascular surgeon, or other physician with a special interest and expertise in the management of amputees.

Therapists. For patients with lower extremity amputation, the physical therapist is responsible for muscular reconditioning, gait retraining, and education in stump management and also provides input for the prosthetic prescription. In a like fashion, the occupational therapist often cares for patients with upper extremity amputation. For patients with both upper and lower extremity amputation, the occupational therapist also provides adaptive equipment and retraining for activities of daily living.

Prosthetist. The prosthetist provides input into the prosthetic prescription, fabricates and fits the prosthesis, and aids in the training for its use.

Nurse. The hospital-based nurse provides ward care during hospitalization and assists in patient and family education. The public health nurse may be required to monitor the patient after dismissal from the hospital.

Social Worker. The social worker is responsible for coordinating the financial and vocational issues pertinent to the patient and frequently provides an interface with the patient's family.

Others. At times, the services of a surgeon, psychologist, psychiatrist, or dermatologist may be required.

The Rehabilitation Process

Preamputation Management. For situations in which elective amputation is contemplated, the team provides valuable assistance for preparing the patient and family for the procedure and the subsequent rehabilitation. The patient and family learn about the various team members and about the expected duration of hospitalization and prosthetic training and a prosthesis is shown to them.

Phantom sensation should be fully explained. It is a painless awareness of the amputated part that persists for a variable time after amputation. The sensation can be very vivid, includes any sensation felt by an intact limb, and gradually disappears. It is important for the patient to understand that phantom sensation is entirely normal; otherwise, the patient may undergo significant psychologic trauma and yet be too embarrassed to discuss it with anyone.

If additional time is available, a visit with an amputee is arranged, crutch-walking is reviewed, and a reconditioning program is initiated. The physician may counsel the surgeon about the amputation level if potential prosthetic problems are uncovered during the evaluation.

Postoperative Management. In the hours and days immediately after the amputation, every effort should be made to dissociate the amputee from pain. Appropriate analgesics are very important because evidence suggests that patients with greater surgical pain are more apt to have problems with phantom pain.

Wound management varies according to the circumstances of the amputation and the surgeon's preferences. At first a soft removable dressing is used if the surgeon is concerned about tissue viability and wound healing. If no complications are expected and the medical center has an active amputee team, a rigid cast dressing will often be placed. Attached to the cast is a metal pylon and prosthetic foot. With this immediate postsurgical fitting, wound edema is controlled, stump healing and molding are accelerated, and the patient is able to begin gait retraining on the parallel bars (toe touch only) or upper extremity retraining almost immediately.

Immediate postsurgical fitting is used frequently with below-knee and upper extremity amputations and occasionally with above-knee amputations. Because the stump shrinks and molds as healing occurs, the casts must be changed every 7 to 10 days. The patient is often dismissed after removal of the sutures. Most patients with above-knee amputations are managed with a similar system, except that a removable thermoplastic socket is used. New wound management approaches include rigid, removable systems for below-knee amputations. Application of the dressings (soft or rigid) is discontinued when good wound healing has occurred, and Ace wrapping is used to mold and shrink the stump further. Throughout this period, muscles proximal to the amputated part are strengthened and joint motion is maintained.

Prescription of Prosthesis. When the wound is healed and the edema has cleared (often at 6 to 8 weeks postoperatively), the patient is evaluated by the entire team for prescription of the prosthesis. Each prosthesis must be tailored to the individual needs of the patient. Considerations include medical and cognitive status, stump characteristics, general level of fitness and coordination, financial status, and vocational and avocational interests. The appropriate prescription is completed, and the patient is then examined by the prosthetist to make a mold of the stump. The prosthesis is then fabricated around this mold.

Fitting of Prosthesis and Training in Its Use. Fitting and training are usually accomplished in 1 to 2 weeks on an outpatient basis. Complicating factors, such as cardiopulmonary disease, a marginally healed wound, or a second amputation, may require the patient to be hospitalized. As the patient undergoes training, the prosthetist continues to modify and adjust the prosthesis until it is comfortable and efficient. Fabrication is then completed, and the patient continues retraining until independent use is ensured. Strengthening exercises for endurance are prescribed at the time of dismissal.

Long-Term Management. Many amputees return to their previous employment without difficulty. Whether they have had an upper or lower extremity amputation, many will require modifications to their automobile. Some patients with upper extremity amputation may require modifications in their workplace, and those with occupations requiring bimanual dexterity or heavy physical labor may require vocational assessment and retraining.

The patient returns to the amputee clinic periodically for monitoring and fitting and to address other problems relating to the amputation.

The frequency of prosthetic replacement varies greatly. Light users may not require another prosthesis for many years, whereas a farmer may need a new prosthesis every 2 years. Because the stump often continues to shrink for many years, periodic socket and prosthetic replacement will be required on an ongoing basis.

Complications. The most frequent complication is loss of prosthetic fit due to changes in the size and shape of the stump. Such changes may result in stump irritation, ulceration, infection, or edema and, if not managed with proper prosthetic modification, may require stump modification.

Stump pain and phantom pain are also frequent and must be carefully delineated. Stump pain is most often caused by problems with the prosthetic fit but may also relate to bony overgrowth, adherent scar, or painful neuroma. Phantom pain is defined as a painful phantom sensation; it is not a universal occurrence. Every effort should be made to identify and correct the cause. Although socket modifications, injections for neuroma, and relaxation with biofeedback training may relieve or modify the pain in some patients, many others are resistant to specific treatment. Whenever possible, the single most important management technique is to return the amputee to regular use of a properly fitting prosthesis.

The rehabilitation process is similar when fitting an orthosis and training a patient in its use, although the duration of intervention is usually much shorter.

SUMMARY

The management of amputees serves as an effective model for comprehensive rehabilitation. These patients present with a major disability. Before rehabilitation intervention, such patients cannot ambulate or perform self-care activities and often cannot accomplish vocational tasks. They have a significant loss of body image and are often depressed and anxious about the future. With comprehensive rehabilitation, they can usually be returned to full functional independence at home and work. This can be done without altering the impairment in any way (the patient still has an amputated extremity). Instead, rehabilitation has an impact on the disability (inability to ambulate or to accomplish activities of daily living) by prosthetic fitting and retraining in gait and activities of daily living and on the handicap (inability to drive an automobile or operate machinery) by modifications to the automobile and workplace.

Early intervention must be stressed. Potentially, amputations caused by vascular disease can be prevented by reducing risk factors such as smoking, a high-fat diet, and poor exercise habits. After the onset of peripheral vascular disease, proper management of ischemic ulcers and timely vascular procedures may avoid or delay the time of amputation. After the amputation, early intervention can avoid complications such as contractures, deconditioning, delayed or improper fitting of the prosthesis, and inadequate training that have an adverse impact on acceptance and use of the prosthesis. Several excellent texts have in-depth discussions of prosthetics and orthotics.[1-3]

REFERENCES

1. Banerjee SN, ed. Rehabilitation management of amputees. Baltimore: Williams & Wilkins, 1982.
2. American Academy of Orthopaedic Surgeons. Atlas of limb prosthetics: surgical and prosthetic principles. St. Louis: CV Mosby, 1981.
3. Redford JB, ed. Orthotics etcetera. 2nd ed. Baltimore: Williams & Wilkins, 1980.

10 LYMPHEDEMA

G. Keith Stillwell, M.D., Ph.D.

Lymphedema occurs because of obstruction or insufficiency of the lymphatic system.[1] It may be congenital or familial, but in most cases it is acquired. The principal function of the lymphatic system is to return water and proteins from the tissue fluid space to the bloodstream. If the capacity of the system is inadequate for the load of lymph being produced, edema results.

PRODUCTION OF LYMPH

Lymph is derived from tissue fluid, although it is believed to differ from it after being in the lymphatics for a time. The Starling hypothesis dealt with factors believed to affect the transudation of water across the blood capillary membrane. This filtration mechanism is responsible for the production of the major part of the interstitial fluid. The production of water as a by-product of metabolic activity would not be a significant factor in the creation of the lymph load.

Increases in the intracapillary hydrostatic pressure, which result from arteriolar dilatation (for example, with local heating, muscular activity, or high environmental temperatures) or from venous obstruction (for example, congestive heart failure or constricting garments), will lead to the passage of more water from the blood to the tissue fluid. A decrease in the tissue fluid hydrostatic pressure is presumed also to encourage the passage of water out of the capillaries, and an increase will resist this. There is controversy over the measurement of this pressure. It may be close to atmospheric, although the embedded perforated capsule method of Guyton et al.[2] yields a value of −7 mm Hg. The presence of edema does stretch and presumably disrupt the fine structure of the tissues so that they become more compliant, less elastic, and less resistant to repetition of the accumulation of fluid.

The osmotic pressure exerted by the plasma proteins resists the passage of water out of the capillaries. Reduction of it tends to cause edema (for example, in hepatic or renal diseases or starvation). Of more frequent importance is an increase in the osmotic pressure from accumulating proteins in the edema fluid. These proteins hold the water in the tissue space. They are, for the most part, plasma proteins. A small proportion of them may normally return to the bloodstream by the capillaries, but the major portion is returned to the blood by way of the lymphatics.[1] Other macromolecular materials present secondary to trauma or inflammation also exert an oncotic pressure. Removal of the proteins, as well as the water, is important for the treatment of lymphedema.

REMOVAL OF LYMPH

Lymph flow from the extremities seems mainly to be caused by active vasomotion of the lymphatics.[3] The action of their smooth muscle in conjunction with their valves is a strong pumping mechanism by which the tissue spaces are normally kept cleared of mobile or "free" fluid and of the proteins. Subsidiary mechanisms, such as the skeletal "muscle pump," the "thoracic pump" (aspiration of lymph into the thorax, especially during respiratory inspiration), the pulsation of blood vessels adjacent to the lymphatics, and the force of gravity, probably are minor factors normally but become more important when the normal lymphatic mechanism is inoperative.

POSTSURGICAL LYMPHEDEMA

After surgical ablation of axillary or inguinal lymph nodes, there is a considerable incidence of lymphedema. The exact frequency with which it occurs is unknown, although it is expected to be less after a modified radical mastectomy than after the standard Halsted radical mastectomy (after which it occurs in about 30% to 50% of cases). Olszewski[4] demonstrated that dogs had a transitory lymphedema for 4 to 6 weeks after the surgical procedure followed by a latent period lasting months to years before the clinical appearance of chronic edema. During the latent period, that part of the lymphatic system that is obstructed progressively deteriorates. This deterioration includes fibrosis with loss of permeability and lymph-concentrating ability, development of tortuosities and varicosities with incompetence of the valves, and increased compliance of the vessels. In 1967, a report showed that about 70% of 321 cases occurred within 1 year after mastectomy, but 11% occurred more than 3 years after mastectomy.

The deterioration of the impeded lymphatic system proceeds insidiously whether or not the patient has edema. Patients should take reasonable precautions to avoid further damage to their lymphatics from trauma or infections and to avoid overloading the system beyond its limited capacity to remove lymph from the limb, such as by local heating or prolonged active use of the limb, especially in a hot environment.

Other types of lymphedema can be appropriately treated along the same lines as postsurgical lymphedema. With long-standing lymphedema, a hyperplasia of the superficial fascia develops that may prove irreversible. Restoration to normal dimensions will not be possible with nonsurgical treatment. However, the presence of "pitting" indicates movable fluid and offers some hope that the edema can be reduced by physical measures.

TREATMENT OF LYMPHEDEMA

Dietary restriction of sodium intake and the use of diuretics are generally of little help in the treatment of chronic lymphedema because removal of the excess protein from the tissue fluid is paramount. Similarly, the routine use of antibiotics is not indicated; however, in patients with evidence of infection in the edematous limb, it is important to control the infection before embarking on vigorous attempts to move the fluid.

Measures to Move the Edema Fluid

When the highly effective normal lymphatic vasomotion pump is rendered inoperative, other methods of moving lymph offer hope of improving the edema. If the fluid cannot be moved through major lymphatic vessels, it can still be moved through the tissues and through the microvascular subdermal lymphatic plexus, which is continuous throughout the body. These methods include most of the time-honored ways to which normal lymph flow was attributed, based on experiments in anesthetized animals. Of course, lymphatics other than those obstructed may drain the limb.

Elevation. Water runs downhill, as does lymph, albeit slowly. The elevated limb need not be vertical. Each period of elevation should be for a half hour or more. Patients are urged to elevate the limb for as much of the night as is compatible with sleep.

Massage. Various pneumatically operated compression devices are available, and all are probably effective. In a study comparing three different devices to the use of no device at all, no significant differences were found, but the patients did have somewhat more improvement with the use of a device.[5] The pneumatic device is usually applied with a pressure of 50 to 70 mm Hg for 45 to 60 minutes at each session.

Manual massage may be helpful for mobilizing pockets of fluid that have been less responsive to the pneumatic device. Questions have been raised about the possibility of damage to the delicate lymphatic terminals, but the significance of this is not established.[6] Massage of an upper extremity usually consumes 10 minutes.

Exercise. Contractions of the skeletal muscles may promote venous and lymphatic flow. When the patient is wearing elastic support, the exercises will also compress the subcutaneous tissues between the muscles and the elastic support. The contractions are performed isometrically or with minimal joint motion, although joint motion is not forbidden. Patients with flaccid paralyses who are unable to perform such exercises have generally not responded as well to the other components of the treatment program.

Measures to Inhibit Accumulation of New Fluid

Because of the increased compliance of the lymphedematous tissue and the skin, there is little natural resistance to recurrence of the swelling. Application of external elastic support is essential if progress is to be made in overcoming the edema. A woven elasticized bandage is preferable for the first few weeks, while the size of the limb is decreasing. Subsequently, the improvement is maintained by the use of an elasticized sleeve or stocking. The bandage should be applied in the morning before arising; it is not worn at night. The bandage must be removed and reapplied about every 2 hours because it does not stay in place indefinitely, particularly around the knee or elbow.

The law of Laplace relates the pressure (P) across the wall of a container, the tension (T) in the wall, and the radius (R) of curvature of the wall, stating that

$$P = \frac{T}{R}.$$

To maintain any given transmural pressure if R is larger, T must be larger too. In the case of the swollen limb, the implication is that it will take less tension in the elastic support (or the skin) to maintain the size of the limb if it can first be made smaller.[7]

RESULTS OF PHYSICAL TREATMENT

Patients with upper extremity lymphedema can generally be treated as outpatients, but it is often preferable that patients with lower extremity lymphedema be hospitalized for more adequate elevation. Treatment, usually applied twice daily, consists of the pneumatic pump, manual massage, and isometric exercise (all used while the limb is elevated) and instruction in the application of the bandage.

After about 4 days of such treatment, a reduction of about 30% of the edema by volume measurement will have been attained in patients with upper extremity lymphedema.[5] The patient then pursues a home program with elevation of the limb for 30 or more minutes every 2 hours, during which time 5 to 10 repetitions of the exercises are done every 5 minutes. At the end of this period of elevation, the bandage is completely removed and then reapplied. After 1 or 2 weeks at home, the interval is lengthened to 3 hours and then 4 hours. The impression is that patients with upper extremity lymphedema obtain a further reduction of about 30% of the edema during 4 to 6 weeks of the home program. They are then fitted with a sleeve.

Because of technical difficulties with measurement of the volume of the lower extremity, there are no comparable data, but the clinical impression is that somewhat less improvement is obtained in the lower extremity. Data on long-term results are spotty, but they suggest that most patients maintain the improvement, a few improve more, and a few have worsening.

CONTINUATION OF EXTERNAL ELASTIC SUPPORT

After the edema has been well controlled for about 3 months, experimenting with removal of the external elastic support is reasonable. By then, the tissue spaces formerly occupied by the edema should have shrunk and the tissues should have regained some of their elasticity. The patient should remove the support 1 hour before going to bed at night. The circumferences of the limb at a few places are measured then and at bedtime. If there is no apparent increase in the size of the limb, the process is repeated an hour earlier each day. In this way, the patient determines how long it is possible to go without the support without having a recurrence of the edema. Most patients with postmastectomy lymphedema can be without support for 4 to 6 hours but cannot abandon the support altogether, but patients who no longer have an underlying cause for edema usually can be without support.

REFERENCES

1. Földi M. Physiology and pathophysiology of lymph flow. In: Clodius L, ed. Lymphedema. Stuttgart: Georg Thieme Verlag, 1977:1–11.
2. Guyton AC, Granger HJ, Taylor AE. Interstitial fluid pressure. Physiol Rev 1971; 51:527–563.
3. Olszewski WL, Engeset A. Intrinsic contractility of prenodal lymph vessels and lymph flow in human leg. Am J Physiol 1980; 239:H775–783.
4. Olszewski WL. Pathophysiological and clinical observations of obstructive lymphedema of the limbs. In: Clodius L, ed. Lymphedema. Stuttgart: Georg Thieme Verlag, 1977:79–102.
5. Tinkham RG, Stillwell GK. The role of pneumatic pumping devices in the treatment of postmastectomy lymphedema. Arch Phys Med Rehabil 1965; 46:193–197.
6. Casley-Smith JR. The structural basis for the conservative treatment of lymphedema. In: Clodius L, ed. Lymphedema. Stuttgart: Georg Thieme Verlag, 1977:13–25.
7. Stillwell GK. The Law of Laplace: some clinical applications. Mayo Clin Proc 1973; 48:863–869.

11 REHABILITATION AFTER STROKE

Mehrsheed Sinaki, M.D.

Hemiplegia due to a cerebrovascular accident (stroke) is common and requires a special rehabilitation program. This program should start early. Stroke creates an important source of dependency in the community that is a considerable burden to medical services. It is important to reduce this burden as much as possible by ensuring that stroke patients with rehabilitation potential reach their maximal level of independence. Hemiplegia is one of the disorders for which patients are most frequently referred for rehabilitation.

CAUSE OF STROKE

The basic processes that account for most strokes are thrombosis, thromboembolism, embolism, and hemorrhage. Hemorrhage may be intracerebral or subarachnoid. Survival is poorest for patients with stroke caused by intracerebral hemorrhage (Table 11–1).[1] The intensity of the rehabilitation program should be adjusted according to the cause of stroke. If the cause is hypertension and hemorrhage, the first goal should be to control the

TABLE 11–1 Survival to 30 Days After Stroke in Residents of Rochester, Minnesota, 1975–1979

Type of Stroke	*Survival (%)*
Cerebral infarction	84
Subarachnoid hemorrhage	63
Intracerebral hemorrhage	42

Data from Garraway, et al.[1]

hypertension. Meanwhile, a mild, slowly progressive rehabilitation program can be initiated (that is, passive range of motion and positioning) until the patient's condition becomes stable. In cases of completed postthrombotic and embolic stroke, range of motion and progressive ambulation should be started as soon as they are tolerated by the patient.

REHABILITATION

The primary concerns of rehabilitation are evaluation of the patient's potential for developing goals (Table 11–2). These goals should be realistic. They should also be flexible because the patient's neurologic status and degree of deficits usually change with time. The best results are obtained when the patient and family participate as team members in setting the rehabilitation goals.

TABLE 11–2 Factors to Consider in Evaluation of a Patient's Potential for Rehabilitation After Stroke

- Exercise tolerance
  - Weakness, stiffness, cardiopulmonary insufficiency, reaction to drugs
- Motivation
  - Level of consciousness, emotional status, behavior, communication, memory
- Motor deficit
  - Weakness, spasticity, contracture
- Sensory deficit
  - Vision, hearing, proprioception, discrimination, cortical integration
- Postural control
  - Sitting, standing, walking

The emotional reactions of the hemiplegic patient to loss of control of the body may be overwhelming; the level of depression, anxiety, fear, frustration, anger, hostility, or sometimes senility may prevent the patient from having a cooperative, receptive, and learning attitude toward rehabilitation. It is important to be aware of the patient's premorbid personality, occupation, and skills and of family and social relationships.

Early Phase (Table 11–3)

The patient may be unconscious, unable to participate actively in care, or uncooperative during the early phase of treatment.

Nursing Care. Pressure sores can be prevented by using a water mattress and changing the patient's position every 2 hours during the day and every 4 hours during the night. Persons involved in the patient's care should be instructed in the principles of posi-

TABLE 11–3 Common Complications After Stroke

Early
Pressure sores
Urinary retention or incontinence
Bowel incontinence or constipation
Urinary tract infection
Depression
Deep venous thrombosis
Pulmonary atelectasis or pneumonia
Language disorders
Late
Spasticity and contractures
Shoulder-hand syndrome
Central pain
Seizure disorders

tioning in bed. The desired positioning principles are as follows: (1) a small pillow is placed by the greater trochanter of the plegic hip when the patient is supine; (2) a pillow is placed in the axilla of the plegic side, abducting the arm up 60° to 90° when the patient is supine, and the hand is elevated higher than the elbow; and (3) the plegic leg is elevated, and the foot is higher than the knee when the patient is supine (a footdrop splint is used when indicated) (Fig. 11–1). Supportive positions should be used to prevent overstretch of the neurovascular plexus and glenohumeral joint of the flail shoulder during sitting or transfer activities. When palmar grasp reflex is present, the resting-hand splint (Fig. 11–2) should be modified in order to avoid increasing the flexor digitorum tone through palmar stimulation (Fig. 11–3).

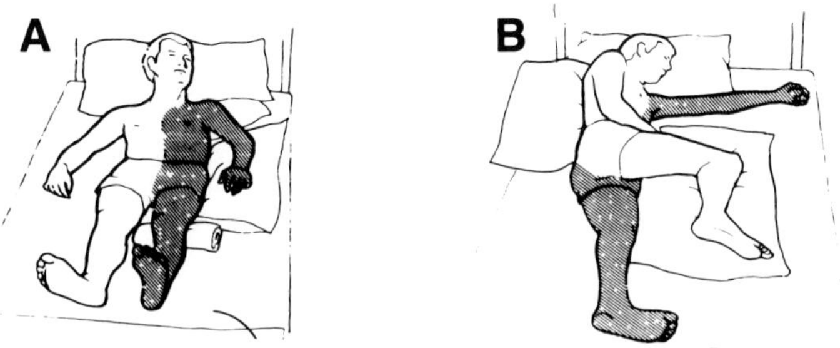

Figure 11–1 Proper positioning principles for patients with hemiplegia. Shaded area is affected side. *A*, When supine. *B*, When lying on affected side. Arm needs to be abducted and extended to avoid rotator cuff injury.

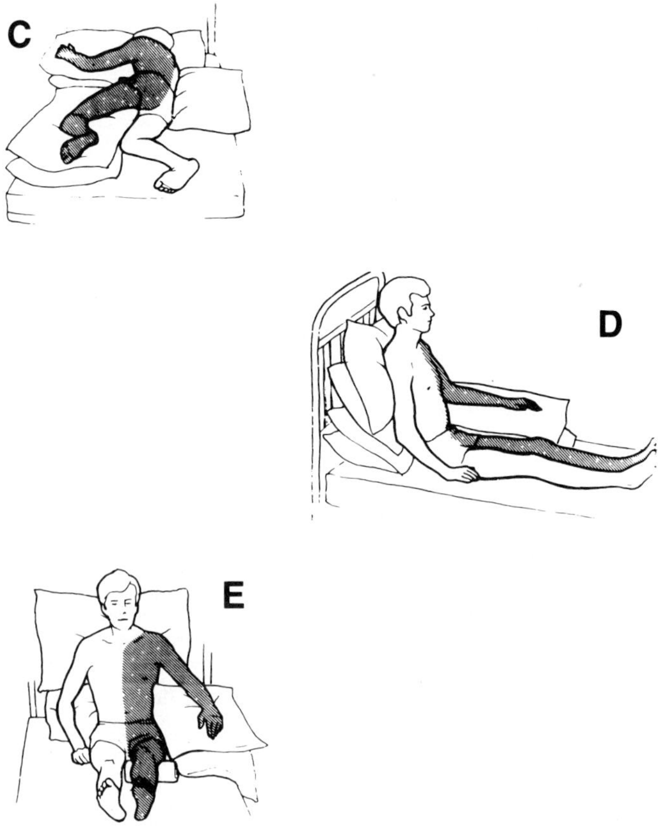

Figure 11–1 Continued. *C*, When lying on unaffected side. *D* and *E*, When sitting in bed. (From Seymour R, ed. Home exercises for the patient with hemiplegia. Lexington, Kentucky: Allied Health Publications, University of Kentucky, 1983. By permission of the publisher.)

Range-of-Motion Exercises. Passive range-of-motion exercises are used to prevent contractures and stiffness. When the upper extremity has marked weakness with severe involvement of the shoulder girdle muscles, the glenohumeral joint needs to be supported during range-of-motion exercises. This prevents glenohumeral subluxation and injury to the rotator cuff by the subluxed head of the humerus.

Urinary Tract and Bowel. Infections of the urinary tract should be prevented. Treatment is required if such infections occur. If the patient is incontinent of urine and if the bladder sphincter is flaccid, an external condom catheter is used in men and an indwelling catheter is used in women. External catheters are changed every day, and indwelling catheters are changed weekly.

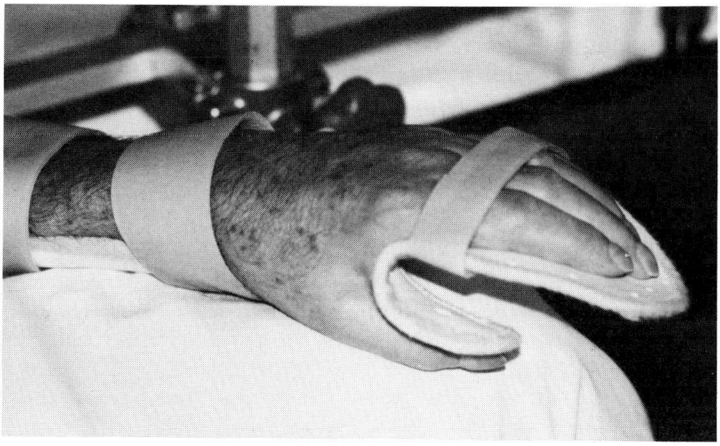

Figure 11–2 Resting-hand splint with palmar contact.

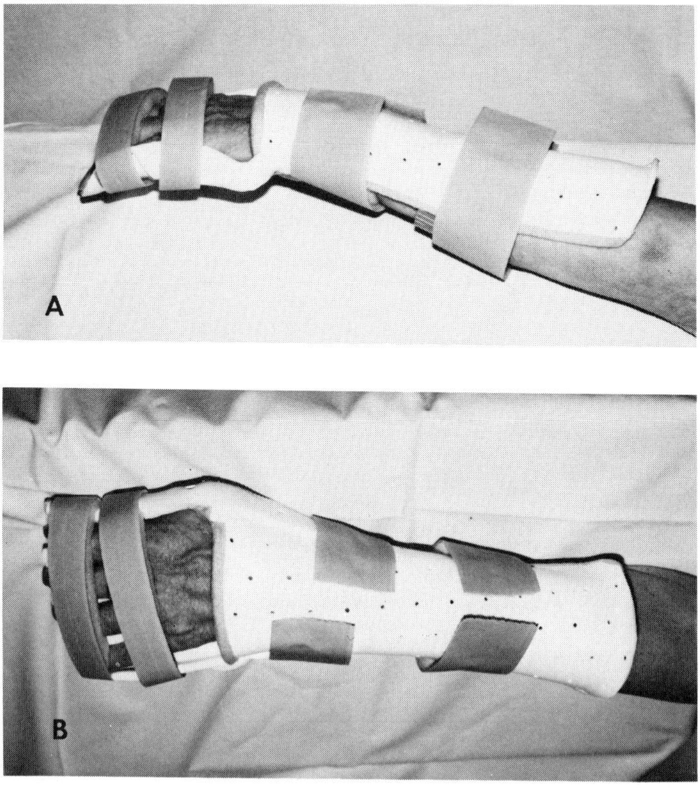

Figure 11–3 *A* and *B*, Resting-hand splint with elimination of palmar contact to avoid palmar grasp reflex during stretching and resting.

If urinary retention is a problem, intermittent catheterization is performed four times a day. Urine specimens for culture need to be obtained weekly until bladder control is achieved (Table 11–4). The amount of residual urine after voiding needs to be determined periodically (perhaps twice a week) to avoid high amounts of residual urine (more than 90 ml) with "overflow" voiding. A fluid intake of 1,600 to 1,800 ml a day improves constipation and urinary output. The care of neurogenic bladder or uninhibited bladder is described in detail in Chapter 21. Bowel movement should be encouraged every other day or even daily if this has been the premorbid pattern. Overall, every effort should be made to prevent fecal impaction. In cases of constipation, a high-fiber diet and a stool softener are recommended. If these measures are unsuccessful, use of glycerin or bisacodyl (Dulcolax) suppositories can be considered.

Emotional Lability. Emotional problems should be recognized and dealt with in order to avoid a delay in the rehabilitation process.

TABLE 11–4 Management of Neurogenic Bladder in Stroke Patients

	Treatment, by Sex	
Findings	*Male*	*Female*
Flaccid bladder sphincter, urinary incontinence	Ambulating: condom catheter In bed: urinal Avoid indwelling catheter if possible Bethanechol (Urecholine), 10 to 15 mg three to four times daily*	Indwelling catheter (change weekly) Bethanechol (Urecholine), 15 mg four times daily*
Spastic sphincter	Intermittent catheterization every 3 hours; later extend to every 4 hours or four times daily Methantheline (Banthine), 15 mg two times daily†	Intermittent catheterization every 3 hours; later extend to every 4 hours or four times daily Fluid intake: 1,600 ml/day Methantheline (Banthine), 15 mg two times daily†
All cases	Urine culture weekly	Urine culture weekly

* Use the lowest effective dose because this drug can increase intestinal peristalsis and bowel incontinence.
† Use the lowest effective dose because this drug can increase constipation.

Deep Venous Thrombosis. Elastic stockings should be worn to prevent deep venous thrombosis of the lower extremities. This is especially important during ambulatory activities. Early detection of phlebitis and application of proper treatment are important. Trauma to the lower extremities should be avoided during transfer activities. The risk of deep venous thrombosis is obviously lower in patients who are receiving anticoagulant treatment for their cerebrovascular disease or for their cardiac disease (in cases of cardiogenic emboli). In other patients, subcutaneously administered heparin (5,000 U every 12 hours) may have a beneficial preventive effect.

Respiratory Care. A dependent position, lack of deep breathing, and accumulation of secretions in the alveoli contribute to the development of pulmonary atelectasis or pneumonia. Incentive deep-breathing exercisers are used when a patient's cooperation permits. Respiratory therapy and postural drainage are indicated in most cases.

Speech and Language. Problems with communication can vary from disturbances of articulation (dysarthria) to disorders of comprehension or programming of language (aphasia). Early evaluation of communication problems and initiation of proper measures and speech therapy are of utmost importance.

Late Phase (Table 11–3)

In this phase, patients participate more actively in physical therapy and occupational therapy training sessions.

Training in Activities on the Mat. Mat activities include turning, rolling, sitting, and kneeling. Motor reeducation should be based on the following points.

(1) The affected side should be activated, and therefore stimulated, with correct postures and with passive and active movements.

(2) The patient should be positioned in postures that inhibit spasticity (for example, a lateral prone position with the involved side up and the head turned to the affected side is useful to inhibit the spasticity of the extensor muscles in the leg and flexor muscles in the arm).

(3) Passive and active exercises of paralyzed limbs should be started early after stroke and continued into the late phase. These are significant sources of exteroceptive and proprioceptive stimuli.

(4) Passive and active movements should be started in the trunk and subsequently be performed in the shoulder and hip. The movements should gradually be extended from these proximal joints to joints that are more distal.

(5) Restoring righting reactions, equilibrium reactions, weight on the affected side, and postural adaptation against gravity should accompany the performance of passive and active exercises. Neuro-

muscular facilitation techniques are used to elicit a refined movement, and eventually that movement can be performed volitionally.[2,3] Once this is accomplished, the movement is repeated and polished until it becomes permanent.[4]

Brachial Plexus and Rotator Cuff Injury in the Flail Upper Extremity. The flaccid hemiplegic shoulder needs to be protected from undue strain in order to avoid rotator cuff injury, which could initiate the development of "hemiplegic shoulder-hand syndrome" and frozen shoulder. The following principles are recommended for the treatment of shoulder-hand syndrome: (1) proper positioning of the upper extremity (Fig. 11–1 and 11–4), (2) antiedema measures (see Chapter 10), (3) passive or active-assisted range-of-motion exercises, and (4) pain reduction by use of analgesics or a trial of transcutaneous electrical nerve stimulation. In some cases, application of a mild, localized heat, such as ultrasound, to the painful shoulder will decrease pain. Heat to the whole upper extremity should be avoided in order to prevent an increment of edema.

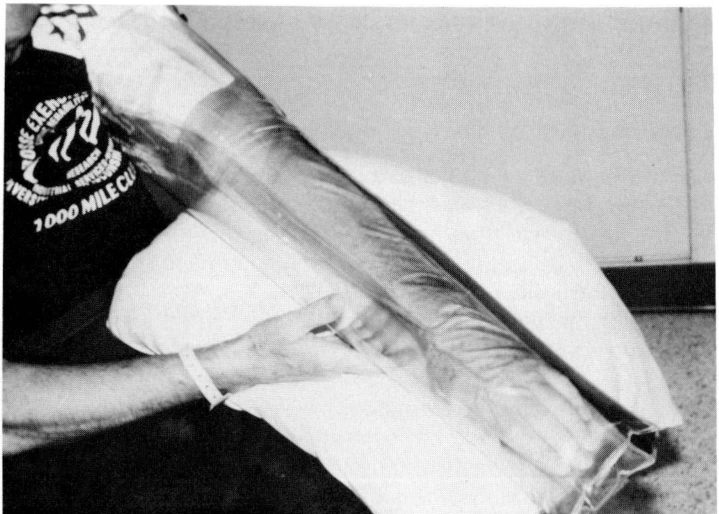

Figure 11–4 Air splint for decreasing edema of upper extremity while stretching it.

Thalamic Pain. Occasionally, some hemiplegic patients who also have suffered injury to the thalamic nuclei complain of disturbing unilateral sensory symptoms. These symptoms are persistent and aggravated by stress and fatigue. They are described as burning, drawing, swelling, tingling, and hurting sensations. When the involved extremities are touched, a disagreeable, unpleasant sensation is produced, and the patient exhibits a "touch-me-not" attitude. The sensory stimuli become blocked or distorted at the damaged thalamus and are perceived as painful and distressing sensations at the sensory cortex. This distressing pain can significantly interfere with rehabilitation efforts. In many patients, this pain syndrome gradually improves. In some patients, pain may be reduced by anticonvulsant medications, such as carbamazepine (Tegretol). Amitriptyline (Elavil) alone or in combination with fluphenazine (Prolixin) is also often helpful, as may be some of the benzodiazepine derivatives. The prolonged use of phenothiazines (such as fluphenazine) should be avoided because it may lead to parkinsonism and, even more disturbingly, to tardive dyskinesias, especially in elderly patients.

Seizure Disorder. A seizure disorder is not a rare complication of cerebral infarction. The residual atrophic region may emanate epileptiform activity leading to partial or generalized seizures. When this occurs, treatment with anticonvulsants should be instituted.

Use of the Upper Extremity for Self-Care and Activities of Daily Living. Patients should be instructed to initiate use of the upper extremity even if the function is not coordinated (Fig. 11–5). Even small accomplishments bring them closer to achieving independence.

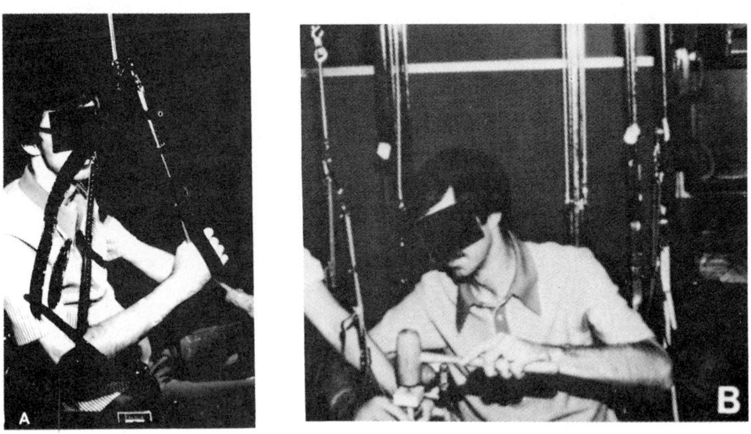

Figure 11–5 *A* and *B*, Patient using deltoid aid (Rancho Los Amigos overhead suspension sling) on hemiplegic side to aid performance of bimanual activities.

Ambulatory Activities. Gait training starts with attaining sitting balance and progresses to standing balance and then walking. Learning to transfer in and out of a bed and chair facilitates self-care and is initiated as soon as it is tolerated by the patient (Fig. 11–6). There are different schools of thought regarding use of ankle-foot orthoses for gait training and also different methods for gait training. Gait training may be applied with the therapist holding and positioning the hemiplegic arm and without use of any devices for ambulation. Gait training may also be secured and applied more safely with use of an ankle-foot orthosis and parallel bars. Later, a broad-based cane or other assistive devices can be introduced.

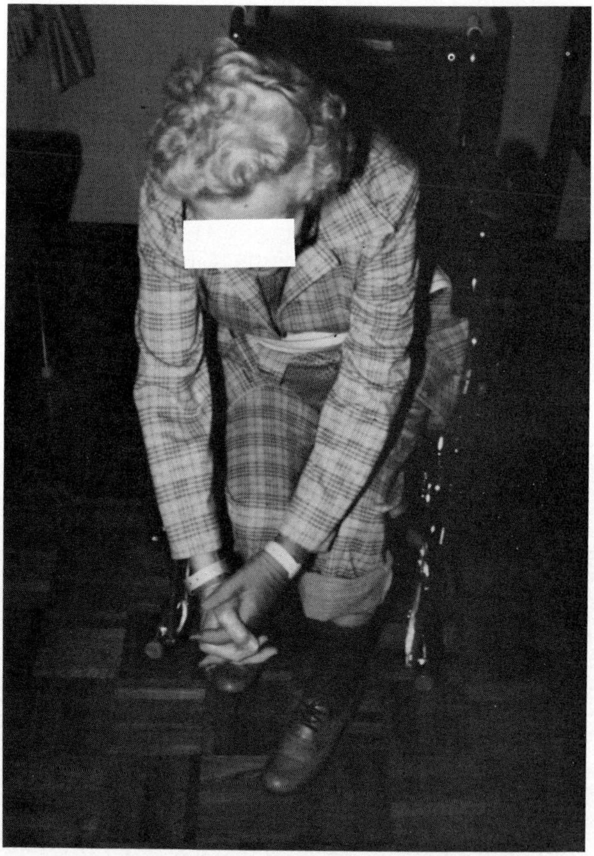

Figure 11–6 Patient, in order to stand, is instructed to extend the hemiplegic left upper extremity with help of unaffected hand. This facilitates extension of affected knee for weight bearing.

Anosognosia, Unilateral Neglect, and Homonymous Hemianopia. Specific methods of treatment are used to try to overcome the deficits of body image, space perception, and unilateral neglect resulting from parietal lobe damage. Intensive training by an occupational therapist is needed. One source of stimulus is placement of a radio or a television beside the neglected side. Perception can also improve with weight bearing after proper splinting of the affected area. Stimulation of the proprioceptors of the joints is a good feedback mechanism. In most cases, the perception of a limb may return if the physical treatment program is geared to its function.[5]

Orthoses in Adults With Hemiplegia

The prognosis for functional use of the upper limb after a severe stroke with hemiplegia is generally poor; however, the prognosis for ambulation is relatively good. Approximately two-thirds of adult patients with hemiplegia after a cerebrovascular accident will have less function of the upper extremities; however, 70% will be able to ambulate with orthotic assistance or external support for the lower extremity. Different types of ankle-foot orthoses are used for ambulatory activities in hemiplegic patients (see Fig. 17–1 *C* and *D*; Fig. 11–7). Ambulation starts with training in sitting

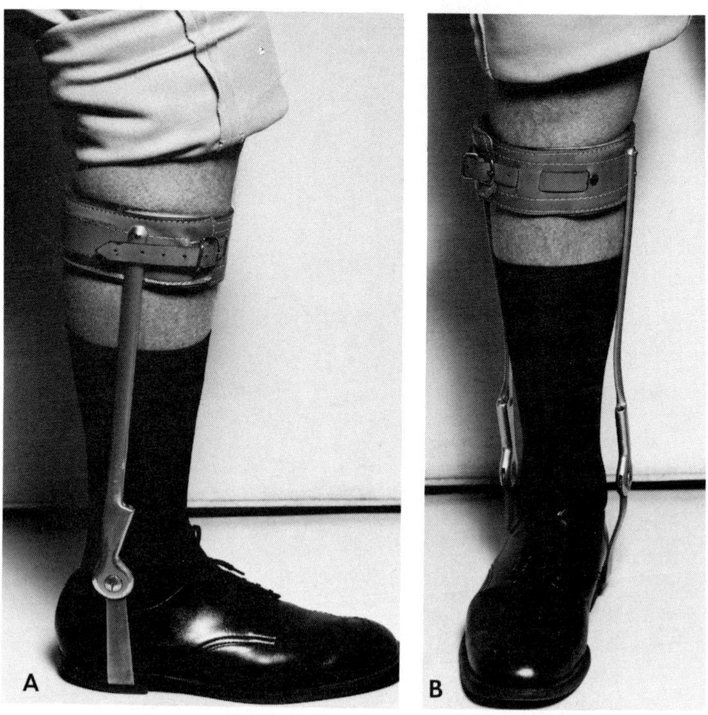

Figure 11–7 Lateral (*A*) and anterior (*B*) views of double-upright ankle-foot orthosis used for moderate to severe weakness of dorsiflexors of ankles. (From Sinaki M. Rehabilitation. In: Mulder DW, ed. The diagnosis and treatment of amyotrophic lateral sclerosis. Boston: Houghton Mifflin Professional Publishers, 1980:169–193. By permission of John Wiley & Sons.)

balance and advances to standing balance and gait training. Hemiplegic patients may or may not need assistive devices for ambulation. Most hemiplegic patients ambulate with use of a cane and an ankle-foot orthosis on the hemiplegic side (short leg splint or brace). In some cases, a shoulder hemisling is used to support the shoulder and arm of a patient with a flail upper extremity; it should be used in selected cases.

If the plegic hand is developing severe spasticity and flexion contractures, splinting needs to be considered. The flail wrist may require only a cock-up splint. The resting-hand and wrist splints are made of molded Orthoplast and may be applied over the dorsal-volar aspect of the extremity, according to the patient's condition. Resting-hand splints with contact on the dorsum of the hand decrease the palmar grasp reflex in spastic upper extremities (Fig. 11–3). Other types of splints are the Bobath digital spreader, hand cone, and Isotoner glove (for certain indications).

The following are some of the most popular arm slings and supports used: (1) Zimmer strap, (2) Zimmer sling, (3) Bobath sling (Fig. 11–8), (4) hemihook harness (Fig. 11–9), (5) deltoid aid (Ran-

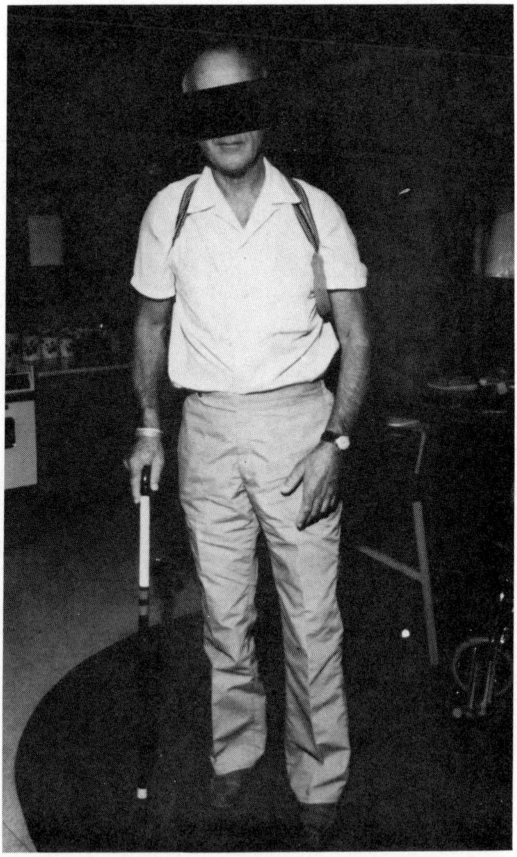

Figure 11–8 Bobath sling, used to decrease pain in left shoulder with moderate weakness of shoulder girdle musculature.

cho Los Amigos overhead suspension sling) (Fig. 11–5), (6) gutter splint (Fig. 11–10), and (7) foam wedge combined with a lapboard (Fig. 11-11).

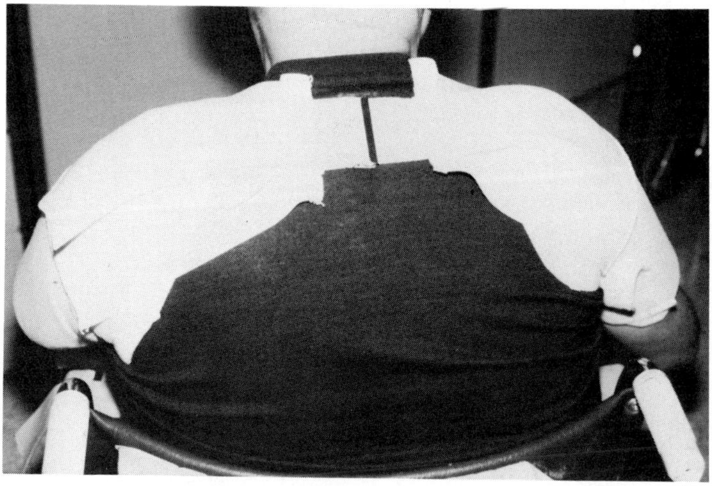

Figure 11–9 Hemihook harness.

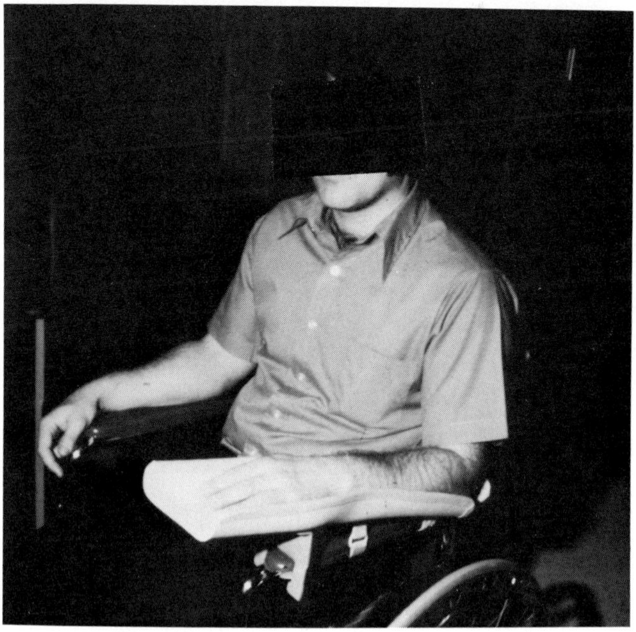

Figure 11–10 Gutter splint, applied to arm of chair.

The following are some of the common wheelchair features and adaptive equipment desired for patients with hemiplegia:[6] (1) desk-type armrests and lapboards with wedge-shaped hand supports to decrease edema in the hand (Fig. 11–11), (2) elevating leg rests, (3) detachable footrests and leg rests, (4) seat cushion or pad, (5) brake handle extension, (6) lapboard, (7) lap belt, (8) low chair or hemichair, and (9) deltoid aid (Rancho Los Amigos overhead suspension sling) (Fig. 11–5).

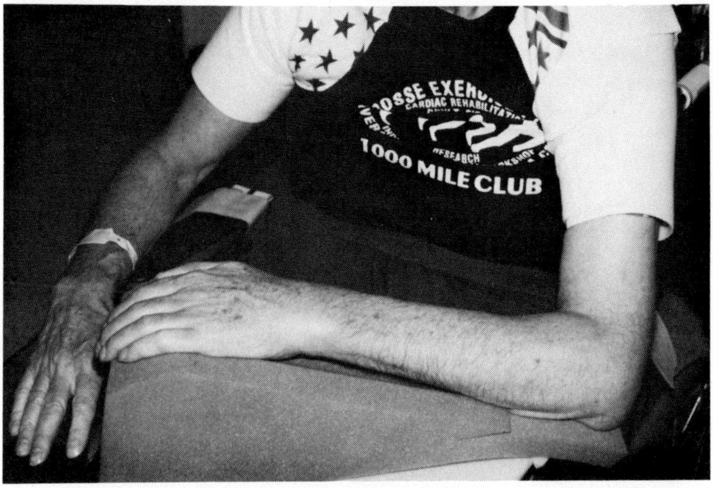

Figure 11–11 Wedge-shaped resting cushion, used to decrease edema in hands of patients with hemiplegia.

Psychometric Tests

Shortly after a stroke, as part of the evaluation of the potential for rehabilitation, the patient's cognitive abilities are evaluated. Detailed psychometric tests are deferred until a patient's medical condition and level of cooperation permit. These tests are useful in most cases.

Dismissal Planning

Before dismissal, a follow-up date should be established and the patient should be referred for vocational rehabilitation if appropriate. Follow-up management may include a neurologic evaluation, a cardiovascular workup, and reevaluation of neurogenic bladder and bowel. A follow-up examination and consultation with the patient and family allow the physicians to remain informed about the implementation and continuation of proper care after dismissal.

REFERENCES

1. Garraway WM, Whisnant JP, Drury I. The changing pattern of survival following stroke. Stroke 1983; 14:699–703.
2. Bobath B. Adult hemiplegia: evaluation and treatment. 2nd ed. London: William Heinemann Books, 1978.
3. Johnstone M. Restoration of motor function in the stroke patient: a physiotherapist's approach. New York: Churchill Livingstone, 1978.
4. Stonnington HH. Rehabilitation in cerebrovascular diseases. Primary Care, March 1980; 7:87–106.
5. Redford JB, Harris JD. Rehabilitation of the elderly stroke patient. Am Fam Physician 1980; 22:153–160.
6. Kottke FJ, Stillwell GK, Lehmann JF, eds. Krusen's handbook of physical medicine and rehabilitation. Philadelphia: WB Saunders, 1982.

12 TRAUMATIC BRAIN INJURY

Robert W. DePompolo, M.D.

Referred to as the silent epidemic by groups such as the National Head Injury Foundation, traumatic brain injury has been little recognized by the general population despite ever-growing numbers of persons suffering from this problem (Fig. 12–1). It is the major cause of death in persons involved in motor vehicle accidents, and it is estimated to cost approximately 4 billion dollars per year for medical care and loss of productivity in the United States. About 50,000 persons each year sustain a head

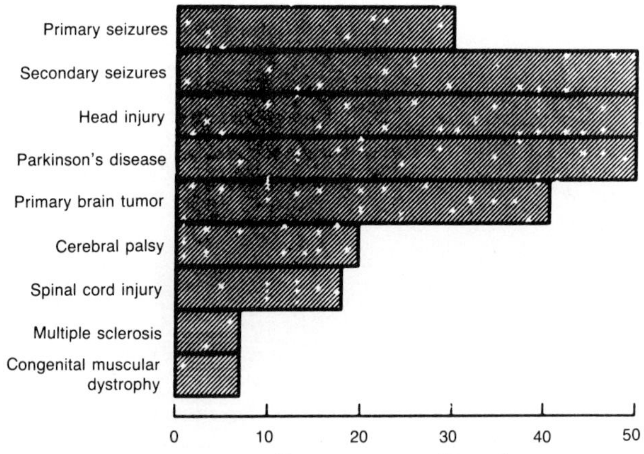

Figure 12–1 Estimated yearly incidence of persons left with disability after head injury compared with incidence of other important neurologic diseases, excluding cerebrovascular disease, which accounts for 450,000 cases yearly. (From National Head Injury Foundation.[1] By permission of the publisher.)

injury that in some way limits their function.[1] In addition, because of continued improvement in the acute care of patients with traumatic brain injury, the number of patients surviving the more severe head injuries has increased. Therefore, the management of patients with traumatic brain injury has become an important issue not only to medical personnel but to society as a whole.

PREVENTION

The first point to be made regarding traumatic brain injury is the issue of preventing new injuries from occurring. Educating the persons at highest risk (those 15 to 30 years of age) as well as the general population to use safety restraints when riding in cars, to wear helmets when riding motorized and unmotorized bikes, and to avoid driving after drinking alcohol may save needless tragedies. Physicians should play an active role in this process and use their position to influence the behaviors of their communities.

PREDICTING OUTCOME

Information regarding outcome based on the injury is useful for planning the appropriate medical intervention as well as for counseling the patient and the patient's family. The need for an accurate prognosis is important. Factors that have been shown to be somewhat predictive of outcome include the patient's age, the duration of coma, the duration of posttraumatic amnesia, the clinical picture, and certain laboratory data.

It has been traditionally believed that given the same extent of brain injury, the patient who is younger than 18 years has a better outcome than the patient who is older than 18 years. The role that age plays in outcome is controversial, but some correlation seems likely, particularly when comparing the extremely young age-groups with the older age-groups.

Both the duration of coma and the duration of posttraumatic amnesia are related to outcome. Jennett and Teasdale[2] found that coma of longer than 2 weeks generally resulted in some physical dependency, coma of longer than 1 month resulted in death or in a persistent vegetative state in 50% of patients, and coma of longer than 2 months resulted in death or a persistent vegetative state in 70% of patients. When they studied the duration of posttraumatic amnesia, they found that if it was less than 14 days 83% of the patients had a good recovery, and if it was more than 28 days only 27% had a good recovery and 30% were severely disabled.

The extent of brain injury obviously is a significant factor in outcome. However, it might be difficult to evaluate the extent of damage early after head injury. Computed tomographic scans may not reveal a more diffuse type of injury to the brain. Brainstem evoked potentials are of some help in predicting outcome.

Certain clinical factors, defined by Jennett and Teasdale[2] in their Glasgow coma scale, are predictive of outcome. The Glasgow coma scale is based on clinical observations of eye movement, motor function, and verbal output. Each category is scored according to the level of performance; the lowest possible score is 3 and the highest is 15 (Table 12–1). Outcome studies based on scores obtained early in the acute phase of traumatic brain injury show that this scale has some predictive value. In addition to predicting ultimate outcome, the Glasgow coma scale also helps standardize the assessments of the different medical and paramedical staff caring for a patient.

TABLE 12–1 Glasgow Coma Scale

Clinical Observation	*Examiner's Test*	*Patient's Response*	*Assigned Score*
Eye opening	Spontaneous	Opens eyes on own	4
	Speech	Opens eyes when asked to in a loud voice	3
	Pain	Opens eyes when pinched	2
	Pain	Does not open eyes	1
Best motor response	Commands	Follows simple commands	6
	Pain	Pulls examiner's hand away when pinched	5
	Pain	Pulls a part of body away when pinched	4
	Pain	Flexes body inappropriately to pain (decorticate posturing)	3
	Pain	Body becomes rigid in an extended position when pinched (decerebrate posturing)	2
	Pain	Has no motor response to pinch	1
Verbal response (talking)	Speech	Carries on a conversation correctly and tells examiner where and who he or she is and the month and year	5
	Speech	Seems confused or disoriented	4
	Speech	Talks so examiner can understand, but makes no sense	3
	Speech	Makes sound that examiner cannot understand	2
	Speech	Makes no noise	1

From Rimel and Jane.[3] By permission of the publisher.

In general, although predicting outcome in patients with traumatic brain injury is important for treatment, establishing firm criteria has been difficult. Certain factors are useful for suggesting outcome; however, assessment of the ultimate outcome is difficult, especially early in the course of the disorder.

MANAGEMENT

Improved acute medical management of patients with traumatic brain injury has resulted in less morbidity and mortality. A few recent texts[2-4] outlined the critical areas of concern. Medical complications that can occur include posttraumatic seizures, hydrocephalus, diabetes insipidus, inappropriate antidiuretic hormone secretion, heterotopic bone formation, and thrombophlebitis.

The specific problems of chronic management of patients with traumatic brain injury vary, depending on the severity of injury. The basic initial rehabilitation problem areas include nutrition, bladder and bowel dysfunction, joint range of motion, skin care, respiratory status, and cognitive stimulation.

The nutritional concerns depend on the patient's level of alertness and ability to swallow. A comatose patient or one with brainstem involvement may be unable to handle oral intake. The initial treatment is usually intravenous maintenance. This probably is adequate for the first few days after injury. If the patient's status remains unchanged, other forms of nutrition need to be considered. The general course is either a nasogastric feeding tube or total parenteral nutrition. Both of these feeding techniques are satisfactory for a few weeks. They allow time for possible recovery and eventual oral feeding. If the patient remains in a coma or persistent vegetative state or continues to be unable to swallow safely, the usual recourse is a feeding gastrostomy or feeding gastrojejunostomy tube. Current techniques allow the gastrostomy tube to be placed using a percutaneous insertion method and local anesthesia.

If the patient shows improvement in the level of alertness and has no major brainstem involvement, oral feedings are possible. If the patient has problems with the oral phase of swallowing, a soft mechanical diet may be preferable to liquids because patients can control soft foods and form a bolus better than they can with liquids.

Bladder and bowel function may be a management problem, again depending on the severity of head injury. Initially, a comatose patient will most likely have an indwelling urethral catheter for bladder drainage. As medical problems stabilize and neurologic status improves, the approach to the bladder will need reconsideration. Depending on the location of the central nervous system damage, spontaneous voiding may or may not occur. The bladder dysfunction that commonly occurs with cortical damage is an uninhibited bladder. However, other types of bladder dysfunction are not unusual, depending on the location of the central nervous system lesion. An uninhibited bladder may not be a management problem if a condom catheter can be worn. Continued episodes of urinary incontinence generally are not tolerated for long periods before the skin in the perineal area breaks down. Bowel control may also be a problem. The extent of the bowel program depends on the patient's level of consciousness, severity of damage, and type of nutritional support.

Maintaining joint range of motion may present a special problem if increased muscle tone exists. A physical therapist may be of significant help in maintaining joint motion through appropriate positioning techniques for the upper and lower extremities and joint range-of-motion exercises. Splinting or inhibitory casting of an extremity may be necessary, depending on the amount of abnormal muscle tone and whether strong synergistic patterns are developing.

Skin care in an immobile patient is also a concern. Such a patient should be repositioned at least every 2 hours by the nursing staff. Skin care also involves preventing irritation from excess moisture resulting from incontinence and sweating. Skin creases that are not kept dry may also be areas of skin breakdown. An air mattress, foam cushion, or water mattress on the bed may prevent bed sores. A sheepskin mattress pad may prevent shear stresses on the skin when the patient is moved around in bed.

Respiratory status may be of concern if the injury involves the brainstem. Cheyne-Stokes respiration, tachypnea, and ataxic respiration can occur with brainstem lesions. Acute respiratory failure requiring ventilation may occur in severe injuries. The respiratory status can also be compromised by aspiration due to poor oral control, and atelectasis may develop secondary to poor ventilation. Patients may require assistance from the nursing staff for coughing. Chest physiotherapy may help prevent pneumonias.

The best approach to the amount and type of stimulation in a patient with resolving coma is somewhat controversial. Providing some degree of visual, tactile, taste, auditory, and olfactory stimulation in a controlled setting is reasonable if only to document the patient's response consistently. In addition, such stimulation may induce a quicker recovery. As coma resolves, cognitive rehabilitation should begin.

It is not unusual for a patient with a closed head injury to move through a state of recovery marked by agitation. When agitation does develop, other possible causes should be ruled out, such as metabolic imbalance, pulmonary embolism, and septicemia. Agitation secondary to head injury can be a difficult management problem. Medications, restraints, and environmental controls are some of the ways to deal with this problem. Appropriate control of the environment is a preferable first step to determine whether it is sufficient to manage the agitation. It is the most difficult but perhaps the most satisfying means of controlling agitation. The patient should be in a structured, consistent, safe environment. If medications are used, the side effects must be clearly understood by the physician. Multiple drugs have been tried, including phenothiazine and haloperidol. Because of concern that these drugs may have a negative impact on cognitive recovery, they are used only when necessary. If restraints are used, they should be appropriate and properly fitted.

REHABILITATION TEAM

Physical Therapy

Often, a patient has a plegic or paretic extremity secondary to the traumatic brain injury. In addition to the role of maintaining range of motion outlined above, the physical therapist is involved in muscle reeducation, strengthening exercises, and exercises directed toward retraining of coordination. Mobility retraining, including gait, transfers, and mobility in bed, may be another area of involvement. Because the deficits vary with the severity of traumatic brain injury, treatment programs must be individualized.

Occupational Therapy

The occupational therapist addresses the areas of activities of daily living such as dressing, hygiene, and feeding and also helps evaluate swallowing difficulties and suggests therapeutic intervention. Cognitive and perceptual functioning can be evaluated and treatment directed toward improvement of a patient's adaptation to these deficits. The occupational therapist may address the issues of disorientation and confusion by helping the team provide the appropriate structure and consistency to the patient's environment. When upper-extremity motor function is impaired secondary to central nervous system damage, the occupational therapist can facilitate maximal use of the arms or hands through functional activities.

Speech Pathology

Patients may demonstrate a speech disorder such as aphasia, dysarthria, or apraxia, depending on the area of central nervous system injury, and require speech therapy. Also, difficulty with prosody can occur. Because communication is a cognitive function, the speech therapist may work in conjunction with the occupational therapist and psychologist to optimize intellectual functioning in many related areas. In some rehabilitation settings, the speech pathologist assesses and treats dysphagia.

Psychology

The psychologist, in conjunction with the occupational therapist and speech pathologist, is the third member of the treatment team who can help direct the rest of the team's efforts in the area of cognitive and perceptual dysfunction. During the recovery stages, the psychologist can provide estimates of cognitive function and, as the deficits stabilize, can administer specific batteries of psychometric tests to define the areas of limitation better. In addition to the standard Wechsler Adult Intelligence Scale, the psychologist can offer other tests to isolate certain areas of cognitive dysfunction. In a patient with a behavioral or emotional problem, the psychologist may counsel the patient or help the rehabilitation team coordinate its efforts more effectively.

Social Service

The social worker may help with arranging financing and obtaining needed equipment. A comprehensive outline of the family structure and the patient's previous work situation and educational experiences can be provided by the social worker. This information can be helpful to the rehabilitation team for setting expectations and goals. The social worker may also provide support to family members and interface among the physician, the therapist, and the family to ensure that questions are being answered appropriately. Other areas of social work involvement include dismissal planning, regardless of the disposition. If the patient is dismissed home, the social worker helps to mobilize the appropriate community resources to provide maximal care for the patient and support for the family. If the disposition is elsewhere, the social worker can help the family locate the best possible alternative housing situation, whether it be a nursing home, sheltered housing, or other chronic care facility. The social worker may also coordinate services with the department of vocational rehabilitation, if appropriate.

Recreation Therapy

Recreation can be used as a tool to facilitate team goals in the areas of motor retraining, cognitive rehabilitation, endurance training, and emotional or behavioral programming. In addition, the recreation therapist helps with issues relating to reentry into the community, including redeveloping avocational interests and social skills. Through trips outside the institution, the patient can be exposed to the community in a protected, gradated fashion.

Rehabilitation Nursing

The nursing staff is an important factor in providing consistency and structure to the patient's daily activities by reinforcing what the patient learns in occupational therapy, in terms of activities of daily living, and in physical therapy, in terms of transfers and mobility. The nursing staff has a significant impact on reinforcing orientation and addressing any behavioral or emotional problems. Finally, the training that might be needed for bowel or bladder function rests heavily on the nursing staff.

Physician

The physician is instrumental not only for managing the medical problems that arise but also for coordinating the efforts of the different team members to establish appropriate goals. The physician has a unique role in counseling the patient and the patient's family to ensure that all questions are answered and that all issues are addressed.

Other

Other possible team members include the dietitian, chaplain, pharmacist, and tutor (for school-age children). No individual team member has exclusive dominion over any particular area of care; the substantial amount of overlap is extremely helpful for reinforcing what is being trained. Therefore, each member should work as part of the team, and the team should set joint goals and approach intervention in a coordinated manner.

CONCLUSION

The rehabilitation of patients with traumatic brain injury demands the teamwork of several different qualified rehabilitation specialists. This may be a devastating injury to both the patient and the patient's family, and the ultimate level of recovery depends to some extent on how aggressively and appropriately rehabilitation services are used. Beyond acute rehabilitation, this patient population has a complex set of needs for community resources, including outpatient rehabilitation, protective housing, vocational retraining, and family and patient support groups.

REFERENCES

1. NHIF Goals. The silent epidemic. Framingham, Massachusetts: National Head Injury Foundation, June 1984.
2. Jennett B, Teasdale G. Management of head injuries. Philadelphia: FA Davis, 1981.
3. Rimel RW, Jane JA. Characteristics of the head-injured patient. In: Rosenthal M, Griffith ER, Bond MR, Miller JD, eds. Rehabilitation of the head-injured adult. Philadelphia: FA Davis, 1983:9–21.
4. Cooper PR, ed. Head injury. Baltimore: Williams & Wilkins, 1982.

13 CEREBRAL PALSY

Ann H. Schutt, M.D.

Cerebral palsy is a nonprogressive disorder of brain dysfunction manifested by abnormalities of movement and posture. It is often accompanied by intellectual defects and language disorders. Aberrant psychosocial behaviors and problems with sensory perception can also occur. This persistent, nonprogressive disorder of qualitative motor abnormalities appears before the age of 3 years. It can affect mobility, self-help, language skills, self-direction, economic self-sufficiency, and capacities for individual living. Two important factors are that cerebral palsy affects children and persists throughout life.

INCIDENCE AND PREVALENCE

The prevalence of cerebral palsy is 500 per 100,000 population, and approximately 500,000 persons in the United States are affected.[1] The life expectancy of these patients ranges from 0 to 82 years (mean, 33.9 years). Approximately 60% of children with cerebral palsy have motor disabilities only, 29% have motor and mental defects, and approximately 2% have other defects such as congenital heart defect, cleft palate, or other congenital abnormalities.

An intervention that seems to have an impact on the outcome of children with cerebral palsy is excellent care in perinatal intensive care units, in which 80% of the children who have brain dysfunctions have mild involvement, 10% moderate, and 10% severe. The incidence of cerebral palsy is decreasing because of preventive measures such as immunizations for rubella and improved obstetric and perinatal care. The morbidity associated with cerebral palsy has decreased because of enrichment programs such as infant stimulation and early infant intervention and mainstreaming in the schools.

ETIOLOGY

When a history is obtained from the parents of a child suspected of having cerebral palsy, some of the salient features are a long labor and a first-born child with a heavy birth weight. The incidence is greater in children whose mothers are older than 35 years or younger than 18 years, and it is more frequent in the white race. Often, the mother has a history of previous miscarriages. Cerebral palsy is known to occur in children with a heavy birth weight, usually more than 4 kg, whose mothers have had multiple pregnancies, and it is more prevalent in multiple births, such as twins.

Some of the common correlates are prematurity, anoxia, breech delivery, and toxemia of pregnancy (especially when the mother has hypertension, proteinuria, or convulsions and requires treatment with magnesium). It is not uncommon when fetal distress or birth trauma occurs. Rh factor, ABO, or MN incompatibilities can be a cause of cerebral palsy, most commonly of the hyperkinesis type; the incidence of this type of cerebral palsy decreased from 20% in 1955 to approximately 2% in 1982. Maternal rubella has been largely eliminated by the immunization programs but is known to be a cause of cerebral palsy. Also, precipitous delivery and cesarean sections are common correlates. The clinical importance of these features lies in the high correlation between specific etiologic factors and clinical syndromes. Unfortunately, only the study of actual brain specimens allows the pathogenesis of these conditions to be well understood. Noninvasive techniques to study the abnormality, such as brain scanning and nuclear magnetic resonance imaging, can be helpful.

CLASSIFICATION

Pathology

Cerebral palsy can be classified according to the site of abnormality. Extrapyramidal tract lesions in the basal nucleus may result in abnormalities of motion such as athetosis, choreas, tremors, ballismus, dystonias, and rigidities. Lesions in the cerebellar area result primarily in the ataxic and atonic forms of cerebral palsy. Pyramidal tract lesions result in spastic forms of cerebral palsy.

Clinical Symptoms

The clinical classification may be subdivided into spastic forms, hyperkinesias, dyskinesias, ataxia, and mixed forms.[1] The spastic forms are characterized by signs of pyramidal tract involvement, specifically by the presence of hyperactive stretch reflexes. They are also characterized by abnormal increases in tone and a release of postural and labyrinthine reflexes and may involve any combination of the limbs and trunk. Affected patients have a tendency for formation of muscle contracture.

Hyperkinesias and dyskinesias are characterized by a movement disorder affecting the trunk and extremities. The muscle tone often varies with the age of the patient. Frequently, patients can be very atonic at birth and then develop abnormal movement disorders around age 2½ to 3 years. These movement disorders have been described as athetosis, choreas, ballismus, tremors, dystonias, and occasionally rigidities. Tremors are uncontrollable and pendular or patternlike. The dystonic movement disorders are characterized by tonic postural attitudes, predominantly in the trunk and neck. They involve intermittent muscle spasms, abnormal imbalances of muscle tension, and spasms, primarily in the trunk musculature. Rigidity is manifested by a non-rate-dependent increase in muscle tone; this feature is in contrast to spasticity, which is a rate-dependent increase in tone. Hyperkinesis and dyskinesis often do not present until the age of 2 years.

The ataxic form of cerebral palsy is characterized by a loss of the sense of balance. Most cases are probably due to involvement of the cerebellum. An intention tremor can result in abnormal depth perception, lack of balance, and extreme incoordination, and patients may stagger as they attempt to walk.

The mixed forms of cerebral palsy are a combination of the spastic and extrapyramidal features.

Site of Involvement

The site of involvement is also used to classify cerebral palsy. *Paraplegia* involves the legs only, and most cases are of the spastic variety. *Diplegia* is the most common form of spasticity; it primarily involves the legs, and the arms are affected to a slight degree. Again, most cases are of the spastic variety. *Tetraplegia* involves all four extremities (Fig. 13–1). Cases in which the greatest involvement is in the legs are usually of the spastic type, and those in which the greatest involvement is in the arms are often of the hyperkinetic or dyskinetic type. Of children with cerebral palsy, 54% have paraplegia, diplegia, or tetraplegia.

Hemiplegia involves primarily the arms and is usually of the spastic variety. Scoliosis can be an associated problem because affected patients may have a shorter arm or leg on the side of involvement. *Double hemiplegia* is a term reserved for cases in which all four limbs are involved, primarily the arms, and one side is often more involved than the other. The hemiplegias most commonly are clinically of the spastic variety. Spasticity can also involve the face, tongue, and mouth. Pseudobulbar-type cerebral palsy involves the muscles of chewing and swallowing and the facial muscles.

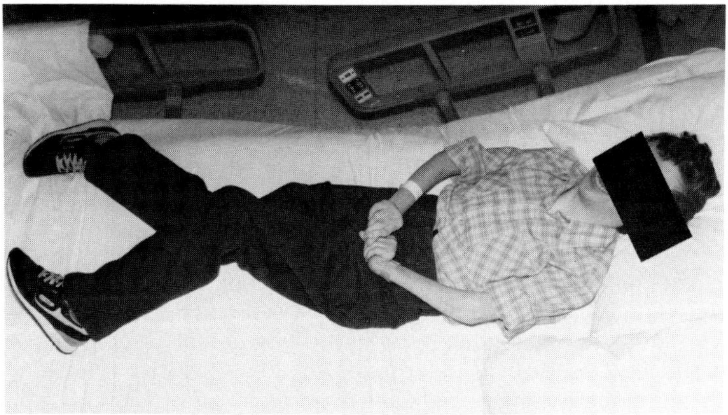

Figure 13–1 Patient with severe spastic tetraplegia.

Severity of Involvement

The severity of involvement can be classified as mild, moderate, or severe. In mild cases, the children are able to ambulate, use their arms, and speak well. They do not need special care. Children with moderate involvement are handicapped in locomotion, self-help, and communication, but they are not disabled entirely. Such patients may need some special care. Severe involvement results in total incapacitation. Affected patients are often bedridden or confined to a wheelchair.

Etiology

Specific etiologic factors often cause characteristic clinical findings. Prenatal circumstances associated with abnormal neurologic functions include abnormalities of placental function, abnormalities in the structure of brain development, exposure to congenital infections or toxins, and chromosome defects.

The natal factors responsible for cerebral palsy occur from the onset of labor to the birth of a viable fetus, and birth trauma, infections, and respiratory distress syndromes can be the underlying abnormalities. Respiratory distress syndrome with obstruction, bronchial dysplasias, and atelectasis is important. Fetal stress from anoxia can result from placenta previa or abruptio placentae. Generally, any anoxia and delivery complications can lead to cerebral palsy. Constitutional factors do play a part in cerebral palsy. These can be prematurity, congenital defects, anemias of newborns, hypoprothrombinemia, fetal hemorrhages, and polygenic familial syndromes.

Factors that occur postnatally, defined as from birth to the age of 3 years, include head trauma, infections, and cardiovascular problems. In trauma, contusions to the brain in a battered child have resulted in an increased incidence of cerebral palsy. Anoxia from infection, vascular lesions, hypoxia, and metabolic factors can also be implicated. Occasionally, cerebral palsy has idiopathic causes, such as cases in which the mother has a normal pregnancy and delivery, no abnormalities are noted at birth, and the nonprogressive defect appears before the age of 18 to 24 months.

EXAMINATION

Examination of the patient with cerebral palsy is important but often difficult, and certain features are specific to the disorder. The type, strength, and tone of muscles must be noted. The basic tone should be observed to determine whether spasticity or rigidity prevails and to what degree when exposed to various stimuli such as speech, noise, and excitement. Pathologic patterns of movement and posture should be noted and observed while the patient is supine, prone, lying on the side, sitting, kneeling, and standing.

Tonic reflex activity should be noted and described as symmetric tonic neck reflex, asymmetric tonic neck reflex, or labyrinthine neck reflex; these are useful reflexes for meeting functional goals. How the child uses his or her hands and whether they cross the midline or are properly positioned should be noted. The associated reactions should also be observed and recorded. Basic automatic reactions such as head posture, balance, and protective movements should be monitored during developmental stages, and gaps in all levels of development should be noted. Primitive motor patterns should be looked for to distinguish between cases of general retardation with little or no pathologic motor activity. Also, contractures and deformities should be noted early in order to provide treatment. The motor patterns responsible for contractures and deformities should be determined.

DIAGNOSIS

One of the diagnostic procedures that can be helpful is computed tomography, with which the presence of hemorrhage or calcification can be visualized. Further investigations such as radionuclide brain scanning, magnetic resonance imaging, and electroencephalography are also useful diagnostic tools.

ASSOCIATED MEDICAL PROBLEMS

An associated medical problem is gastroesophageal reflux. This can occur in approximately 50% of severely handicapped, brain-injured children. A potential complication of this problem is failure to survive aspiration pneumonia. Seizure disorders are more common in spastic types than dyskinetic types, and from a third to a half of children with cerebral palsy will have a seizure or recurrent seizures.[1] Mental retardation does not necessarily accompany the motor handicaps of cerebral palsy.[2] It is most common in children with bilateral and widespread cerebral injury, and it is less common in children with extrapyramidal forms of cerebral palsy and spastic diplegia.

When appropriate, psychologic testing and communication evaluation should be completed. Pseudoretardation may be apparent when the handicaps are so severe that they interfere with both communication and self-help skills. Speech dysarthrias can occur in approximately three-fourths of patients with cerebral palsy. The sensory defects in hemiplegic persons can be more disabling than the motor weakness. Associated dental abnormalities are bruxism (grinding of the teeth), enamel defects, jaw deformities, and drooling. Emotional problems are common, and about 80% of adults with cerebral palsy are unemployed because of these emotional problems.[1]

AIMS OF TREATMENT

Functional self-care is the first aim of treatment. Ambulation is often desired by the parents. In terms of the handicapping condition, ambulation can mean by wheelchair (Fig. 13–2 and 13–3) or with aids such as walkers, canes, crutches, or bracing. Communication is extremely important in patients with cerebral palsy, and augmentative communication is often necessary by computer, word boards (Fig. 13–4), or sign language. Without communication, affected children are locked into their own world. Vocational or

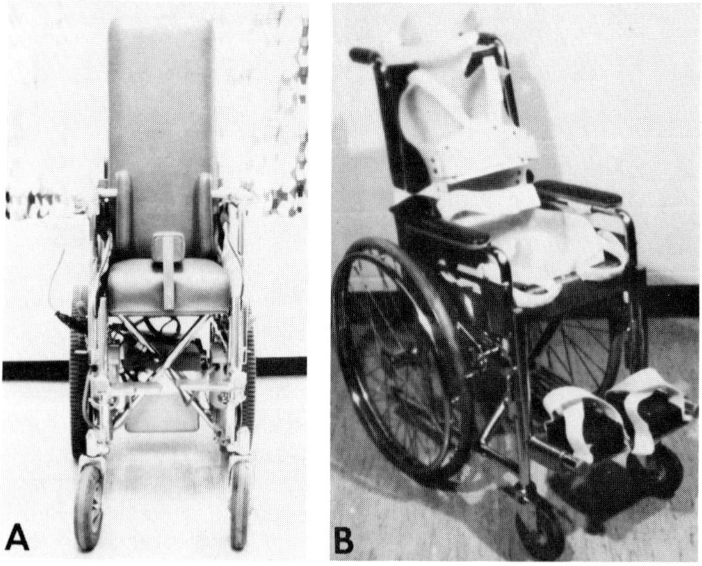

Figure 13–2 *A*, Electric wheelchair with adapted seat insert. *B*, Wheelchair with molded sitting orthosis.

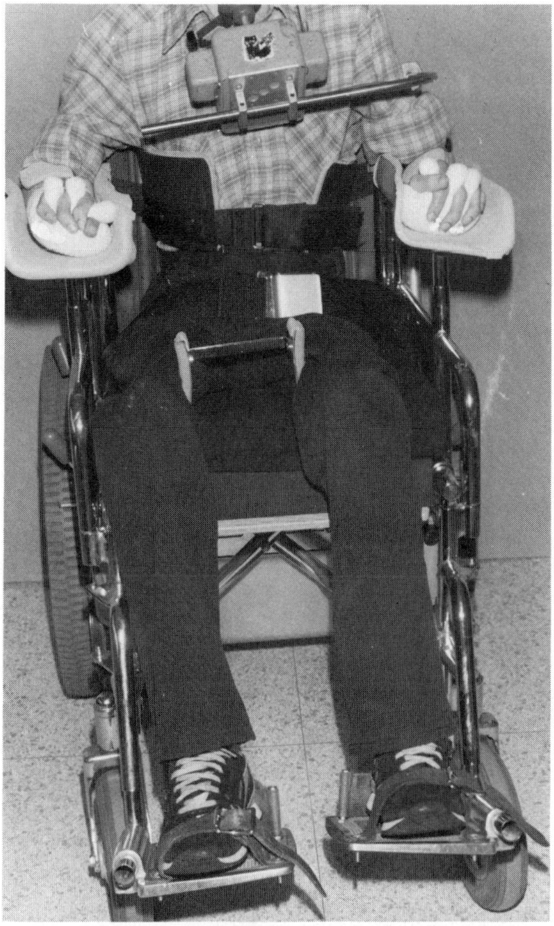

Figure 13–3 Chin-operated electric wheelchair with hand splints, adductor bar, lateral trunk supports, and wedge seat.

avocational skills should be addressed. In school-age children and teenagers, it is particularly important to strive for a near-normal appearance. Recreational capabilities should not be overlooked. Emotional stability is important. In the area of exercise, it is important to work for substitution of weak muscles, stabilization of joints, and alignment of the trunk for extremity posture. Prevention of contractures is most important in an exercise program. Relief of abnormal weight-bearing surfaces such as the sacrum or the curvature of the spine is important. The exercise program should train for function. Also, positioning for function is extremely important.

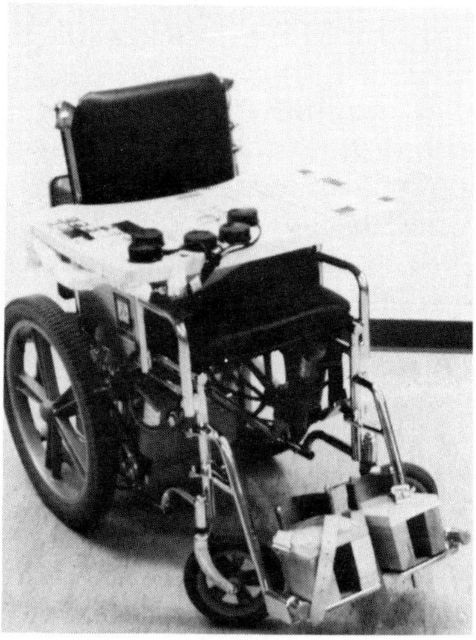

Figure 13–4 Specially adapted electric wheelchair with word board on tray table.

THE MEDICAL TEAM

The team approach is needed for the care of children with cerebral palsy. Fragmentation of care should be avoided but can happen because of the need for colleagues in multiple medical disciplines, such as physiatrists, orthopedists, neurologists, pediatricians, neurosurgeons, dentists, psychologists, and psychiatrists. Physical therapists, occupational therapists, speech therapists, teachers, nurses, psychologists, parents, and vocational counselors must also be members of the team. Interrelationships and full cooperation are essential in a multidisciplined team approach to treatment.

TREATMENT

Treatment in early infancy is used to stimulate normal motor activity and prevent deformities. Abnormal muscle activities must be suppressed or inhibited. Facilitation of postural adjustment reactions is important in early treatment, as are positioning and handling techniques during daily activities, and one should consider correction of disturbances of reciprocal inhibition.[2]

The basic approach is to teach motor skills that affected children cannot acquire spontaneously.[3] This treatment must include social experiences, sensory motor stimulation, and provision of activities of daily living.[4] Early treatment goals are to accomplish rolling, raising the head, scooting, sitting, feeding, and creeping and to develop an ongoing home treatment program. The Bobath method of treatment is aimed at reducing spastic patterns. Activities in the lower extremity that should be avoided are stimulation of extensors and extension, inversion of the foot, retraction of the pelvis, and external rotation of the thigh. Activities in the upper extremity that should be avoided are retractions of the shoulder, depression of the shoulder girdle, adduction, and internal rotation of the shoulder. Also, prolonged flexion of the elbow, wrist, and fingers should be avoided if at all possible. Pronation and ulnar deviation of the wrist and adduction of the thumb and fingers should be prevented.

PERSISTENT PROBLEMS

Some of the persistent difficulties in children with cerebral palsy are psychosocial problems, intellectual stimulation, and uniform education. Sexuality, independence, and employment can also be problems. The numbers of adolescent mothers with cerebral palsy and the abuse of children with cerebral palsy are increasing.

BRACING

The philosophy of the Mayo Clinic is to use braces as little as possible and only when necessary. Many types of shoes, used with or without bracing, are available. Wedges can be attached to the shoes; these can be medial, lateral, heel, or sole wedges. Longitudinal arch pads can also be used. Metatarsal bars can be applied. The many varieties of short leg braces can be most helpful. Often, a solid plastic (polypropylene) ankle-foot orthosis is helpful (see Fig. 17–1), in which inhibition of extensor spasm is built into the foot areas. The long leg braces consist of calf and thigh bands, molded lacers, and fastening-tape (Velcro) closures. Scott-Craig braces, Legg-Perthes braces, and ischial weight-bearing braces are needed in specific cases.

Many knee and ankle mechanisms approach normal anatomy. Prone standers or standing tables can be used for standing. Scoliosis can sometimes be managed with polypropylene (Fig. 13–2 *B*) or Orthoplast jackets.[5] The Milwaukee brace is helpful in children with progressive scoliosis or kyphosis. Before surgical stabilization, the sitting orthosis is often helpful. Casting for tight heel cords and hamstrings is occasionally advocated. With casting, precautions should be taken to prevent ulcers from pressure areas. Casting is time consuming. Inhibiting casting for severe spasticity of the gastrocnemius-soleus muscles is often done early.

SPLINTING

Splinting in the lower extremity can be with night splints, gutter splints, or Denis Brown splints for stretching and abduction.

Dislocated hips can be managed with Scottish-rite splints or Frejka pillow splints. In the upper extremity, dorsal cock-up and volar cock-up splints can be helpful for wrist flexion. Splints to hold the thumb in opposition and for webbed-space stretching can be helpful for adducted, flexed thumbs. Night-resting splints are used to maintain proper wrist and hand positioning (see Fig. 25–1). Dorsal dynamic resting splints are alternatives. Foot splints are used to maintain dorsiflexion. Neck splints, such as the Philadelphia and foam collars, are usually not needed.

DRUGS

Atropine or propantheline bromide can be used for excessive drooling. Frequently, anticonvulsant drugs are necessary. Spasticity can be pharmacologically managed with diazepam, dantrolene, or baclofen.[1] For increased concentration in school, dextroamphetamine sulfate or methylphenidate has often been proposed. Chlorpheniramine maleate is used for nasal congestion. Dextroamphetamine sulfate has also been proposed for psychologic disturbances.

OPERATIVE PROCEDURES

Orthopedic surgical procedures for patients with cerebral palsy are often tenolysis and tendon lengthenings. Occasionally, bone reconstructions such as osteotomies or rotational or derotational osteotomies are done for dislocated hips.[1] Fusion of wrists, fingers, or ankles may be needed. Tendon transfers promote ankle dorsiflexion and wrist extension.[6]

The neurosurgical procedure advocated for children with cerebral palsy is often destruction of the dentate nucleus and a stereotactic operation.[1] Hemispherectomies have been done for intractable seizures. Neurectomies such as obturator neurectomy, tibial neurectomy for spasticity, and Jacobson's plexus neurectomy for drooling are helpful. Equally, nerve or motor point blocks can be used.

PARENTS AND THERAPY

Parental instruction in and understanding of the physical therapy program are essential. To achieve the best results, parents must work with the therapist. They must understand the program and its objectives. They must be aware of the limitations imposed on their child by specific types and degrees of handicaps. Everyone treating a child with cerebral palsy must work toward common aims and have some understanding that the physical therapy is ongoing, changing, and progressive.

The parents must learn that the fundamentals of movement have to be learned by the child before complicated motor activities can be accomplished. Parental understanding and help are important factors in treatment. Overzealous parents must be cautioned that they are not going to alter the rate of development but are providing opportunities for development to occur. Motor skills are best done manually with muscle reeducation. Muscle reeducation is necessary through successful voluntary efforts, and repetition is important. Repetition of proper volitional motor patterns is extremely important. Developmental sequencing must occur. Simplicity of environments, regardless of chronologic age, avoids distractions. Toys must be stored and used only as needed. The therapy setting should be quiet.

Principles of behavior modification and reinforcement of positive behaviors are important. In physical therapy, the general treatment routine is stretching, range of motion, relaxation, muscle reeducation, coordination, conditioning, dominance, and repetition. Occupational therapy addresses eye-hand coordination, skills in activities of daily living, two-handed activities, sensory reeducation and development, and proprioceptive motor development.

REFERENCES

1. Molnar GE, ed. Pediatric rehabilitation. Baltimore: Williams & Wilkins, 1985:420–467.
2. Finnie NR. Handling the young cerebral palsy child at home. 2nd ed. London: Heinemann Medical Books, 1974.
3. Köng E. Very early treatment of cerebral palsy. Dev Med Child Neurol 1966; 8:198–202.
4. Mead S. The treatment of cerebral palsy: presidential address 1967. Dev Med Child Neurol 1968; 10:423–426.
5. Alexander MA. Orthotics, adapted seating, and assistive devices. In: Molnar GE, ed. Pediatric rehabilitation. Baltimore: Williams & Wilkins, 1985:158–175.
6. Bleck EE. Orthopaedic management of cerebral palsy. Philadelphia: WB Saunders, 1979.

14 MYOPATHIES

Stephen F. Noll, M.D.

The neuromuscular diseases account for a myriad of diagnoses that are not infrequently encountered by physicians in rehabilitation medicine. An important subset of the neuromuscular diseases is primary muscle disease, which of itself includes a vast array of disorders (Table 14–1). Although each of these disorders has its peculiarities, certain characteristics are common to their presentation, and certain principles are common to their management.

A common fallacy associated with neuromuscular disorders, including muscle disease, is that if they are not curable, neither are they treatable. Although rehabilitation does not alter the pathophysiologic course of these diseases, it certainly, and often significantly, alters their functional impact.

PRESENTATION

Whatever other characteristics may be present, the hallmark of primary muscle disease is muscle weakness. But rather than complain of general fatigue, patients with true muscle weakness often volunteer specific difficulties, and the difficulties vary depending on where weakness is most apparent.[1] For example, patients commonly complain of the inability to place objects on a high shelf, to hammer overhead, or to comb their hair. These particular complaints indicate proximal more than distal upper extremity weakness. Patients with hand weakness, however, complain of difficulty opening jars or buttoning shirts. Alternatively, weakness in the proximal lower extremities results in complaints of difficulty getting out of chairs or off the toilet or perhaps with ascending and descending stairs. Yet, if patients have weakness of the distal lower extremities, they complain of tripping and stumbling, especially when walking on uneven surfaces.

TABLE 14–1 A Brief Classification of Myopathies*

Categories	*Examples*
Dystrophies	Duchenne Facioscapulohumeral Limb-girdle Myotonic
Congenital myopathies	Central core disease Nemaline (rod) myopathy Centronuclear myopathy Sarcotubular myopathy
Metabolic myopathies	Glycogen storage diseases (for example, acid maltase deficiency) Lipid storage myopathy (for example, carnitine deficiency)
Endocrine myopathies	Hyperthyroidism or hypothyroidism Hyperparathyroidism Corticosteroid-induced
Toxic myopathies	Alcohol-induced Chloroquine
Inflammatory myopathies	Polymyositis Dermatomyositis

* This table is not meant to be an all-inclusive list of myopathies.

Just as the complaint of weakness is important to the diagnosis of muscle disease, so too is the demonstration of weakness. Formal manual muscle testing is the accepted method to determine muscle weakness. Equally as helpful, however, is functional or task-oriented muscle testing. Table 14–2 itemizes several functional tasks or tests and the major muscle or muscles with which they are associated.

Gait analysis is another functional evaluation that may give clues to muscle weakness. Several typical gait alterations occur with weakness. For example, weakness of the gluteus medius results in a waddling appearance referred to as a Trendelenburg gait. Likewise, with weakness of the gluteus maximus, gait is characterized by a sudden forward lurch and marked lumbar lordosis that provide for stability at the hip. If the quadriceps are weak, genu recur-

TABLE 14–2 Functional Tasks Used to Determine Muscle Weakness

Functional Task	*Key Muscles Tested**	*Strength*
Toe walk	Gastrocnemius, soleus	+
Heel walk	Tibialis anterior	+
Deep knee bend	Quadriceps	+
Gower's maneuver	Gluteus maximus, quadriceps	–
Froment's sign	Adductor pollicis	–
Arms overhead	Supraspinatus, deltoid	+

* Several other muscles must often work synergistically to accomplish such tasks.

vatum will be prominent during the stance phase of walking to provide stability at the knee. Finally, weakness of the tibialis anterior results in a "steppage" gait, so called because, in order to clear the foot during the swing phase of walking, patients must actually lift the leg high as if to step up.

CONSIDERATIONS FOR REHABILITATION

As stated above, primary muscle disease includes multiple types of disorders. However, rehabilitation is not as specific to a diagnosis as it is to functional disability. With any muscle disease, it is important to ask certain questions that pertain to decision making in rehabilitation, irrespective of the diagnosis.

Is it reversible or irreversible? Most primary muscle diseases are irreversible, but not all. Steroid myopathy or polymyositis may be amenable to treatment—steroid myopathy to withdrawal of steroids, and polymyositis to their introduction. The answer to this question has a bearing on what is to be done. For example, if an ankle-foot orthosis is needed, prescribing an off-the-shelf orthosis may be most practical when the condition is temporary, and a more expensive and durable custom-fitted orthosis may be a better choice if the process is permanent.

Is it stable or progressive (and if progressive, at what rate)? The course of a disease has a significant influence on decision making. In classic Duchenne's muscular dystrophy, for example, loss of ambulation can be predicted to occur approximately 6 to 12 months after the loss of ability to climb stairs.[2] Consequently, the need for a wheelchair can be easily anticipated. In contrast, the need for a wheelchair is more delayed in Becker's variant of muscular dystrophy, which is much slower to evolve.

Is it genetic or acquired? The impact of a primary muscle disease is related not only to the person with the disease but also to other family members and to their environment. As part of the rehabilitation effort, incorporating a genetic counselor, psychologist, and social service worker into the team approach is often imperative.

REHABILITATION EFFORTS

The goal of rehabilitation in muscle diseases is the same as that for any other disease: to maximize independent functional capacity. This process may involve attempts to restore lost function (for example, with an orthosis) or to prevent further loss of function (for example, with regular therapeutic exercise). Several rehabilitation measures are available to improve function.[3]

Physical Modalities

Physical methods are sometimes useful for the management of primary muscle disease. Hot or cold applications, whether packs or a radiant heat lamp, may effectively relieve the pain sometimes associated with inflammatory myopathies. Use of a Hubbard tank is often helpful for facilitating range-of-motion exercises in the case of severe muscle weakness and for providing comfort for the myalgias that may be associated with muscle disease. Treatment with ultrasound is particularly effective when used in conjunction with prolonged stretching exercises for joint contractures that often plague patients with chronic myopathies. Finally, biofeedback can enhance muscle reeducation efforts in a recovering but weakened muscle.

Therapeutic Exercise

In any muscle disease, contracture formation is a major concern. Weakness often prevents full active range of motion, and resting postures tend to become fixed. Although all muscles can tighten, at most risk for this complication are those that cross more than one joint, such as the hamstrings, the gastrocnemius, and the tensor fasciae latae. Thus, a common pattern for contractures in the lower extremities is hip flexion and abduction, knee flexion, and plantar flexion. Likewise, because of a predisposition for contracture formation, special attention should be given to the shoulder adductors, elbow flexors, pronators, and metacarpophalangeal extensors in the upper extremities.[4] Regardless of the stage of disease, range of motion of all joints related to weakened muscles is important, as is gentle, prolonged stretching of key muscles such as those mentioned above.

The applicability of strengthening exercises in myopathies remains controversial. The fear associated with exercising to the point of muscle fatigue has been that the exercise will actually exacerbate weakness rather than promote strength. In a small, controlled study of a group of boys with Duchenne's muscular dystrophy, submaximal isokinetic exercise resulted in no overwork weakness and a statistically nonsignificant increase in strength.[5] More extensive study is needed in several of the myopathies to clarify this matter. Currently, if strengthening is considered necessary, a practical approach seems to be (1) strengthening early in the course of the disease rather than late and (2) strengthening at submaximal exercise levels.[6] Corollaries to this approach might also be to strengthen muscles that are only minimally affected rather than those that are severely affected and to strengthen primarily the muscles of functional importance such as the hip extensors and quadriceps.

Specific training in functional skills, such as transfers from bed to a chair, onto the toilet, or into a car, is often the most important component of an "exercise" program for patients severely impaired with primary muscle disease. Aids may be necessary to augment these skills, such as a sliding board, an overhead trapeze, or ultimately even a Hoyer lift.

Mobility Training

Independent mobility is an important goal. Although this goal is usually thought of in terms of ambulation, wheelchair mobility may be best functionally. Both assisted ambulation and wheelchair mobility have their advantages. Walking, for example, has an advantage in overcoming some architectural barriers; however, wheelchair propulsion usually is more energy efficient.

Assistive Devices. Ambulation can be maintained, in part, by means of assistive devices, such as a cane, quadripod cane, hemiwalker, crutches, or walker. These devices provide various amounts of stability. Their use, however, implies fair to good strength in the so-called crutch muscles of the upper extremities, some of which include shoulder depressors, shoulder abductors and adductors, and triceps. For patients with diffuse or proximal muscle weakness of the upper extremities, such as occurs in Duchenne's muscular dystrophy or facioscapulohumeral dystrophy, crutch or cane-assisted ambulation may not be feasible.

Bracing. Another means of assisting ambulation is with orthotic devices. Bracing serves several functions that assist gait. A brace may protect a joint. A jointed knee brace, for example, may prevent progression of genu recurvatum and provide knee stability in a patient with significant quadriceps weakness. A brace also positions the joint and may prevent contracture formation. A person with marked weakness of the tibialis anterior muscle can be placed in a molded polypropylene ankle-foot orthosis that will hold the foot and ankle in near neutral position. In doing so, the orthosis stabilizes the joint, prevents tripping and falling from footdrop, and prevents equinus-positioned contractures at the ankle. Finally, an orthotic device may, in fact, augment function. For example, the reciprocating hip-knee-ankle-foot orthoses provide assisted hip flexion and extension by means of passive movement of a cable.[7] Likewise, the elastic qualities of materials used in a posterior leaf-spring ankle-foot orthosis may provide dynamic ankle dorsiflexion.

Orthoses may also have merit unrelated to mobility itself. Standing and walking are thought to decrease disuse osteoporosis, retard the development of scoliosis in some cases, and provide a psychologic lift to the patient.

Unfortunately, orthoses are not without disadvantages. The use of an ankle-foot orthosis in Duchenne's muscular dystrophy, for example, may in fact, collapse the patient. Passive stability of stance[8] is dependent on maintaining the center of gravity weight line posterior to the hip and anterior to the knee. This task is, in part, accomplished by toe walking. Therefore, if the foot and ankle are braced independent of other joints, this compensatory posture is broken and the patient may collapse. Another disadvantage is the energy requirement for braced ambulation. Braces significantly increase the energy expenditure of walking.[9] The rate of ambulation is often decreased to compensate for this increased workload. Thus, because of the increased workload and the decreased efficiency, in some instances bracing may not be worth the effort required.

Wheelchairs. Although there is often a hesitancy to use it, a wheelchair is a reasonable alternative to ambulation for mobility and may offer the most efficient means of mobility. The energy cost of propelling a wheelchair is approximately the same as that of normal ambulation. Furthermore, a wheelchair need not be the sole means of mobility. For example, a patient with facioscapulohumeral dystrophy may walk well on smooth surfaces for short distances (a household ambulator) but may benefit from the use of a wheelchair for mobility around the community and for sports activities.

Because of their expense, electric wheelchairs are often viewed as luxury items. In fact, however, they should be prescribed as would any other medical device to provide for lost function, just as one would prescribe a catheter for urinary drainage or a cast for stability of a fracture. The electric wheelchair provides for lost independent mobility.

The wheelchair provides more than mobility.[10] Through proper positioning, it has the potential to retard scoliosis and contracture formation, especially in young persons. Therefore, it is important to prescribe a wheelchair with certain specifications, as shown in Figure 14–1: (1) a firm seat, with or without a cushion, to discourage pelvic obliquity; (2) removable and adjustable desktop armrests to prevent "slumping" (a lap tray is also often helpful for positioning); (3) a lumbar support and firm backrest to position the spine in extension in an attempt to stabilize facets and discourage scoliosis; and (4) swing-away, detachable footrests to prevent equinus posturing at the ankles. Lateral pads, or even a custom-molded seating orthosis, may be additional needs.

Activities of Daily Living

Because of weakness, whether proximal or distal, the ability to accomplish basic self-care activities may be significantly impaired by primary muscle disease. With specific training in techniques, energy conservation, and the use of adaptive aids (Table 14–3 and Figure 14–2), the safe performance of activities of daily living is often possible.

In addition to assistive devices, static or dynamic splints can be fabricated to prevent contractures and to promote or improve function. For example, a wrist cock-up splint in a patient with distal myopathy may improve grasp by means of stabilizing the wrist and providing a tenodesis effect.

Other Concerns

Prevention of contractures, maintenance of muscle strength, mobility, and independence in self-care are the usual and tradi-

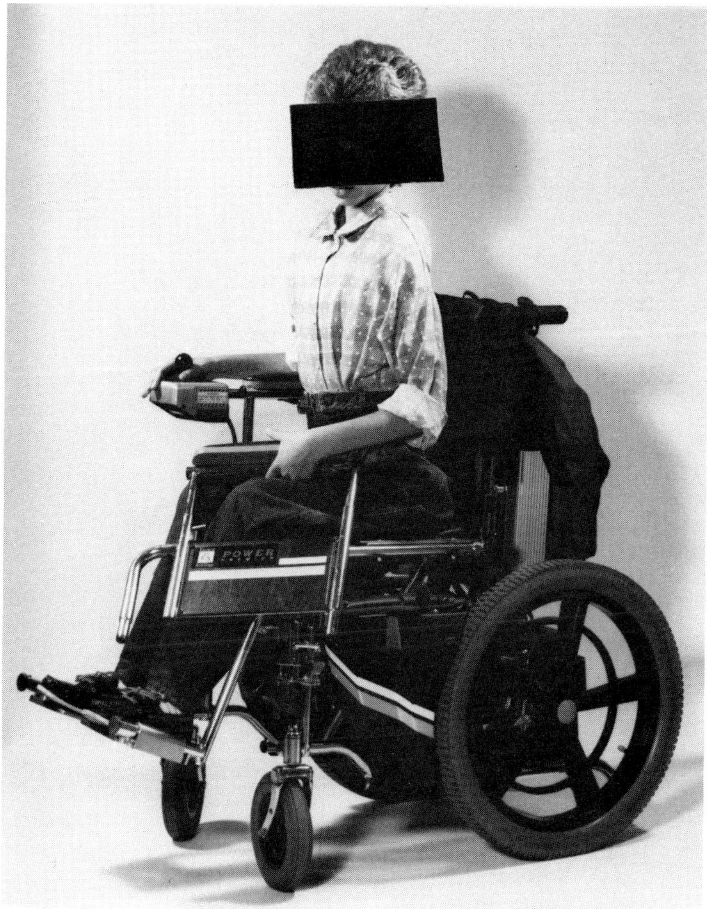

Figure 14–1 Prescribed electric wheelchair for an adolescent with facioscapulohumeral dystrophy.

TABLE 14–3 Examples of Assistive Devices for Activities of Daily Living

Dressing aids
Fastening-tape (Velcro) closures
Buttonhook
Sock loops
Eating aids
Universal cuff
Built-up grips
Balanced forearm orthosis
Hygiene aids
Bath bench
Grab bars
Toilet seat riser
Long-handled sponge and brush

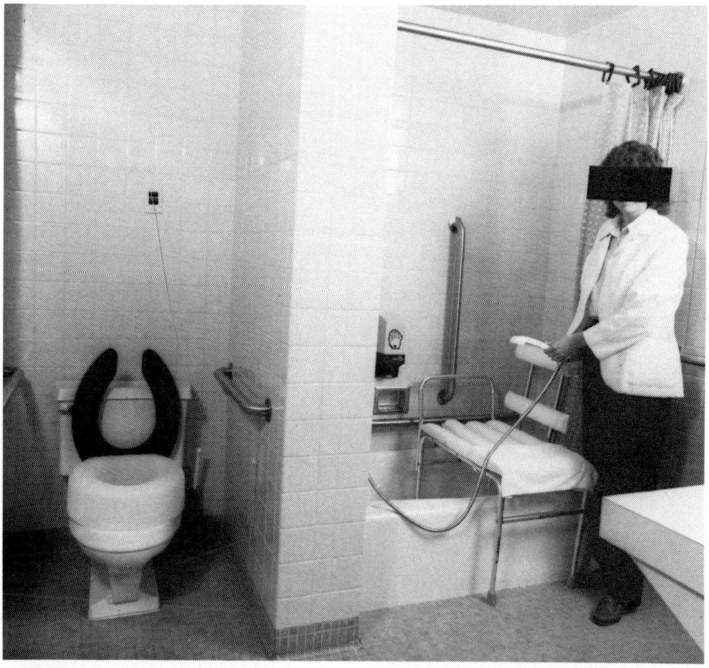

Figure 14–2 Adapted bathroom and hygiene aids for patients with muscle disease.

tional goals in the rehabilitation of patients with primary muscle disease. Other problems arise, however, that require rehabilitation efforts, and, although there can be many, two of these problems deserve special comment.

Dysphagia is a disorder that plagues patients with certain primary muscle diseases, such as myotonic dystrophy. Swallowing difficulties may be significant and result in malnutrition or aspiration pneumonia. Proper positioning, modification of food consistencies, and compensatory and facilitation techniques for swallowing may, in fact, resolve this problem. If not, home enteral feeding programs are feasible. Dysarthria often accompanies dysphagia. It, too, at times, is amenable to treatment (for example, with a palatal lift).

Respiratory failure is the most feared complication of primary muscle disease. Options now exist for patients with advanced disease and impending respiratory failure.[11] For example, life may be prolonged in Duchenne's muscular dystrophy by using an iron lung or a chest cuirass at night for temporary respiratory support. Tracheostomy with portable ventilatory support is also an option for some patients. Such treatments have both advantages and disadvantages for patients and their families. Therefore, decisions regarding respiratory support must be reached far in advance of the "crisis" of respiratory failure.

SUMMARY

Management of primary muscle disease from a rehabilitation standpoint varies considerably with the particular disease entity, its course, and its extent. In some cases, rehabilitation may involve only the prescription of an exercise program to prevent contractures. In other cases, it may demand a comprehensive program involving a full complement of services, including medical or surgical consultations, rehabilitation nursing, physical, occupational, and recreational therapy, speech therapy, orthotics, genetic counseling, educational and vocational counseling, and psychologic and social service work evaluations. Regardless of the extent of involvement, treatment must be directed not only at the disease process itself but also at the restoration and preservation of a patient's functional capacity for as long as possible.

REFERENCES

1. Brooke MH. A clinician's view of neuromuscular diseases. 2nd ed. Baltimore: Williams & Wilkins, 1986:1–35.
2. Vignos PJ Jr. Rehabilitation in progressive muscular dystrophy. In: Licht S, ed. Rehabilitation and medicine. Baltimore: Waverly Press, 1968:584–642.
3. Fowler WM Jr. Rehabilitation management of muscular dystrophy and related disorders: II. Comprehensive care. Arch Phys Med Rehabil 1982; 63:322–328.
4. Johnson EW, Alexander MA. Management of motor unit diseases. In: Kottke FJ, Stillwell GK, Lehmann JF, eds. Krusen's handbook of physical medicine and rehabilitation. 3rd ed. Philadelphia: WB Saunders, 1982:679–690.
5. de Lateur BJ, Giaconi RM. Effect of maximal strength of submaximal exercise in Duchenne muscular dystrophy. Am J Phys Med 1979; 58:26–36.
6. Fowler WM Jr, Taylor M. Rehabilitation management of muscular dystrophy and related disorders: I. The role of exercise. Arch Phys Med Rehabil 1982; 63:319–321.
7. Douglas R, Larson PF, D'Ambrosia R, McCall RE. The LSU reciprocation-gait orthosis. Orthopaedics 1983; 6:834–839.
8. Johnson EW. Pathokinesiology of Duchenne muscular dystrophy: implications for management. Arch Phys Med Rehabil 1977; 58:4–7.
9. Fischer SV, Gullickson G Jr. Energy cost of ambulation in health and disability: a literature review. Arch Phys Med Rehabil 1978; 59:124–133.
10. Alexander MA. Orthotics, adapted seating, and assistive devices. In: Molnar GE, ed. Pediatric rehabilitation. Baltimore: Williams & Wilkins, 1985:158–175.
11. Alexander MA, Johnson EW, Petty J, Stauch D. Mechanical ventilation of patients with late stage Duchenne muscular dystrophy: management in the home. Arch Phys Med Rehabil 1979; 60:289–292.

15 ACUTE POLYMYOSITIS

Janet M. Cogoli, M.D.
Mehrsheed Sinaki, M.D.

Polymyositis has been defined as a nonhereditary inflammatory myopathy of unknown cause affecting skeletal muscle, to which the term "dermatomyositis" is applied in the presence of the characteristic rash.[1] Although much has been written about this disorder, there is a dearth of literature concerning the application of physiotherapy for its management. The disease varies in severity; therefore, a rehabilitation program that addresses the variability of the illness needs to be established. This chapter discusses the essential components of a physiotherapy program directed at the physical and functional problems of this illness.

Many investigators have attempted to classify polymyositis. Winkelmann et al.[2] proposed a classification based on the clinical course of the disease and divided it into acute, chronic, recurrent, and cyclic forms. We have found that, for purposes of organizing our rehabilitation techniques for acute polymyositis, it is helpful to group patients according to the course of their illness; the three rehabilitation phases are early acute, middle, and remission (Table 15–1).

EARLY ACUTE PHASE

In this stage of the disease, myalgia may be a prominent symptom.[1] Pain may be minimized by the application of mild heat; superficial heat can be applied with an infrared heat lamp. Hydrotherapy may also be used for the relief of pain; immersion in a Hubbard tank (temperature, 36.7° C to 37.2° C) or a warm tub bath for 20 to 30 minutes may be used. The alleviation of myalgia by these simple methods is effective for decreasing secondary muscle spasm. However, before and during the use of these

TABLE 15–1 Comprehensive Program for the Three Rehabilitation Phases of Acute Polymyositis

Early Acute Phase	*Middle Phase*	*Remission Phase*
Proper positioning Prevention of DVT* Respiratory care Tilt table Skin care Mild heat, hydrotherapy Stroking massage Passive ROM† Assistive devices (occupational therapy evaluation)	Active or active-assisted ROM† Mild strengthening exercises Progressive ambulation Assistive devices (occupational therapy evaluation) Avoidance of exertional physical activities	Active ROM† Strengthening exercises Assistive devices (occupational therapy evaluation) Vocational counseling Dismissal planning

* DVT, deep vein thrombosis.
† ROM, range-of-motion exercises.

methods, the cardiac status of the patient must be determined. Electrocardiographic abnormalities have been noted in polymyositis.[1,3,4] In the presence of cardiomyopathy, serious rhythm abnormalities, or heart block, these treatments are contraindicated. A gentle, stroking massage over the bony prominences of bedridden patients has a relaxing, sedative effect. Massage would be inappropriate in patients who manifest dermatomyositis because of the presence of fragile, atrophic skin.

To maintain the tone of the cardiovascular system in the early acute stage with severe weakness, we recommend the use of a tilt table once or twice daily, before which the lower extremities of the patient are wrapped in elastic bandages to provide support against venous pooling and resultant orthostatism.

In patients with involvement of the respiratory muscles, respiratory function should be determined at least once daily. Some patients will need respiratory assistance with a positive-pressure respirator. The danger of pneumonia exists in debilitated patients with acute polymyositis,[5] and treatment should include adequate postural drainage and chest physical therapy.

Because remission of this disease may occur,[2,6] patients should not be left with disabling residua that could have been avoided with proper daily care. Therefore, a major emphasis of the treatment program should be the maintenance of flexibility. Muscle contractures may develop as the weak muscles are unable to move the respective joints through their normal range of motion and as intrinsic changes within the muscle, such as fibrosis, occur.[7] Tightness occurs early in the two-joint muscle groups, such as the gastrocnemius-soleus muscles, the hip flexors, and the hamstrings. In the upper extremity, the forearm pronators and the elbow, wrist, and finger flexors are often tight. Examination for tightness should be a part of the evaluation of all patients with polymyositis during all stages.[7]

Gentle range-of-motion exercises that avoid the production of pain but gradually increase the arc of motion are a necessity. During the early acute stage, only passive range-of-motion exercises should be applied to the joints. They should be done by an experienced therapist once or twice daily, and care should be taken to avoid pain and fatigue. Range-of-motion exercises performed by the patient are not recommended during the early acute stage because they may cause overuse of the muscles involved by an active inflammatory process. Properly performed range-of-motion exercises help to decrease myalgia and to protect against the early development of contractures. If allowed to develop, contractures are a painful, disabling, time-consuming, and expensive complication to correct. Other measures that should also be taken to prevent contractures are proper positioning of the joints when the patient is in bed and maintaining the joints in their functional positions to avoid ankylosis and deformities. This effort is greatly helped by splinting the wrists, digits, and ankles, as needed. The principles of proper positioning are discussed in Chapter 11.

A common problem with immobility is constipation or bowel impaction, which can be prevented with a proper fluid intake and use of stool softeners (docusate sodium, Colace), bulk formers, or suppositories (bisacodyl, Dulcolax) on an as-needed basis. One needs to avoid frequent use of laxatives (see Chapter 11).

The skin must be scrupulously cared for in order to prevent the development of pressure sores. It should be inspected daily, and the patient should be provided with a water mattress or an alternating air mattress and synthetic sheepskin. If unable to turn himself or herself, the patient should be turned by the nursing staff every 2 hours during the day and every 4 hours while sleeping. The heels should be prevented from resting on the mattress by placing a pillow under the calves.

Deep vein thrombosis in the lower extremities of severely weakened patients must also be prevented. Subcutaneously administered low-dose heparin may be helpful toward this end, as in the treatment of patients with spinal cord injuries.[8,9]

MIDDLE PHASE

This stage is evidenced by cessation of the active progression and perhaps by a reduction in the level of serum muscle enzymes and, later, a decrease in muscle weakness. In the presence of any significantly weakened proximal muscles, therapy should be aimed at transfers and gradual ambulation with the use of an appropriate gait aid, if needed. Involvement of the distal extremities has also been documented, in both polymyositis[5] and dermatomyositis.[10] The use of lightweight ankle-foot orthoses may be beneficial because weakness of the distal extremities significantly interferes with gait. Bracing should be kept to a minimum to avoid limitation of the patient's functional ability.

During this stage, as serum enzyme levels improve, the range-of-motion exercises can be safely progressed to active-assisted and then to active, in which the patient performs the motions on his or her own power. Each session, at least once but preferably twice daily, should consist of three to five consecutive full-range movements of each joint. Initially, to avoid fatigue, we prefer to limit the patient's participation in the performance of range-of-motion exercises on the major peripheral joints (that is, the shoulders, hips, and knees).

REMISSION PHASE

As the patient continues to improve and serum enzyme levels decrease toward normal, active range-of-motion exercises may be performed. Mild strengthening exercises may also become a part of the treatment program. The exercise program may advance from simple isometric contraction to resistive exercises. Charting the strength in several key muscles (which could be estimated with manual muscle testing and done consistently by the same examiner) is helpful to follow the patient's course.

During all stages of acute polymyositis, occupational therapy is invaluable. Functional assessment by evaluating the patient's ability to perform activities of daily living is of vital importance. This information must be known to determine treatment goals and to help with the planning for dismissal. Adaptive equipment may be needed to help the patient translate motor residuals into practical function.

When dismissal is planned, the patient's occupation needs to be considered. Some modification may be needed to avoid overuse of the muscles in exertional activities. In some cases, a major change in career becomes necessary.

All patients with polymyositis should be carefully followed up for reactivation of the myositis.[2] Those receiving maintenance doses of corticosteroids[11] should also be watched for the development of side effects, which could include a steroid-induced myopathy or osteoporosis predisposing to compression fractures of the spine. If osteoporosis occurs, measures outlined in Chapter 23 and application of a back support during physical activities are recommended.

REFERENCES

1. Bohan A, Peter JB. Polymyositis and dermatomyositis. N Engl J Med 1975; 292:344–347, 403–407.
2. Winkelmann RK, Mulder DW, Lambert EH, Howard FM Jr, Diessner GR. Course of dermatomyositis-polymyositis: comparison of untreated and cortisone-treated patients. Mayo Clin Proc 1968; 43:545–556.

3. Fernandez-Herlihy L. Heart block in polymyositis. N Engl J Med 1971; 284(Letter):1101.
4. Hill DL, Barrows HS. Identical skeletal and cardiac muscle involvement in a case of fatal polymyositis. Arch Neurol 1968; 19:545–551.
5. Malpe RR, Lee MHM, Alba A. Rehabilitation technics in polymyositis. NY State J Med 1973; 73:1208–1210.
6. Pearson CM. Polymyositis and dermatomyositis. In: Hollander JL, ed. Arthritis and allied conditions: a textbook of rheumatology. 8th ed. Philadelphia: Lea & Febiger, 1972:940–961.
7. Kottke FJ, Stillwell GK, Lehmann JF. Krusen's handbook of physical medicine and rehabilitation. 3rd ed. Philadelphia: WB Saunders, 1982:334, 683.
8. Watson N. Anti-coagulant therapy in the prevention of venous thrombosis and pulmonary embolism in the spinal cord injury. Paraplegia 1978–1979; 16:265–269.
9. Cotton LT, Roberts VC. The prevention of deep vein thrombosis, with particular reference to mechanical methods of prevention. Surgery 1977; 81:228–235.
10. Resnick JS, Mammel M, Mundale M, Kottke FJ. Muscular strength as an index of response to therapy in childhood dermatomyositis. Arch Phys Med Rehabil 1981; 62:12–19.
11. Gilroy J, Meyer JS. Medical neurology. 3rd ed. New York: Macmillan Publishing Company, 1979:733–736.

16 NEUROPATHIC DISEASE

Jon B. Closson, M.D.

This chapter reviews the management of neuropathic diseases. No attempt is made to classify these entities; standard neurology textbooks dealing with these topics generally contain a classification. Therapeutic principles and options for both sensory neuropathies and motor deficits are discussed. Also, specific approaches to a representative neuropathic disease, the Guillain-Barré syndrome, are reviewed. Those for amyotrophic lateral sclerosis are outlined in Chapter 17.

Some basic principles apply to all patients with one of these entities. First, use of the interdisciplinary team is helpful. Some of the diseases strike during the peak of economic and family responsibilities, and some are fatal within a short time. Therefore, all possible resources and support need to be marshaled to help the patient and family. Second, every effort should be made to maintain or regain function and to strive for as much independence as possible, both in mobility and in activities of daily living.

THERAPY FOR SENSORY INVOLVEMENT

Patients with peripheral neuropathies generally have both sensory and motor involvement, although not to an equal degree. The sensory involvement is likely not to be the same in all the senses. Most commonly, patients complain of some form of decreased sensation (numbness) or some type of pain.

The therapeutic approach may need to be multifaceted. The benefits of oral analgesics are usually less than optimal, and narcotics are rarely, if ever, indicated.

The use of heat or cold for pain relief requires great caution, especially when sensation is decreased. Radiant heat provides superficial heat and is probably the safest form because the skin can be observed during the therapy. Methods that provide deeper heat, such as short wave diathermy or ultrasound, may be unsafe because the feedback about pain that is needed for their regulation is diminished. Tepid, swirling water may be helpful. The use of cold is of limited value for pain control.

Massage techniques, especially desensitization massage, may be helpful, particularly in the presence of positive symptoms in the distal extremities.

Transcutaneous electrical nerve stimulation is effective in some cases. There are no hard-and-fast rules regarding the use of either "high" or "low" stimulation; a trial of both may be warranted. Likewise, placement of the electrodes proximally or distally is a matter of trial.

One of the most important tasks when dealing with a patient with decreased sensation is that of education. This includes providing information not only about the disease, its course, and prognosis but also about how to protect the skin from damage due to environmental factors. The patient needs to be reminded that damage can occur from temperature changes (hot or cold) as well as from trauma.

THERAPY FOR MOTOR INVOLVEMENT

The effects of peripheral neuropathy on motor function can be the result of one problem or a combination of problems. Muscular weakness can be due to an abnormality in the motor pathway. Weakness also results from immobility; normal persons confined to bed rest lose about 3% of their initial strength per day.[1] Patients can also lose joint mobility due to either a lack of muscle power or the development of contractures of soft tissues about the joint; either one of these problems or a combination can result in decreased flexibility and mobility.

Therapy can be instituted at any point in the course of the disease. However, reversing the limitations imposed by joint contractures is difficult because it is prolonged and there may be less than full return of motion or function. Therefore, prophylactic measures (that is, range of motion) should be used, even when the involvement is mild.

The methods described in the section on sensory neuropathies can be used to treat motor involvement. However, in addition to providing pain relief (if present), some of these measures can be used to improve flexibility and mobility.

As long as sensation is intact, the deeper heat treatments (short wave diathermy and ultrasound) can be beneficial. Because of the effect of heat on collagen, short wave diathermy and ultrasound are especially helpful for treating joint contractures. Specifically, the application of ultrasound to an affected area accompanied and followed by prolonged stretch of the contracted tissues is the most effective noninvasive technique available.[2]

If spasticity is present, application of cold or heat may reduce muscle tone.

Exercises can be an important part of the treatment of patients with peripheral neuropathies and primary motor involvement. Maintaining flexibility is important. Each peripheral joint should be put through its full range of motion once daily. Depending on the degree of weakness, the range should be applied either by the therapist (passive) or with assistance from another person (active assisted).

In the presence of joint contractures, prolonged stretch by traction or proper positioning should be tried. Depending on the response, it may need to become a lifelong habit.

The question of strengthening in the presence of neuropathic disease is currently of considerable controversy. Submaximal strengthening (avoidance of fatigue during exercise) is believed to be generally safe. Maximal strengthening during the acute phase and early convalescence is to be avoided. Therefore, a specific, well-supervised program is important.

As strength improves, muscle reeducation should be instituted. This can be accomplished under the specific guidance of a physical therapist. Biofeedback techniques may be effective.

Orthoses may be needed during the course of the illness or after it. Many orthoses are available for both the upper and lower extremities to help maintain proper alignment and to help compensate for weakness in muscle groups. These can be either static (no motion in the orthosis) or dynamic. In dynamic orthoses, power to move the appliance is provided, at least in part, by some external source (for example, rubber bands or springs).

Likewise, gait aids may be needed to provide stability or to compensate for a lack of muscle strength. Gait aids include canes, crutches, walkers, and wheelchairs.

SPECIFIC APPROACHES

There are many neuropathic diseases, and no attempt has been made to detail a program for each. However, a suggested program is outlined for two—the Guillain-Barré syndrome and amyotrophic lateral sclerosis (see Chapter 17).

The Guillain-Barré syndrome is a sensory-motor polyneuropathy that can affect any striated muscle in the body. Because about two-thirds of patients recover completely and 25% have some residual deficit, intervention with principles of physical medicine and rehabilitation is important.

When paralysis is present, particular attention needs to be paid to positioning and posture. Resting splints can help maintain proper alignment. All peripheral joints should be put through their full range of motion daily to prevent contractures. Preventive measures to avoid pressure sores must be instituted. Special attention needs to be directed toward bowel and bladder function (see Chapter 21).

As recovery progresses, all the skills of the rehabilitation team are needed—physical therapist, occupational therapist, recreational therapist, medical social worker, psychologist, and physiatrist. Recovery depends, to some extent, on the severity of the initial involvement and can take up to 2 years. Attempts to strengthen too rapidly can result in relapses. Pain is sometimes a significant problem, and if the measures outlined above are ineffective, medications may be needed. Other authors have outlined rehabilitation principles for neuropathic diseases.[3,4]

In conclusion, knowledge of the basic course and prognosis of neuropathic diseases is essential for deciding what needs to be done and when.

REFERENCES

1. Kottke FJ. The effects of limitation of activity upon the human body. JAMA 1966; 196:825–830.
2. Lehmann JF, de Lateur BJ. Diathermy and superficial heat and cold therapy. In: Kottke FJ, Stillwell GK, Lehmann JF, eds. Krusen's handbook of physical medicine and rehabilitation. 3rd ed. Philadelphia: WB Saunders, 1982:275–350.
3. Vignos PJ Jr. Physical models of rehabilitation in neuromuscular disease. Muscle Nerve 1983; 6:323–338.
4. Fowler WM Jr, Taylor M. Rehabilitation management of muscular dystrophy and related disorders. I. The role of exercise. Arch Phys Med Rehabil 1982; 63:319–321.

17 MOTOR NEURON DISEASE

Mehrsheed Sinaki, M.D.

Disorders of the motor neurons or anterior horn cells consist of many diseases that affect the lower motor neurons or, as in amyotrophic lateral sclerosis (ALS), both upper and lower motor neurons. These diseases are insidious at onset and are progressive. The progression is often slow. Motor neuron diseases are classified according to the age of the patient at onset of disease, clinical course, and outcome (Table 17–1). Werdnig-Hoffmann disease is the infantile form of motor neuron disease involving the lower motor neurons. It has a poor prognosis. Kugelberg-Welander disease is the juvenile form of motor neuron disease. Its progression is much slower and clinically may mimic limb girdle muscular dystrophy. Sometimes, involvement of the anterior horn cells is limited to certain segments of the spinal cord (segmental spinal muscular atrophy of Sobue). Sometimes, bulbar innervated musculature is primarily involved (progressive bulbar palsy, juvenile progressive bulbar palsy of Fazio-Londe). Primary lateral sclerosis is a syndrome

TABLE 17–1 Primary Motor Neuron Diseases

Infantile progressive muscular atrophy (Werdnig-Hoffmann disease)
Chronic proximal muscular atrophy (Kugelberg-Welander disease)
Scapuloperoneal atrophy
Juvenile progressive bulbar palsy (Fazio-Londe atrophy)
Progressive bulbar palsy
Segmental spinal muscular atrophy (Sobue)
Amyotrophic lateral sclerosis
Sporadic
Familial
? Primary lateral sclerosis

manifested by signs of corticospinal tract involvement without evidence of lower motor neuron involvement. The most common form of motor neuron disease, however, is ALS—the focus of this chapter. Postpolio weakness has many similarities to ALS. Thus, many of the rehabilitation measures used for ALS can also be applied to patients with postpolio weakness.

EPIDEMIOLOGY AND INCIDENCE

The incidence rate of ALS is between 0.4 and 1.8 per 100,000 population. It accounts for about 1 in every 1,000 deaths. For reasons that are thus far unclear, the disease occurs 50 to 100 times more frequently among the Chamorros of Guam. ALS occurs more frequently in men (the male:female ratio in the United States is 1.7:1). The disorder is inherited as an autosomal dominant trait in 5% to 10% of patients.[1] ALS is a disease of middle and later life and rarely occurs in young adults. The average age at onset is about 60 years, and the average age at death is about 64 years.

SYMPTOMS AND SIGNS

The initial manifestations are often asymmetric. They vary depending on the distribution and extent of lower motor neuron involvement and the proportion of upper and lower motor neuron involvement. The manifestations of lower motor neuron involvement include muscle weakness and atrophy, fasciculations, and diminished muscle stretch reflexes. The manifestations of upper motor neuron involvement include spasticity, exaggerated muscle stretch reflexes, clonus, and Babinski signs. Corticobulbar involvement may cause pseudobulbar features. Muscle cramps are common early symptoms. Gait disorder and progressive limb weakness are often present. Dysphagia and dysarthria (flaccid, spastic, and mixed flaccid and spastic) are frequently noted. Tongue atrophy and fasciculations sometimes occur. Sphincter control is intact, eye movements are unaffected, sensation is not disturbed, and intellect is spared.

In most cases, ALS is rapidly progressive. It is an incurable disorder. Many physicians and also patients and their families equate the diagnosis with a loss of hope for the future, an attitude that results in a nihilistic approach to therapy.

LABORATORY DATA

Electromyographic examination characteristically shows normal nerve conduction studies or only slightly slow conduction velocities. Needle electrode examination usually shows "neurogenic" changes, including irritability, fibrillation potentials, fasciculation potentials, and large polyphasic, rapidly firing motor unit potentials. The degree of the changes noted depends on the stage of progression of the disease. Ordinarily, denervation should be noted in at least three extremities before a definite electromyographic diagnosis of motor neuron disease is made. The serum creatine kinase value is elevated in about half of patients, but its elevation does not correlate with the stage, the severity, or the rate of progression of the disease.[2] ALS is usually diagnosed by careful clinical and electromyographic examinations. Thus, a muscle biopsy is needed only infrequently to diagnose ALS.

SYMPTOMATIC TREATMENT

The variability in the distribution of weakness in patients with ALS requires that rehabilitation techniques be individualized.[3,4] The progression of the illness requires continuous modification of treatment for each patient. We have found it useful to classify patients according to the rapidity of the illness, the site of onset of the disease, and the stage of disability. Patients with a long clinical course have a remarkable capacity to compensate for motor unit loss,[5] which may enable them to continue daily activities for years. Patients with a slow clinical course continue to have slow progression throughout their illness, whereas those whose illness has been rapidly progressive can be expected to continue to deteriorate rapidly. It is helpful to differentiate patients according to whether the symptoms began in the bulbar or in the axioappendicular musculature. For patients with axioappendicular symptoms, we have found it particularly useful to "stage" the severity of the illness when outlining a therapeutic program. Different stages of ALS and the rehabilitation measures required at each stage[6] are outlined in Table 17–2.

Brainstem involvement with so-called bulbar symptoms may occur during any stage of ALS. These symptoms are usually prominent terminally. However, they have been noted in patients who have the chronic, slow form of the disease as well as in those with the more rapid form; thus, their occurrence does not necessarily indicate a brief clinical course. Accordingly, the prognosis should be based on the rapidity of the clinical course and not on the site of onset of the symptoms. Because of the involvement of the bulbar musculature about the throat, speaking and swallowing are difficult, and respiration is eventually compromised.

Breathing difficulty is the most serious complication of ALS. It is often concomitant with bulbar symptoms but is not necessarily a part of these symptoms; it may, in fact, be the initial complaint. The diaphragm and all of the muscles of breathing, including the auxiliary muscles, become involved. The problem may be compounded by obstruction of the airway because of bulbar symptoms. A simple chest respirator may be sufficient if the illness is slowly progressive. The use of more extensive respiratory measures, such as tracheostomy and permanent respirators in patients who are

TABLE 17–2 Exercise and Rehabilitation Programs for Patients With ALS, According to Stage of Disease

Stage, Characteristics	*Treatment*
I Patient is ambulatory, independent in ADL* Mild weakness, clumsiness	Encourage ROM* exercises, normal activities Encourage nonstrenuous strengthening of unaffected muscles to compensate for weakened muscles Discourage strenuous exercise to strengthen already weakened muscles (leads to increased fatigue and disability) Provide psychologic support †
II Patient is ambulatory Moderate selective weakness Slightly decreased independence in ADL (difficulty climbing stairs, raising arms, buttoning clothing)	Substitute fastening tape (Velcro) for buttons Encourage use of ankle-foot orthoses (Fig. 17–1), wrist and thumb splints Encourage cautious, selective nonstrenuous strengthening for unaffected muscles and stretching exercises to avoid contractures
III Patient is ambulatory Moderately decreased independence in ADL Easily fatigued with long-distance ambulation Severe selective weakness in ankles, wrists, hands, or neck extensors (Fig. 17–2 through 17–5)	Keep patient physically independent as long as possible Encourage deep-breathing exercises to strengthen auxiliary muscles of respiration Prescribe wheelchair (standard or battery operated with proper modifications) Apply nuchal support (Fig. 17–6) to improve patient's posture and gait
IV Patient is confined to wheelchair Still able to perform ADL Severe LE* weakness, moderate UE* weakness (± spasticity)‡ Hanging-arm syndrome with shoulder pain and sometimes edema in the hand (Fig. 17–8)	Apply heat, massage, shoulder sling (Fig. 17–7), and measures to prevent edema Apply passive ROM to the weakly supported joints Encourage nonstrenuous strengthening of the few remaining uninvolved muscles
V Patient is in wheelchair Increasingly dependent in ADL Severe LE weakness,§ moderate to severe UE weakness Possible skin breakdown	Encourage family to learn proper transfer and positioning principles Encourage modifications at home to aid patient's mobility and independence Suggest water mattress or water bed
VI Patient is bedridden Completely dependent in ADL	For dysphagia, use soft diet, long spoons, or tube feeding For accumulated saliva, use suctions, medications, or surgery to decrease flow For dysarthria, use palatal lifts, electronic speech amplification For breathing difficulty, clear airway, perform tracheotomy, use respirator

* ADL, activities of daily living; LE, lower extremity; ROM, range of motion; UE, upper extremity.
† Sedatives and tranquilizers (such as diazepam) may cause depression.
‡ Spasticity may serve as a splinting effect for ambulation; if severe, try the least dose of baclofen that is effective.
§ For prevention of thrombophlebitis in flaccid lower extremities, avoid trauma and apply passive ROM (twice a day), elastic stockings, dorsal and plantar flexion every 2 or 3 hours, thromboguards (device that provides intermittent pneumatic pressure to aid circulation), and a trial of subcutaneous heparin (5,000 U every 12 hours) in selected cases.
From Sinaki, et al.[6] By permission of the publisher.

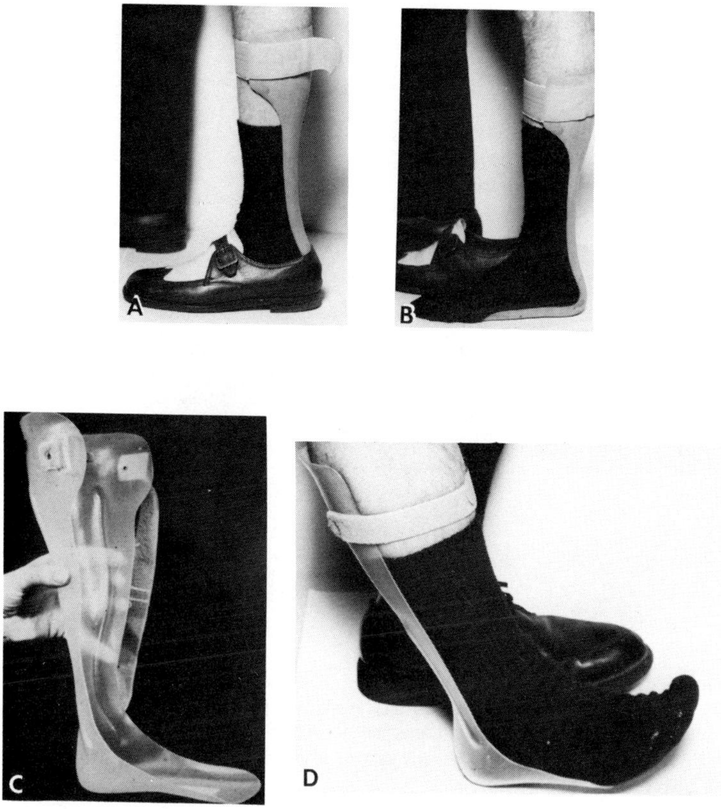

Figure 17–1 Examples of lightweight ankle-foot orthoses. *A* and *B*, Custom-made posterior leaf-spring brace. *C*, Alimed orthosis, commercially available in small, medium, and large sizes. *D*, Alimed splint can be used by patients who have footdrop but incomplete paralysis of foot dorsiflexor muscles. Patient can attempt some dorsiflexion. Alimed splints are not as strong a support as posterior leaf-spring braces. (*A* and *B*, From Sinaki.[4] By permission of John Wiley & Sons. *C* and *D*, From Sinaki and Mulder.[3] By permission of Mayo Foundation.)

already totally paralyzed, must be discussed in detail with the patient and the family to determine their appropriateness.

Involvement of the pyramidal pathways, another component of ALS, results in hyperreflexia and spasticity.[6] These symptoms, surprisingly, account for only a small portion of a patient's complaints, if the dysphonia that occurs with pronounced spasticity is excluded. Simple rehabilitation methods are usually sufficient for their management (Table 17–3).

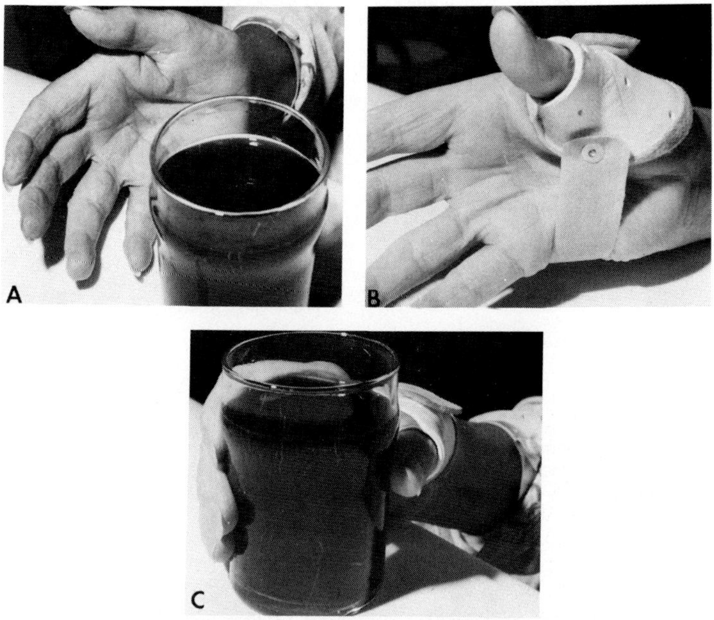

Figure 17–2 Patient with weakness and atrophy of thenar muscles. *A*, Patient is unable to hold a glass. *B* and *C*, Application of thumb-shell splint stabilizes thumb in oppositon (*B*) and enables patient to have effective cylinder grasp (*C*). (From Sinaki and Mulder.[3] By permission of Mayo Foundation.)

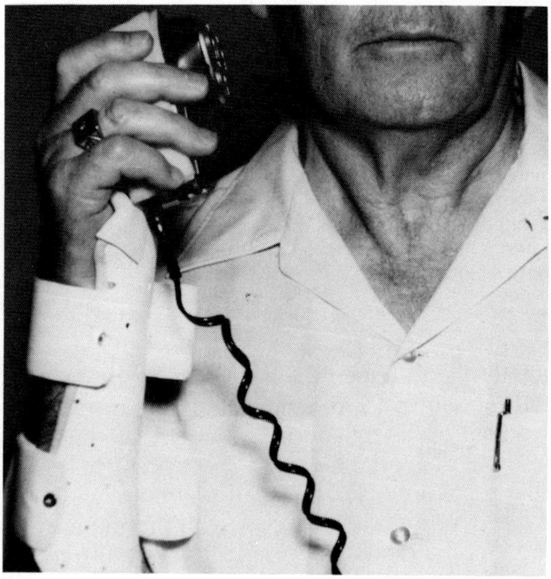

Figure 17–3 Application of wrist-extension splint with thumb-shell addition enables patient to hold electric razor effectively with one hand. (From Sinaki and Mulder.[3] By permission of Mayo Foundation.)

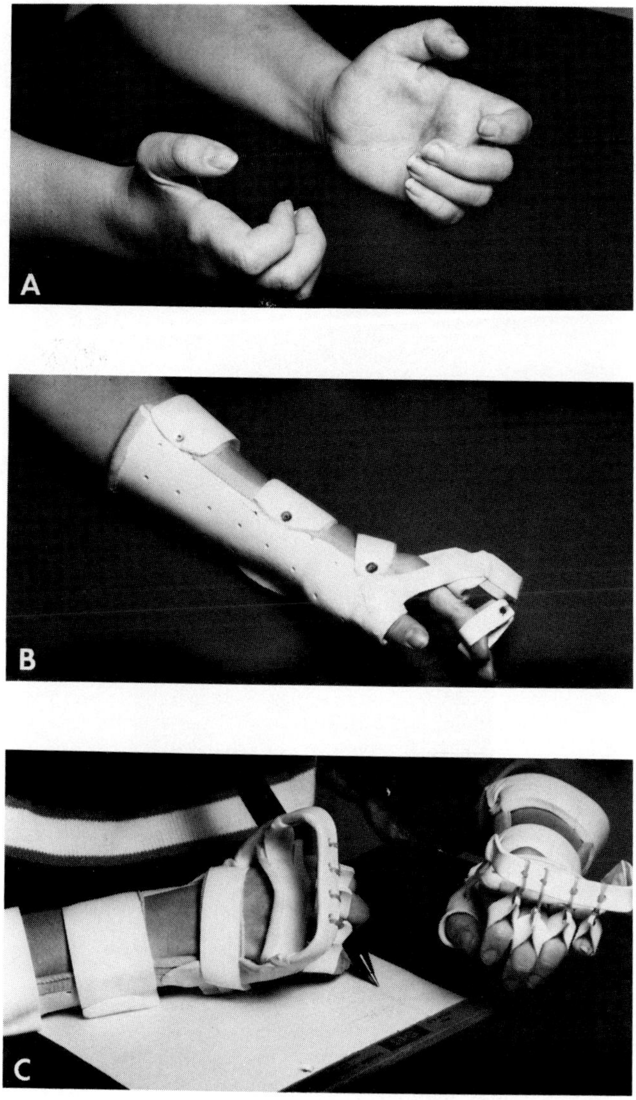

Figure 17–4 *A*, Patient with severe atrophy and weakness of thenar muscles and of finger and wrist extensors. *B*, Static wrist-extension splint with thumb-shell addition coupled with dynamic finger-extension device. *C*, Complex but practical splint enables patient to do certain (even fine) movements, such as writing. (From Sinaki.[4] By permission of John Wiley & Sons.)

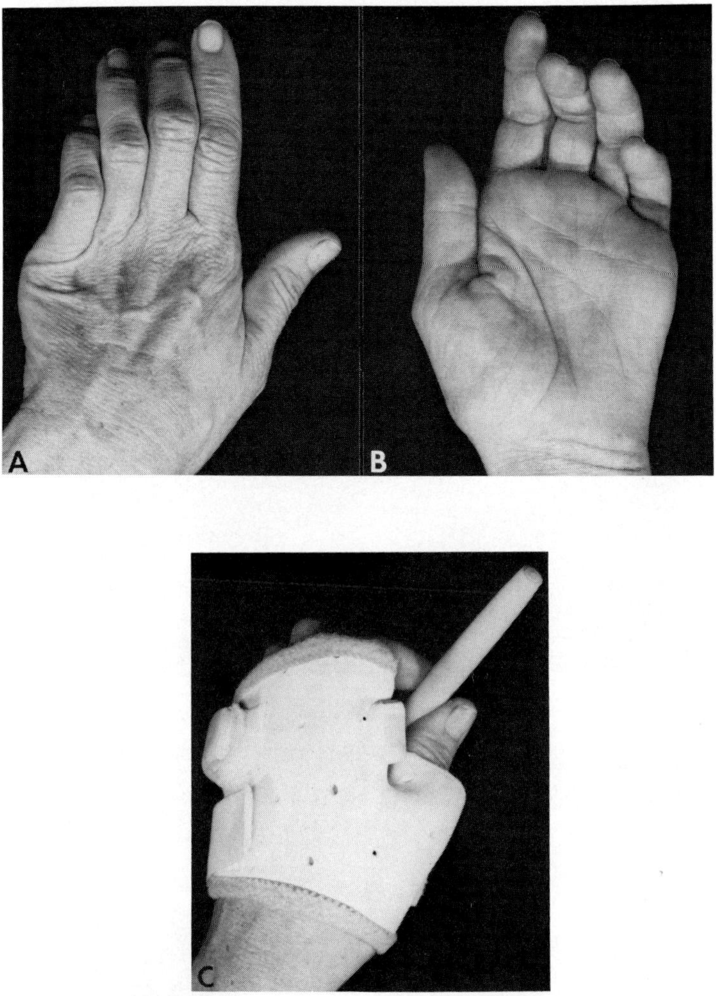

Figure 17–5 *A* and *B*, Claw-hand deformity in a patient with ALS. *C*, Hand splint used for rehabilitation.

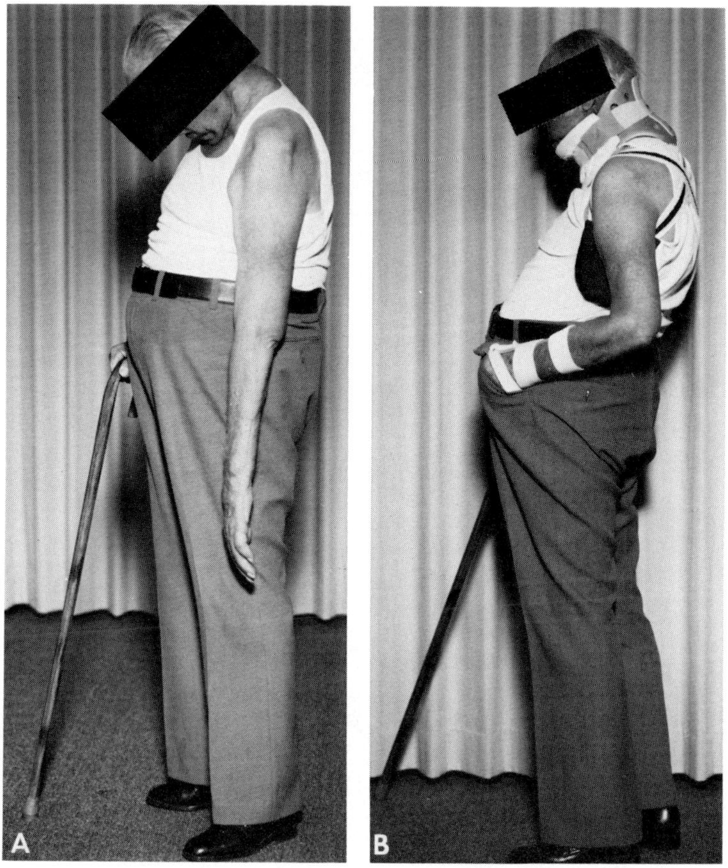

Figure 17–6 *A*, Patient with weakness of extensor nuchal muscles. *B*, Application of cervical collar (Philadelphia collar) to improve posture and independence in activities of daily living.

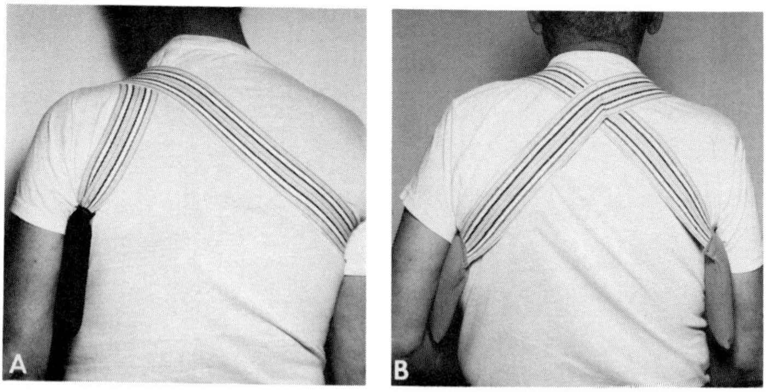

Figure 17–7 Shoulder slings. *A*, Bobath shoulder sling used to decrease sagging of shoulder and to reduce stretch on brachial and axillary neurovascular bundle. *B*, Modified Bobath sling used for bilateral shoulder-girdle weakness (so-called hanging-arm syndrome). (From Sinaki.[4] By permission of John Wiley & Sons.)

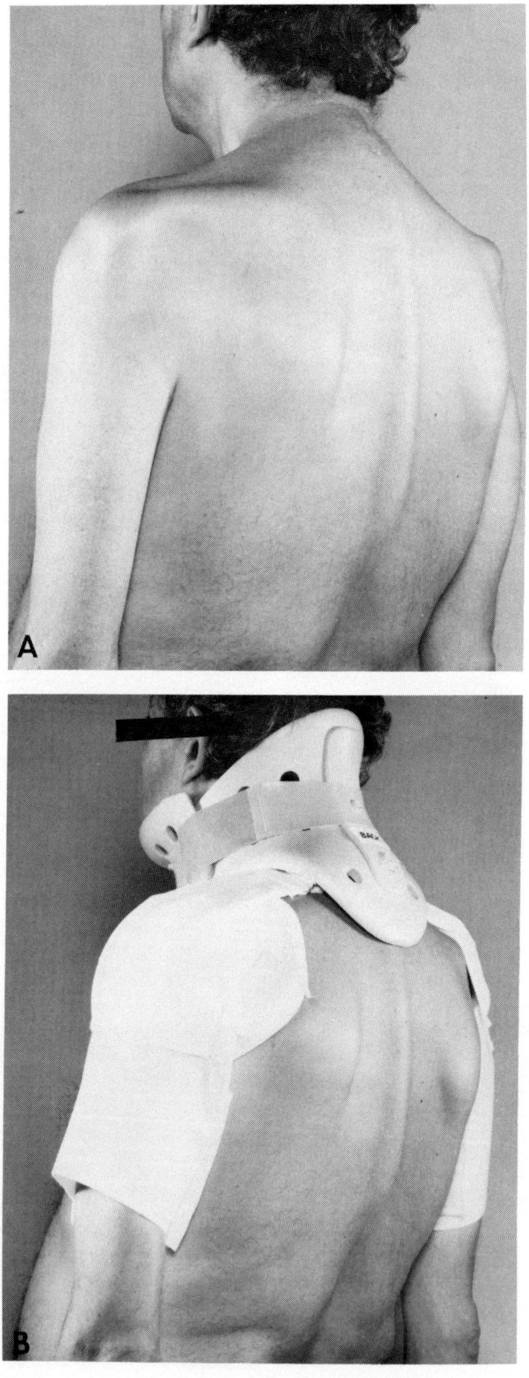

Figure 17–8 *A*, Patient with weakness of shoulder girdle and extensor nuchal musculature. *B*, Combined application of hemihook shoulder sling and cervical collar (Philadelphia collar) to compensate for weakness and to decrease discomfort.

TABLE 17–3 Treatment of Common Symptoms of Motor Neuron Disease*

Symptom	*Treatment*
Constipation	Hydration
	High-fiber diet
	Stool softener (e.g., docusate sodium [Colace])
	Suppositories (e.g., bisacodyl [Dulcolax], glycerol)
Cramps	Quinine (200 mg at bedtime)†
	Phenytoin (Dilantin)†
Spasticity	Baclofen (Lioresal)
Sialorrhea	Amitriptyline (10 mg four times daily)†
	Hyoscyamine sulfate (0.125 mg four times daily)†
	Trihexyphenidyl hydrochloride†
Dysphagia	Slow eating
	Food that is easy to swallow
	Frequent meals
	Caloric supplementation (e.g., Ensure, Isocal)
	Pureed food
	Percutaneous gastrostomy
Dysarthria	Speech therapy
	Writing (e.g., Magic Slate)
	Alphabet cards
	Typewriters (Canon Communicator)
	Computerized communication devices

* For patients with motor neuron disease, we use medications cautiously because of untoward side effects.

† Titrate to effective dose.

From Sinaki, et al.[6] By permission of the publisher.

Emotional support of the patients and their families must be addressed at any stage of the disease. Reactive depression is not uncommon, but suicide is rare. Counseling and planning for the future must begin at the early stages. Chapters of the ALS Society and the Muscular Dystrophy Association are helpful not only for providing emotional support but also for extending specific help to both the patient and the physician.[6]

REFERENCES

1. Mulder DW. Commentary. In: The diagnosis and treatment of amyotrophic lateral sclerosis. Boston: Houghton Mifflin Professional Publishers, 1980:79–82.
2. Sinaki M, Mulder DW. Amyotrophic lateral sclerosis: relationship between serum creatine kinase level and patient survival. Arch Phys Med Rehabil 1986; 67:169–171.
3. Sinaki M, Mulder DW. Rehabilitation techniques for patients with amyotrophic lateral sclerosis. Mayo Clin Proc 1978; 53:173–178.
4. Sinaki M. Rehabilitation. In: Mulder DW, ed. The diagnosis and treatment of amyotrophic lateral sclerosis. Boston: Houghton Mifflin Professional Publishers, 1980:169–193.

5. Mulder DW, Howard FM Jr. Patient resistance and prognosis in amyotrophic lateral sclerosis. Mayo Clin Proc 1976; 51:537–541.
6. Sinaki M, Litchy WJ, Mulder DW. Motor neuron disease. In: Bayless TM, Brain MC, Cherniack RM, eds. Current therapy in internal medicine - 2. Philadelphia: BC Decker, 1987:1325–1329.

18 PARKINSONISM

Gail L. Gamble, M.D.
Mehrsheed Sinaki, M.D.

Parkinson's disease is described as a progressive neurologic disturbance of motor function characterized by the presence of rigidity, resting tremor, and bradykinesia. The common and progressive nature of this disease mandates that primary care and rehabilitation physicians be familiar with the disease and its consequences. Parkinson's disease has an estimated incidence of 20 per 100,000 population and a prevalence rate of 100 to 150 per 100,000 population. It is rated third after stroke and dementia as a severely disabling neurologic disease in the elderly population. The quality of life of both patient and family is affected by this disease. When instituted early, rehabilitation techniques can be effective for helping patients maintain maximal function.

PATHOPHYSIOLOGY

The symptoms of parkinsonism are known to occur in connection with several different pathologic states (Table 18–1). The clinical manifestations are ascribed to lesions that involve the substantia nigra and its efferent pathways. Parkinson's disease (paralysis agitans) accounts for most cases of parkinsonism. Of great interest is a recently identified form of parkinsonism in young patients with an associated history of drug use. A neurotoxin in street drugs (1-methyl-4-phenyl-1,2,3,6-tetrahydropyridine) has been found to cause progressive signs of the disease and associated pathologic findings.[1,2]

The common abnormality is progressive degeneration of nerve cells of pigmented nuclei of the brainstem, especially the substantia nigra. These are dopamine-containing neurons whose cell bodies are primarily in the substantia nigra and whose axons project to the putamen and globus pallidus.[3]

TABLE 18-1 Conditions That May Exhibit Parkinsonian Features

Degenerative diseases
Parkinson's disease (paralysis agitans)
Shy-Drager syndrome
Progressive supranuclear palsy
Infections
Postencephalitic parkinsonism
Drug- or toxin-induced diseases
Neuroleptics (phenothiazines, haloperidol)
Carbon monoxide poisoning
Chronic manganese poisoning
MPTP*-induced parkinsonism
Vascular conditions
Lacunar infarcts
Other chronic neurologic disorders
Alzheimer's disease
Huntington's disease
Wilson's disease
Normal-pressure hydrocephalus

* 1-Methyl-4-phenyl-1,2,3,6-tetrahydropyridine.

On gross examination, the substantia nigra appears pale and depigmented. Microscopically, neuronal dropout and gliosis are noted, as are intracytoplasmic inclusions called Lewy bodies. Thus, pharmacologically, there is dopamine deficiency as the result of degeneration of the dopaminergic neuronal system.[2] The greater the cell loss in the substantia nigra, the lower the concentration of dopamine in the striatum and the more marked the parkinsonian manifestations.[4]

CLINICAL PRESENTATION

Parkinson's original description appeared in 1817 and included tremor but not rigidity or bradykinesia. The clinical manifestations in parkinsonism may be variable, particularly depending on the stage of the disease. Advanced Parkinson's disease is immediately recognizable, even from a distance. However, early cases of the disease may not be so easily diagnosed, especially when the typical tremor is absent and the disease presents with rigidity or bradykinesia. Most constant among the manifestations of the disease is the classic triad of tremor, rigidity, and bradykinesia.

Tremor

One of the most visible symptoms, tremor is the most common reason affected patients present to a physician. It is usually a resting tremor that is increased with anxiety, emotion, or tension. The tremor characteristically exhibits a rate of 4 to 8 Hz, and it can and should be distinguished from the intention tremor of cerebellar dysfunction and from essential familial tremor. The tremor, which can be bilateral or unilateral, most often affects the distal parts of the limbs. It can also involve the face, jaw, and even the tongue.

Rigidity

One clinical sign found on examination of nearly all affected patients is rigidity.[5] It is described as a consistent plasticlike resistance exhibited in both flexion and extension with attempted passive range of motion. It is present constantly and is interrupted only by the cogwheel phenomenon, which is thought to be the transmission of tremor through the rigidity.

Bradykinesia

This important feature is manifested in many ways. It has been shown to be different from pure rigidity by specific surgical ablation and can be described as a poverty of movement or lack of initiation of movement. It is distinctly not muscle weakness (which is not a characteristic of this disease). Patients may exhibit the typical masked facies, with paucity of facial expression and facial movements. Blinking is usually infrequent. Speech is often hypokinetic and monotonous. Handwriting becomes small (micrographia). Automatic movements of the limbs are sparse and hard to initiate. In general, patients are unable to perform any movement that requires the quick reciprocal muscle actions that are so important for the coordinated movements of normal living. Many of the activities of daily living can be affected by a significant bradykinesia (Table 18–2).

TABLE 18–2 Functions Affected by Bradykinesia

Swallowing (dysphagia)
Communication (hypokinetic dysarthria)
Transfers ("freezing")
Gait (propulsion, retropulsion)
Balance (en bloc movements)
Self-care activities

Posture

Associated with the difficulty of motor initiation is the loss of appropriate posturing. Patients tend to assume a stooped posture with flexed trunk, neck, hip, and knees (Fig. 18–1). The inability to maintain erect posture has a significant effect on balance and gait. Patients find walking difficult to initiate because of the bradykinesia, and their forward-balanced posture makes gait extremely hard to control.[6] Arm swing is decreased or absent, and the postural and righting reflexes may also be affected. The tendency to fall is markedly increased. When this occurs, it is often without an attempt to protect oneself, and the movement can be truly "en bloc."

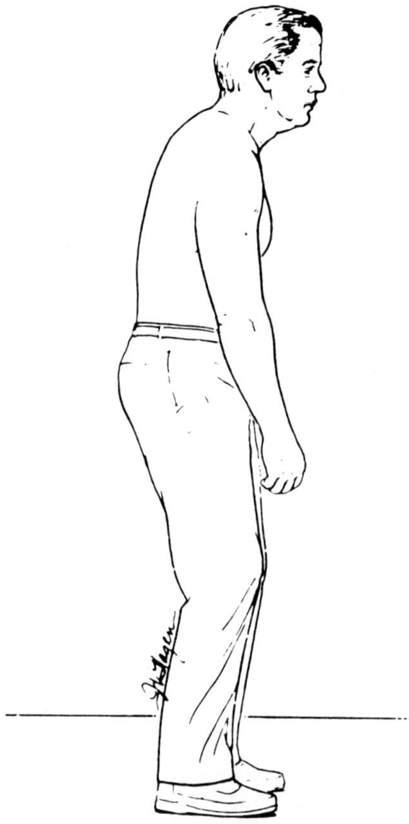

Figure 18–1 Flexed posturing of patient with parkinsonism.

Autonomic Symptoms

Flushing of the skin may occur and is sometimes associated with increased sweating. Excretion from sebaceous glands may increase and the skin may feel greasy. Excessive salivation is common. Blood pressure is usually low, and many patients have orthostatic hypotension, which in some cases can be severe and disabling. Urinary retention has been described, but in many cases this can be attributed to the effect of anticholinergic drugs. Constipation is common, and questions regarding bowel and bladder function should be included in the rehabilitation evaluation.

Neuropsychologic Changes

Various psychologic manifestations may also be exhibited, including depression and personality changes. Patients with parkinsonism tend to isolate themselves from their normal social environment because of embarrassment about resting tremor, difficulty with movements, impaired speech, or excessive drooling. This behavior must be distinguished from a clear change in personality characteristics. Additionally, a mildly progressive dementia can be associated with the disease.[7] It is not present in all cases, however, and any suspected cognitive deficits need to be assessed closely because the frozen facial expression and poor ability to communicate may be the major problems.

PHARMACOLOGIC TREATMENT

Parkinson's disease is a gradually progressive degenerative disease, and a slow decline will occur despite adequate pharmacologic and physical management. However, the life expectancy of patients with this disease remains normal despite the considerable functional disability. The goals of any rehabilitation program, which include preservation of function and maintenance of independence, remain important in the care of patients with parkinsonism.

Various drugs have been used to treat Parkinson's disease (Table 18–3). A closely followed, well-adjusted dosage schedule for carbidopa-levodopa is the preferred method of pharmacologic management in most cases.[8] Levodopa combined with carbidopa (a peripheral dopa decarboxylase inhibitor) has allowed for decreased dosages of levodopa, minimization of side effects, and improved levodopa levels in the central nervous system. The rehabilitation physician should be aware of the effects and side

TABLE 18–3 Drugs Used for the Management of Parkinson's Disease

Neurotransmitter replacement therapy
Levodopa
Carbidopa-levodopa (Sinemet)
Receptor agonists
Bromocriptine (Parlodel)
Amantadine (Symmetrel)
Anticholinergics
Trihexyphenidyl (Artane)
Benztropine (Cogentin)
Ethopropazine (Parsidol)
Antihistamines
Diphenhydramine (Benadryl)
Chlorphenoxamine (Phenoxene)

effects of these medications, that dosages do need to be adjusted, and that the effects of the medications act over a period of hours. Physical therapy should be administered at a time when blood levels, and therefore performance, are optimal. With use of carbidopa-levodopa particularly, an on-off effect may occur. Also, increased doses of this medication may cause dystonic movements. In some patients, particularly those who are elderly, antiparkinsonism drugs (especially anticholinergics) may cause hallucinations, disorientation, and confusion.

PHYSICAL THERAPY

Patients who are even moderately affected with parkinsonism will benefit from a daily program of both physical and occupational therapy. Speech therapy, if needed, may be helpful. At first, the intervention should be supervised, and then a daily home program can be developed.

The onset of disease is usually insidious, and family roles may have changed as discreetly as disease progression itself. Family members should be counseled to encourage the patient to assume the most active role possible in all areas of home life in order to preserve an inner sense of dignity. Efforts must be made to include the patient in decisions about family affairs and also the rehabilitation program. Enough time should be allowed for completion of daily tasks as long as the patient's independence can be maintained.

Exercises are particularly useful and should become part of a patient's daily routine.[9] Exercises are more effective when they are used consistently and early in the course of disease to maintain a functional level rather than to restore function in an unused limb affected with contracture. Multiple types of exercises are used in a comprehensive therapy program (Table 18–4).

TABLE 18–4 Therapeutic Exercises for Parkinson's Disease

Range of motion
Stretching
Posture
Coordination
Deep breathing
Facial
Transfers and gait

Range-of-Motion Exercises

These should be performed daily on all peripheral joints and may be done actively or on an active-assistive basis when a patient is unable to perform them independently. These simple movements will help minimize joint stiffness and will decrease the progressive tendency toward contracture.

Stretching

One of the major components of all exercise programs for parkinsonism is stretching. A gentle, prolonged, passive stretch program is frequently necessary to work against the effects of progressive rigidity and to maintain full range of motion. Proper posture is the major goal, and stretching of multiple muscles, including pectoral and upper chest wall, neck flexors, abdominal flexors, and hip and knee flexors, should be included (see Fig. 28–3 and 28–4). Stretching the hamstring is important because it affects the ability to assume an erect posture. The stretching program must become part of the daily routine of a patient and spouse and should preferably be done twice a day. A simple gravity-assisted stretch may be done by merely having the patient lie supine without pillows for an extended time (Fig. 18–2).

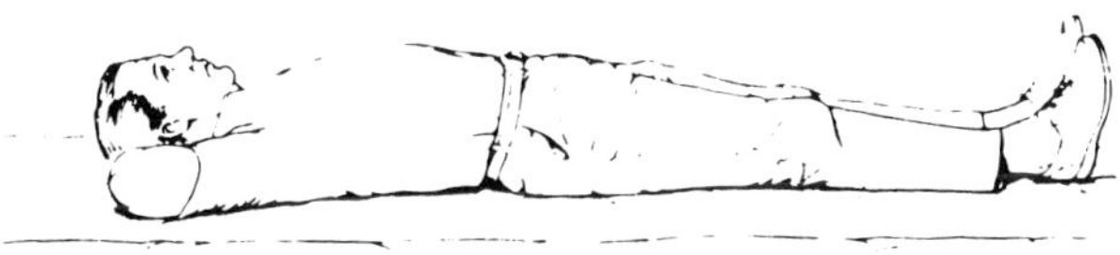

Figure 18–2 Supine stretch to avoid flexion.

Posture

Nearly all patients with parkinsonism have a tendency for stooped posturing, and avoidance of this posture is imperative. The patient should continually work toward avoiding downward gaze by learning correct cervical posture in sitting and standing positions. In addition to flexor cervical muscles, the pectorals frequently become contracted, and a program of pectoral stretch by doing pushups against a wall should be undertaken (see Fig. 28–5). Extension exercises for the upper thoracic spine are also helpful and can be done in either the prone or erect sitting position (see Fig. 28–2). The patient must also be instructed to avoid both hip flexor and knee flexor posturing.

Coordination

The combined effects of rigidity and bradykinesia limit the ability to move in a smooth and well-controlled pattern. In an attempt to retain coordinated reciprocal movements, coordination exercises for both the upper and the lower extremities should become part of a daily regimen. Lower extremity coordination exercises should stress reciprocal movements and postural balance. Rhythmic exercises such as use of a stationary bicycle may improve ambulatory activities. Patients with parkinsonism live with an increased fear of falling, and exercises should be directed at overcoming this fear and insecurity. Upper extremity exercises should also be undertaken using reciprocal motions when possible.

Gait

The typical gait of parkinsonism is frequently present and is often socially embarrassing for patients. Rapid small steps, forward flexed posturing, and shuffling of feet are characteristic. Gait mechanics can be improved when attention is given to widening the gait base and directing the patient to take a longer stride. Because of the rigidity, patients are frequently unable to correct a minor imbalance with slight movement and, therefore, falls are frequent. As mentioned previously, righting reflexes can be impaired and the quick movement necessary to sustain balance is often lacking.

Truncal and rotational exercises are also important for gait reeducation. Rotatory movements are often impaired, but they are an essential component of independent gait and transfer activities. Rising from a chair can also be difficult. Attempts can be made to teach a "rocking" activity—leaning the body forward and backward until the patient can rise out of the chair.

An assistive device such as a cane is usually not helpful for gait stabilization because patients tend to carry it rather than use it smoothly as a balancing mechanism. Walkers can also tend to complicate gait patterns. However, a wheeled walker may be useful if it is spring loaded for a pressure stop on the two posterior feet. With this assistive device, the forward propulsion of gait is allowed without the necessity of picking up the walker with each step.

OCCUPATIONAL THERAPY

Early efforts with an intensive program of occupational therapy are also important for patient and family. Patients should be taught the skills that allow independent function, when possible.

An occupational therapy evaluation will document a patient's present level of functioning. Instruments such as the nine-hole peg test and bilateral upper extremity coordination tests and evaluation of hand strength, pinch, and grasp may prove helpful. Additionally, an evaluation of a patient's ability for self-care will identify areas in which improvements might be made (Table 18–5).

Occupational therapy activities include rhythmic prehension and coordination skills, both gross and fine. Upper extremity range-of-motion activities should be continued, with an emphasis on reciprocal rhythm. Exercises may be developed that specifically address a patient's handwriting abnormalities, particularly if handwriting is an important part of vocational capabilities.

Training in activities of daily living is an important area of occupational therapy. Skills for dressing, including the small move-

TABLE 18–5 Occupational Therapy for Parkinson's Disease

Activities of daily living
Adaptive equipment
Cognitive evaluation
Safety and judgment
Fine motor coordination
Handwriting

ments of buttoning, and the coordinated movements of feeding should be closely evaluated. Adaptive equipment options should be made available to patients. Items such as buttonhooks (see Fig. 24–8 *C*), feeding utensils, and a toilet-seat riser may allow patients to maintain independence (see Fig. 14–2). Periodic reevaluations should be scheduled because self-care abilities gradually change during the course of the disease. A relative may assume that a patient remains capable of performing daily activities, but periodic evaluation may reveal a subtle decline in physical and intellectual capabilities, which may require an alteration of home care.

SPEECH THERAPY

Altered speech may be an important and disabling effect of parkinsonism and, in many cases, it may have a significant effect on vocation. The characteristic speech pattern has a low volume with high monotonous pitch and a hurried unpunctuated rate. Loss of the ability to vary intonation and cadence is defined as prosody.[10] These deficiencies were not thought to be amenable to speech therapy until recent years. Now, however, intensive efforts with speech therapy may help the patient vary intonation and control the rate of speech.[11,12]

In conjunction with speech therapy, patients should be taught deep-breathing exercises, which may help to add increased volume to speech. A form of dysarthria may be present if facial and tongue movements are poorly controlled. Facial, oral, and lingual exercises are also an important part of a speech therapy program. The ability to phonate may vary over the clinical course of the disease, and periodic evaluations by a speech pathologist are helpful.

REHABILITATION: AN INTEGRATED APPROACH

The rehabilitation needs for patients with parkinsonism vary widely, and an integrated program should be developed by the coordinator of care. The psychologic impact on patient and family may be a major disability factor, and the involvement of a psychologist or social worker can be important. The physician coordinator or social worker should also inform patients of local community resources and national support groups.[13] Parkinsonism is a chronic and progressive disease, but independence and quality of life may be better maintained through appropriate pharmacologic management and involvement of rehabilitation team members.

REFERENCES

1. Adams RD, Victor M. Principles of neurology. 3rd ed. New York: McGraw-Hill, 1985:872–881.
2. Current concepts and controversies in Parkinson's disease. Proceedings of a symposium held at Montebello, Quebec, October 21–22, 1983. Can J Neurol Sci 1984; 11 suppl 1:89–237.
3. Meyers FH, Jawetz E, Goldfien A. Review of medical pharmacology. 7th ed. Los Altos, California: Lange Medical Publications, 1980.
4. Yahr MD. Parkinsonism. In: Rowland LP, ed. Merritt's textbook of neurology. 7th ed. Philadelphia: Lea & Febiger, 1984:526–537.
5. Selby G. The Graeme Robertson Memorial Lecture, 1983: the long-term prognosis of Parkinson's disease. Clin Exp Neurol 1984; 20:1–25.
6. Cailliet R. Rehabilitation in parkinsonism. In: Licht S, ed. Rehabilitation and medicine. Baltimore: Waverly Press, 1968:430–445.
7. Dakof GA, Mendelsohn GA. Parkinson's disease: psychological aspects of a chronic illness. Psychol Bull 1986; 99:375–387.
8. Gilroy J, Meyer JS. Medical neurology. 3rd ed. New York: Macmillan, 1979.
9. Palmer SS, Mortimer JA, Webster DD, Bistevins R, Dickinson GL. Exercise therapy for Parkinson's disease. Arch Phys Med Rehabil 1986; 67:741–745.
10. Ross ED, Mesulam M-M. Dominant language functions of the right hemisphere? Prosody and emotional gesturing. Arch Neurol 1979; 36:144–148.
11. Scott S, Caird FI. Speech therapy for Parkinson's disease. J Neurol Neurosurg Psychiatry 1983; 46:140–144.
12. Robertson SJ, Thomson F. Speech therapy in Parkinson's disease: a study of the efficacy and long term effects of intensive treatment. Br J Disord Commun 1984; 19:213–224.
13. Duvoisin RC. Parkinson's disease: a guide for patient and family. 2nd ed. New York: Raven Press, 1984:137–190.

19 MULTIPLE SCLEROSIS

E. Lyle Gross, M.D., F.R.C.P. (C)
Mehrsheed Sinaki, M.D.

Rehabilitating the patient with multiple sclerosis requires the maximal efforts of the rehabilitation team and taxes the rehabilitation armamentarium. This neurologic disease not only affects white matter of the central nervous system but also does so in varying degrees at different times. The patient with multiple sclerosis needs to deal with an interruption in career and family life and to face a disease process that typically has remissions and exacerbations but could also be steadily progressive.

PATHOLOGY

Multiple sclerosis affects the central nervous system. Histologically, there is loss of the myelin sheath and infiltration by phagocytes engulfing degenerating myelin. The myelin sheath is affected to various degrees by partial to complete destruction, and axons, glia, and other structures are relatively spared. With chronic lesions, proliferation of glial cells and fibers results in typical "sclerotic plaque."

ETIOLOGY AND EPIDEMIOLOGY

The cause of multiple sclerosis has escaped researcher and clinician. The presence of increased levels of gamma globulins in both cerebrospinal fluid and surrounding tissue is strong evidence of an immunologic abnormality. A viral basis has been speculated, but attempts to identify an infectious agent have repeatedly failed. It is recognized that persons who relocate to a high-risk area before the age of 15 years take on the risk of the new geographic location. Epidemiologic evidence reveals a high prevalence (more than 30 per 100,000 population) in the temperate zones of southern

Canada, northern United States, and Europe, a moderate prevalence (5 to 25 per 100,000) in the Mediterranean, southern United States, and most of Australia, and a low prevalence (less than 5 per 100,000) in the tropical zones. Genetic immunologic characteristics of patients also seem equally, if not more, important. The disease is far less common in black Americans than white Americans, and it is rarely if ever noted in American Indians or Eskimos. Characteristically, this disease affects young persons. Among those who are affected, two-thirds are between 20 and 45 years of age, and 75% are between 10 and 50 years of age. The female: male ratio is 3:2.

COURSE

The course of multiple sclerosis follows one of four patterns. The *benign course* occurs in about 20% of affected patients, and usually they have a remitting pattern with very long periods of stability. The *relapsing-remitting course* occurs in the greatest proportion of patients. Relapses commonly occur at a rate of one every 6 months to one every 3 to 4 years. The *chronic progressive course* affects 30% of patients (particularly elderly patients) and is characterized by slow onset of spastic weakness or ataxia and progression without remission. The result is early severe disability, generally within 10 years. Few patients have a *malignant course*. For those who do, however, total disability and death can occur within months.

MANIFESTATIONS

Clinically, a myriad of deficits may occur. Demyelination within the central nervous system may manifest in several ways within the motor system, causing sensory, motor, and visual symptoms. Exposure to a hot environment (hot bath or shower) may increase the neurologic symptoms or signs. At times, neck flexion may cause a vibrating-tingling sensation down the spine and the extremities (Lhermitte's phenomenon). Dizziness and vertigo are not rare.

SPASTICITY

The neurophysiologic basis of spasticity is beyond the scope of this text, but the ramifications are of frustrating concern. Spasticity can affect all aspects of mobility, beginning with mobility in bed and progressing to more difficult tasks such as sitting, ambulating, self-care, and performing one's vocation. When severe spasticity prevails, the foot may fix in an equinovarus position, resulting in a relative "leg-lengthening" problem. Patients must circumduct the limb in order to carry the leg forward, and this requires more energy. In order to minimize the amount of energy expenditure and allow a more efficient gait, an ankle-foot orthosis will restrict this plantar flexor position and result in a more "anatomic" limb position that enhances gait potential. Spasticity can also be decreased by using physical treatment measures, pharmacologic intervention, and various surgical procedures.

Methods such as ice treatment or functional electrical stimulation can modify spasticity. Ice treatment does not result in a permanent decrease in spasticity but may provide enough decrease in tone to allow for range of motion. Pharmacologic management, although it can be effective, is not without repercussions. Diazepam can affect higher cognitive functioning, and baclofen or dantrolene can have metabolic repercussions or result in excessive fatigue. Baclofen, a centrally acting gamma-aminobutyric acid agonist, is currently considered the drug of choice for the management of spasticity. The initial dosage is often small, 5 mg three times per day, and can be gradually increased, if needed, up to 80 mg per day in divided doses. Elimination of the "splinting" effect of spasticity, however, may further unmask the weakness in some patients.

Motor point block is a technique in which pharmacologic agents such as phenol or alcohol are injected into the site where the motor end-plates exist. This useful technique is appropriate for cases in which spastic individual muscles interfere with specific function.

Spasticity also results in abnormal limb and trunk posturing. Soft tissue having constant pressure from spastic muscles in combination with a distorted sensation can result in skin ulceration.

The effects of spasticity, however, are not all detrimental. Muscle activity maintains stress on bone, thereby minimizing the degree of osteoporosis. Spasticity may also allow support of an otherwise weak limb.

WEAKNESS

The decreased motor power may range from fatigue to a feeling of heaviness to total paralysis. Although the exact physiologic basis is unknown, the weakness associated with this disease can have a major impact. Energy expenditure can be minimized and security enhanced by ambulating with aids such as Lofstrand crutches or a standard wheeled walker. Bracing is often unsuccessful because of the extent of lower extremity spasticity, and the weight of an orthosis is often prohibitive. Specially designed shoes, such as those with a rocker bottom, can decrease energy use during gait.

Some patients prefer a cool bath or ice packs in the early morning because such measures may lessen the spasticity and make them feel stronger. With this pattern in mind, the activities of daily living need to be done during periods of peak performance.

Strengthening exercises can counter disuse weakness and

maintain peak performance. Excessive exercise can result in a further loss of strength. Regular rest intervals are important. Patients should be encouraged to maintain range of motion and functional activities such as those of daily living and ambulation. Fatigue is often a major complaint. Patients may need more rest, preferably at regular periods.

ATAXIA

Cerebellar dysfunction can dramatically influence all levels of functional independence from mobility to eating. Ataxia occurs in 60% of patients and is often difficult to manage.

DYSARTHRIA

Dysarthria in multiple sclerosis is common. An abdominal binder can help increase the volume of speech. Breathing exercises to maintain thoracic excursion and the strength of respiratory muscles should be used.

SENSORY DEFICITS

Sensory deficits, which affect 40% of patients, result in obvious difficulties. Ulcer formation can result from pressure points secondary to ill-fitting splints and poor bed positioning in combination with the constant pressure induced by spasticity. Dexterity becomes a problem, and buttoning is difficult, to name only one function that is taken for granted. Adaptive devices, sensory reeducation, and accommodative techniques for activities of daily living can be provided by the occupational therapist. Rehabilitation management for sensory deficits relies heavily on education of patient and family, but biofeedback training is another viable alternative.

PSYCHOLOGIC EFFECTS

Emotional lability may manifest as either depression or euphoria and may be based on organic involvement. Equally, it is not unreasonable to be depressed when affected with this disease. Of the various psychologic changes associated with multiple sclerosis, depression may be the most common. It is believed to be reactive depression rather than a direct result of the disease process. Some patients manifest euphoria. This excessive emotional response may occur in the advanced stages, when significant physical and intellectual deteriorations occur. Dementia probably occurs more often than admitted or appreciated. It is sometimes masked by a patient's euphoria or depression.

REHABILITATION

Hospitalized patients receive daily care and close observation from the rehabilitation team; as a result, this intervention minimizes the chances of developing skin irritation, contractures, and urinary tract infection. Once at home, however, patients are often at the mercy of their environment. A proper examination before dismissal is a priority.

Skin ulceration can prolong hospitalization and delay rehabilitation. Skin ulcers can result from excessive prolonged pressure, called decubital ulceration, or from forces resulting from friction, which are shear forces. The skin should be kept clean and dry, and appropriate skin checks should be made. Skin should be checked every 2 hours initially after patients receive new splints or are confined to bed rest. The duration the splints are worn or the intervals between positioning in bed can be increased by ½ hour twice daily if the skin remains clear. Superficial redness lasting more than 24 hours is by definition a pressure sore, which can be the beginning of a decubital ulcer. The treatment of choice is prevention of prolonged pressure and avoidance of shear. A superficial ulcer (grade 1) can take weeks to resolve. Synthetic sheepskin over select areas minimizes the shear effect of bed positioning and transfers, but it does not decrease the pressure phenomenon that results in ulceration.

Application of range-of-motion exercises twice a day and proper positioning prevent contracture formation. Footboards and splints will help maintain proper positioning. Spasticity and weakness may be so restrictive that contractures can occur early if not recognized.

Trained occupational therapists or speech therapists can provide necessary diagnostic trials to assess swallowing difficulties. Liquids are often tolerated poorly, and a mechanical soft diet is recommended.

Pain occurs in about 20% of patients, usually in the low back. It remains a difficult problem to treat. Frequently, if spasticity is managed, the pain complaints lessen. Use of a transcutaneous nerve stimulator may prove useful.

The neurogenic bowel and bladder dysfunction associated with multiple sclerosis may require a tremendous amount of attention in overall rehabilitation management. The clinical presentation and management differ from those associated with spinal cord injury in that multiple sclerosis is not static. The clinical presentation can change depending on the disease severity. Therefore, rigid protocols cannot be followed.

For management of the *neurogenic bladder*, which occurs in 50% to 80% of patients, the main feature to remember is attainment of a balanced bladder. The bladder problems noted in patients with multiple sclerosis frequently result from a low-volume, irritable, spastic bladder. The related symptoms are usually frequency, urgency, and urgency incontinence. Anticholinergic therapy may improve these symptoms. Propantheline, 7.5 mg three or four times daily, can be used and, if needed and tolerated, the dose can be increased, even up to 30 mg four times daily. Sometimes the urinary symptoms are related to detrusor-external sphincter dyssynergia and can lead to urinary symptoms such as hesitancy, diminished size and force of stream, postvoiding dribbling, and the feeling of fullness. A trial of oxybutynin chloride (Ditropan), 5 mg two to four times daily, is often helpful. Sometimes patients with multiple sclerosis may have a high-volume flaccid bladder (see Chapter 21).

As in all patients with neurogenic bladder, urinalysis and urine culture should be performed and urinary tract infection should be searched for. The daily fluid intake should be limited to an average of 1,800 ml. Intake should be evenly distributed throughout the day. The bladder should be catheterized for retention or residual volume beginning with a 4-hour protocol. If combined voided and residual or retention volumes are less than 400 ml on the 4-hour schedule, a 6-hour program can be used. Voiding trials using the Credé or Valsalva maneuver can trigger a detrusor response in some patients. These trials should be attempted before catheterization for retention of urine. An immediate catheterization will give a true residual volume after voiding. The acceptable level is 20% of the normal bladder capacity or up to 100 ml.

Neurogenic bowel dysfunction, if poorly managed, may not result in life-threatening situations; however, lack of proper control does interfere with meeting rehabilitation goals and with an active social life. The following prescription is based on the idea that bulk is of prime importance for maintaining continence. This includes a high-fiber diet, bulk agents (psyllium hydrophilic mucilloid, Metamucil), a stool softener, a laxative when necessary, and adequate fluid intake. Defecation attempts should be timed to use the gastrocolic reflex, and suppositories may be needed for effective evacuation.

Sexual dysfunction occurs in 92% of male and 72% of female patients. Although sensory disturbances are a factor in both sexes, male patients also have unpredictable erection and ejaculation. Physiopathologic and psychologic factors are both important. Fostering understanding by a patient's partner is an important step. Some male patients may find a penile prosthesis helpful.

OUTCOME

There are no exact methods for prognosticating outcome. Courses of treatment with steroids and particularly with ACTH may shorten the duration of exacerbations of the disease but may have no effect on the overall long-term course. The following list provides a general framework for projecting and determining general disability. Again, however, even though most patients have a slowly progressive course, the unpredictability of the disease prevails. The positive predictive factors for patients are (1) less than 35 years of age at onset, (2) ambulatory at onset, (3) one symptom during the first year, (4) sudden onset of symptoms, (5) early disappearance of symptoms (less than 1 month), (6) little or no residual effect after each exacerbation, (7) absence of plantar extensor reflexes, (8) optic neuritis as the only symptom, and (9) minimal cerebellar or pyramidal signs after 5 years.

In summary, patients with multiple sclerosis may need the expertise of the entire rehabilitation team. Two-thirds of patients remain ambulatory and many can be productive throughout their life.[1-5]

REFERENCES

1. Matthews WB, Acheson EO, Batchelor JR, Weller RO. McAlpine's multiple sclerosis. New York: Churchill Livingstone, 1985.
2. Rudick RA, Herndon RM, guest eds. Disorders of myelin. Semin Neurol 1985; 5:85–193.
3. Vinken PJ, Bruyn GW, Klawans HL, Koetsier JC, eds. Handbook of clinical neurology. Vol 47. Demyelinating diseases. New York: Elsevier Science Publishing, 1985.
4. Antel JP, ed. Symposium on multiple sclerosis. Neurol Clin 1983; 1 no. 3:571–785.
5. McFarlin DE, McFarland HF. Multiple sclerosis. N Engl J Med 1982; 307:1183–1188; 1246–1251.

20 SPINAL CORD INJURY

Mark M. Mitros, M.D.
Joachim L. Opitz, M.D.

The causes of spinal cord injuries are many. Approximately 70% of cases are due to *trauma*.[1] Frequent traumatic causes of spinal cord injuries include vehicular accidents, falls, sports accidents, and gunshot or stabbing wounds. Although the ages of patients with traumatic spinal cord injury range from birth to the oldest of the general population, about 80% are younger than 40 years; their mean age is 29 years.[2] Eighty percent of the patients are male.[2] The 30% of spinal cord injuries that are *nontraumatic* result from many possible causes: vascular insufficiencies or malformations, infectious processes, mechanical processes such as disk prolapse or bony spinal stenosis, multiple sclerosis, metastatic or primary cancer, and aftereffects of radiation. The mean age of patients at onset of nontraumatic spinal cord injury is about 55 years. The male:female ratio in the population with nontraumatic spinal cord injury is about 1:1.

TERMINOLOGY

The spinal cord is organized in a rostral to caudal manner such that there is a segmental representation of neuronal function. Each segment is referred to as a *"level"* of the spinal cord. Each level has a characteristic distribution of sensory function (a *dermatome*) and motor function (a *myotome*) (Fig. 20–1 and Table 20–1).

At the Mayo Clinic spinal cord injury center, the level of the spinal cord injury is defined as the last completely normally functioning motor and sensory level of the spinal cord. The level of injury does not refer to the level of bony injury (if there is any in a given patient). The term *"zone of injury"* refers to the up to three neurologic levels at the point of damage to the spinal cord where there is frequently some preservation, to varying degrees, of motor

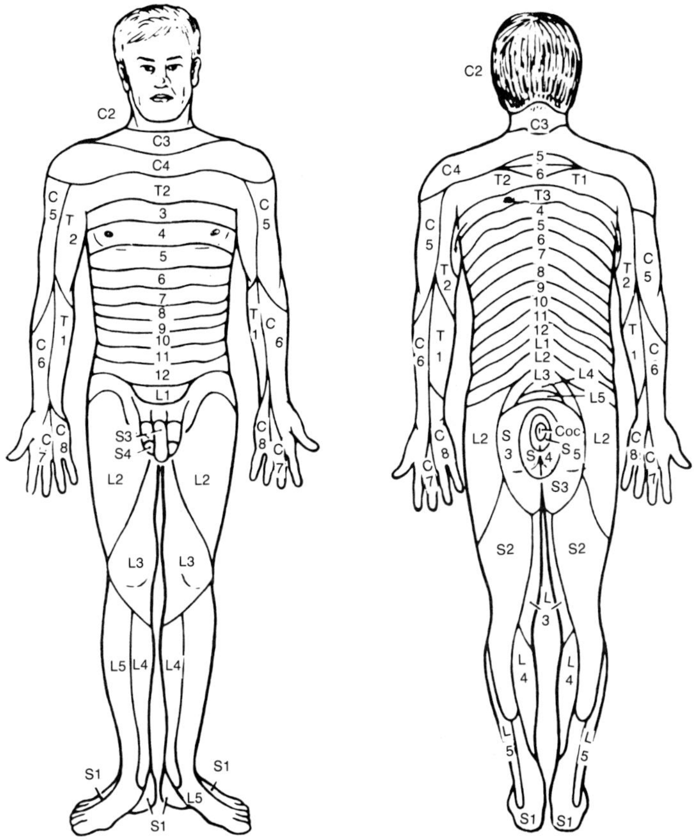

Figure 20–1 Sensory dermatomes. *Left*, Front view. *Right*, Back view. (From Standards for neurological classification of spinal injury patients.[3] By permission of the publisher.)

TABLE 20–1 Key Muscles for Motor Level Classification

C4 Diaphragm	L2 Iliopsoas
C5 Deltoid or biceps	L3 Quadriceps
C6 Wrist extensors	L4 Tibialis anterior
C7 Triceps	L5 Extensor hallucis longus
C8 Flexor profundus	S1 Gastrocnemius
T1 Hand intrinsics	S2–S5 Use sensory level
T2–L1 Use sensory level, abdominal reflexes, and Beevor's sign to help localize lowest normal neurologic segment	

From Standards for neurological classification of spinal injury patients.[3] By permission of the publisher.

or sensory function or both.[3] This zone may represent a gradation of damage that would be clinically manifested as a gradual decrease in, for instance, sensory function across several dermatomes.

A *complete* injury is one in which there is no voluntary motor or sensory function below the zone of injury. This results in either *paraplegia* or *tetraplegia*. An *incomplete* injury is one in which there is some sparing of useful motor or sensory function below the zone of injury. Some useful voluntary motor function throughout the entire remaining spinal cord below the zone of injury is referred to as paraparesis or tetraparesis.

Paraplegia or *paraparesis* results from injury in the thoracic (below T–1), lumbar, or sacral spinal segments. Arm function is normal.

Tetraplegia or *tetraparesis* results from injury in the cervical spinal segments (or uppermost thoracic level); therefore, arm function is involved to various extents, in addition to involvement of the trunk and legs.

ACUTE MANAGEMENT

An integrated multispecialty team approach is essential in order to provide appropriate care for the many problems (surgical, medical, psychologic, social, and vocational) of persons with spinal cord injuries.

Emergency medical technicians are specially trained in the proper methods to identify persons with actual or potential bony spinal or spinal cord injuries, their extrication, and their transport.

Typically, a trauma surgeon cares for the abdominal, thoracic, or vascular injuries and continues as the primary physician until these conditions are stable. A neurosurgeon takes primary responsibility when there is a spinal cord deficit or one has to presume that a spinal cord deficit is imminent and no polytrauma exists. The patient is initially in the intensive care unit and is followed regularly by the orthopedic surgery and rehabilitation medicine services. A physiatrist, in association with other members of the spinal cord injury rehabilitation team, introduces the concept of rehabilitation to the patient, family, and significant others. The physiatrist coordinates the rehabilitation efforts throughout the hospitalization and during subsequent outpatient follow-up. The physiatrist also reviews the acute medical management of the patient and places special emphasis on preventive medical care in the areas in which the patient is at especially high risk.

The orthopedic surgeon, in association with the neurosurgeon, provides for reduction of the spinal fracture by external or internal fixation and for management of other fracture sites. In cases of cervical injury, temporary stability is often provided first by halo traction and later by halo vest to provide firm fixation until the skeletal lesion is healed. The indications for open reduction and internal fixation of spinal fractures or management of significant soft tissue injuries that render the cervical spine unstable have been increasing during the past 10 years. The advantages of early open reduction and internal fixation include fewer physical and psychologic complications from prolonged immobilization and greater success within less time for reintegrating the patient into society.

In the thoracic and lumbar regions of the spine, temporary stability is usually achieved by placing the patient on a rigid frame. The frame allows for early turning of the patient. In the thoracolumbar area of the spine, skeletal disruption and partial neurologic deficit are common. In thoracolumbar fractures, early open reduction and internal fixation of the spine with Harrington rods and fusion allow early mobilization with the use of a molded body jacket, which allows early participation in intensive rehabilitation.

After the spinal fracture or soft tissue injuries have been managed to provide stability (or at least managed to provide eventual spinal stability), associated polytrauma has been treated, and markedly unstable medical conditions have stabilized sufficiently to allow transfer from the intensive care unit, the patient is transferred to the care of the physical medicine and rehabilitation service on the rehabilitation unit. A physiatrist serves as the primary physician during the remainder of the hospitalization. After dismissal from the hospital, the patient's general medical care is coordinated by the home physician. Subsequent follow-up visits for rehabilitation concerns are coordinated by the physiatrist. Guidelines for preventive care have been developed,[4] some of which are outlined below.

AREAS OF INCREASED RISK IN SPINAL CORD INJURIES

Pulmonary

Early mortality after acute traumatic tetraplegia is primarily due to retention of bronchial secretions and subsequent development of atelectasis and pneumonia. Other sources of pulmonary morbidity and mortality include respiratory failure secondary to impaired function of the diaphragm and intercostal and abdominal muscles and to pulmonary embolism.

Pulmonary assessment, in addition to a history and physical examination, includes a chest roentgenogram and measurement of arterial blood gases, vital capacity, and maximal inspiratory and expiratory pressures. Management includes (1) oxygen supplementation with humidification to maintain $Po_2 > 70$ mm Hg; (2) placement of a nasogastric tube for relief of gastric distention, prevention of aspiration of gastric contents, and easier movement of the diaphragm (adynamic ileus often present initially); (3) for the prevention of secretion retention and atelectasis, turning the patient regularly, performing deep breathing, incentive spirometry, assisted coughing, and chest wall percussion and vibration, and externally rotating the humeri (unless contraindicated by shoulder injuries); (4) not allowing smoking; and (5) measuring pulmonary function twice weekly in the early stages and immediately before and after the application of potentially constrictive body casts or vests.

For the treatment of secretion retention and atelectasis, the following measures are used: (1) intermittent positive-pressure breathing with a bronchodilator solution (Bronkosol) and assisted coughing immediately before pronation, (2) bronchoscopy in the presence of radiologic evidence of lobar collapse, and (3) microbiologic examination of sputum and appropriate antibiotic management.

Eventually, the pulmonary regimen can be reduced in midthoracic paraplegia to a minimum of assisted coughing and incentive spirometry three times a day.

Vascular

Patients with acute spinal cord injury are at a significantly increased risk for deep venous thromboses and pulmonary emboli. The following methods of prevention are instituted in all patients with spinal cord injury who have weakness that does not allow for antigravity mobility of the lower extremities.

(1) Passive range-of-motion exercises for joints below the level of injury are performed twice a day. (2) Passive ankle dorsiflexion and plantar flexion maneuvers are performed, 10 repetitions every 2 hours. (3) Meticulous care is used to avoid trauma to the lower extremities and, therefore, avoid damage to the endothelial lining of the blood vessels. (4) Antithrombotic stockings are applied; they are removed three times a day to examine the skin. (5) The crossed-leg position is avoided. (6) Intermittent pneumatic compression devices are used. (7) [^{125}I]Fibrinogen uptake scanning is performed; however, this test is generally not recommended for patients younger than 18 years or for pregnant women. If the scan indicates thrombus formation limited to the calf veins only, full-dose anticoagulation therapy is not indicated, and scanning is continued; if the scan indicates active thrombus in the popliteal or iliofemoral vein, full therapeutic anticoagulation is indicated. Plethysmography, Doppler studies, or venography may be helpful to confirm and define the extent of the deep venous thrombosis. If anticoagulation is specifically contraindicated, a venous filter or umbrella may be used. If a deep venous thrombosis is present above the calf, bed rest for 7 to 10 days, leg elevation, Ace wraps (rewrapped every 3 hours to prevent sequential swellings and to inspect the skin) for the affected leg, and full-dose anticoagulation are prescribed;

during this time, no range-of-motion exercises are applied to this leg. Administration of full-dose anticoagulation is then continued for 6 months.

For patients with no evidence of deep venous thrombosis or pulmonary embolus, low-dose subcutaneously administered heparin may be instituted as early as deemed safe after injury or after 2 weeks of negative [^{125}I]fibrinogen uptake scanning—unless contraindicated by bleeding or a history of bleeding diatheses. Therapy with low-dose heparin should be continued through the initial rehabilitation stay.

Skin

Because of the lack of pain sensation, patients with spinal cord injury are at high risk for developing pressure sores. Measures used to prevent these sores are as follows. (1) While the patient is on a Foster frame, sheepskin is kept beneath the shoulder area and the sacrum. When the patient is placed on a regular bed, a full-length sheepskin is placed over a water mattress or an alternating air mattress. (2) When the patient is supine, whether on a frame, a water mattress, or a regular bed, a pillow should be placed under the calves to remove pressure from the heels ("bunny boots" or similar padding is not adequate for heel protection). (3) Until the patient can be turned, nursing personnel should reach under the patient and massage the bony prominences every 2 hours. (4) Once the patient is able to be turned, a schedule of turning every 2 hours should be initiated and continued 24 hours a day. (5) The skin should be inspected each time the patient is turned. (6) Bony prominences should be especially diligently monitored. (7) If the patient is wearing a halo vest, a flashlight should be used to assist in inspecting the skin beneath the vest. (8) Care of the halo pin site involves swabbing with hydrogen peroxide and applying an antibiotic ointment (Neosporin) twice a day. (9) When the patient is sitting, a proper wheelchair cushion should be used (for example, a "Bye Bye Decubiti Cushion"). Regular pillows do not provide adequate protection.

Urinary Tract

The goals of urinary tract management are (1) to avoid urinary retention in excess of 500 ml, (2) to prevent upper and lower urinary tract infection, (3) to avoid noxious stimuli to the spinal cord from urinary tract complications, and (4) in 65% of patients, to achieve catheter-free voiding.

As long as intravenously administered fluids are necessary, continuous urinary drainage is maintained with an indwelling catheter and a closed system of urine collection. When an indwelling catheter is used, the following measures apply. (1) In male patients the catheter should be taped to the abdomen to avoid pressure ulcers within the urethra that may lead to penoscrotal fistulas. (2) In female patients the catheter should be taped to the inner aspect of the thigh to prevent pulling on the tube that may damage the bladder or urethra. (3) Fluid intake should be maintained between 2,500 and 3,000 ml per 24 hours, an amount that will allow adequate washout of rapidly multiplying bacteria from the bladder. (4) Because bacteriuria cannot be prevented and occurs within 6 to 10 days after catheterization, antibiotics are not indicated unless the patient is symptomatic or has sepsis. (5) The catheter should be changed every 2 weeks. (6) Urine specimens should be obtained weekly for culture and determination of susceptibilities. If relatively resistant organisms are present, proper isolation procedures should be instituted.

Intermittent catheterization should be started once the intravenous infusions have been discontinued, the urine is sterile, and urine output is approximately 1,400 ml per 24 hours. A urine specimen should be obtained for a Gram stain and a specimen for culture should be obtained from a newly inserted (within 3 days) Silastic Foley catheter (16-F) to determine whether urine is sterile. If either test result is positive, appropriate antibiotic full-dose treatment is initiated before the catheter is removed. If the result of a repeat Gram stain is negative, intermittent catheterization may be initiated. Weekly urine specimens for culture are obtained during the remainder of hospitalization.

The routine 1,800-ml daily fluid intake schedule is instituted when intermittent catheterization is begun. Preventive measures during intermittent catheterization include bacteriostatic medications such as trimethoprim-sulfamethoxazole (Septra or Bactrim, 1 single-strength tablet orally at bedtime), which has been shown to be more effective than methenamine mandelate (Mandelamine, 1 g four times a day) or methenamine hippurate (Hiprex, 1 g twice a day). (See Chapter 21 for more information on the management of neurogenic bladder.)

Bowel

Once bowel sounds return and the patient is able to tolerate regular foods, the patient should receive a high-fiber diet and docusate sodium (Colace, 100 mg orally once or twice daily). At the same time every day or every other day, a glycerin or bisacodyl (Dulcolax) suppository is used 30 minutes after a meal (this schedule maximizes the use of the gastrocolic reflex). If the patient does not expel stool within 20 to 30 minutes, a lubricated gloved finger may be inserted into the rectum for digital stimulation.

Autonomic Hyperreflexia

Autonomic hyperreflexia is a potentially life-threatening syndrome of severe paroxysmal hypertension that can occur after spinal shock has ended in patients who have injuries with lesions above T–6.[1] It occurs to various extents in upwards of 80% of such patients. Noxious stimulation below the level of the lesion produces massive sympathetic discharges (as part of cord spasticity) that result in marked arteriolar constriction. The result is a marked elevation of blood pressure that cannot be adequately counter-regulated because of the interruption of inhibitory neuronal pathways by the spinal lesion.

Typical inciting factors include bladder distention, rectal distention or manipulation, decubital ulcers, urinary tract infection, urinary calculi, a surgical procedure, tight-fitting clothes, pressure on the testicles or glans penis, sexual intercourse, braces, acute abdominal conditions, labor in pregnant women, voiding and bowel movements, or any noxious input to the markedly hyperreflexic cord.

The patient usually experiences sudden marked hypertension, a pounding headache, anxiety, sweating, piloerection, and bradycardia (which results from strong vagal attempts at counterregulation). Other manifestations may include blurred vision, a feeling of impending doom, chest pain, nausea, and respiratory distress.

Immediate management includes elevation of the head of the bed to decrease intracranial pressure, monitoring of blood pressure and pulse every 5 minutes, removal of all tight clothing, braces, or leg bags, and checking for bladder and bowel distention. Because a distended bladder is frequently the cause, the urinary catheter should be routinely irrigated immediately; if the catheter is plugged, it should be changed immediately. If these procedures do not produce a satisfactory response, the patient should be checked for rectal impaction by applying an anesthetic ointment (Nupercainal) into the anal canal and to the perianal skin. Then, a well-lubricated gloved finger may be inserted slowly to check for a fecal impaction. Blood pressure should be monitored during the rectal examination. If an impaction is present and the blood pressure increases to 200/130 mm Hg, ganglionic blockage should be obtained before removal of the impaction.

If the patient does not respond to the above measures, drug treatment should be initiated while a primary cause is being identified. This could include mecamylamine (Inversine), hydralazine, or diazoxide, depending on the circumstances. Admission to the intensive care unit for monitoring and intravenous administration of nitroprusside may be necessary.

Orthostatic Hypotension

Not infrequently, patients with spinal cord injury are subject to precipitous drops in blood pressure, often without premonition. The patient may suddenly lose consciousness. Activities associated with the falls in blood pressure are usually related to postural changes such as going from supine to sitting or exceeding sitting tolerance, with a drop in blood pressure being the limiting factor. Blood pressure must be carefully monitored, especially in the earliest attempts to sit a newly injured patient. Other associated activities may include eating and drinking. The mechanism seems to be pooling of blood in the abdomen and the dependent extremities associated with the absence of reflex vasoconstriction with lesions above the sympathetic outflow (T–5 to T–8).[1]

If the patient complains of light-headedness, dizziness, or a feeling of faintness, he or she should be placed in a recumbent position with the lower extremities elevated. If the patient is in a wheelchair, the brakes should be locked and the chair should be tipped backward immediately to lower the patient's head and elevate the lower extremities.

Preventive measures include (1) the use of thigh-length support garments or Ace wraps (the skin is inspected and the wraps are reapplied every 3 hours), (2) the use of a lumbosacral corset with sheepskin lining, designed for spinal cord injuries, (3) gradual changes from the supine to the upright position, and (4) judicious increments in the time spent "up."

Spasticity

Spasticity is a condition of excessive reflex activity of the spinal cord below the level of the lesion, often associated with involuntary movements. In patients who are unable to initiate voluntary movement, marked involuntary movement sometimes evolves. Spasticity develops in most patients with injury above the sacral aspect of the spinal cord. The type and magnitude may vary greatly from patient to patient.

Spasticity is not present at the onset of spinal cord injury. The period immediately after injury is termed "spinal shock." It is characterized by diminished muscle tone and absent stretch reflexes. The duration of spinal shock varies from a few days to several months. As spinal shock subsides, the activity of the stretch reflexes and muscle tone gradually increase. Spasticity may cause discomfort, may interfere with daily functioning (for example, by interfering with stability during transfers), or may result in secondary complications such as contractures, decubital ulcers, bladder hypertrophy with vesicoureteral reflux, and fractures.

Identification, elimination, and diligent prevention of nociceptive input to the spinal cord and participation in a reasonable twice-daily stretching program are the basics of therapy. A hierarchy of treatment methods may be used. In addition to stretching, medications, intramuscular neurolysis of key muscle groups, intrathecal and peripheral neurolysis, tenotomies, neurectomies, rhizotomies, myelotomies, cordotomies, and cordectomies may be used.

Heterotopic Ossification

The deposition of para-articular bone occurs in from 10% to 50% of patients with newly acquired spinal cord injuries.[1] This bone formation typically appears within the first 6 months after injury and usually affects the hips, but other joints below the level of the spinal lesion may be involved. The clinical presentation is often a slight decrease in hip range of motion that may progress to severe loss of motion about the affected joints. The early clinical appearance may mimic that of a deep venous thrombosis with warmth and swelling in one or both lower extremities. Early roentgenograms may not demonstrate the calcium deposition, but a bone scan may be diagnostic. Typically, the bone fraction of alkaline phosphatase is elevated.

Vigorous passive range-of-motion exercises are necessary to maintain range. Etidronate (Didronel) may retard the development of this condition, but it is generally thought to be of little value once calcium deposition is evident roentgenographically. For cases in which the loss of range of motion has become so severe that it limits daily functioning (for example, an inability to flex the hips sufficiently to sit), surgical resection followed by radiation therapy may become necessary. Wedge resection of the heterotopic ossification should not be done until the bone has ceased to grow. An indication of cessation of bone growth is reduction of the bone fraction of serum alkaline phosphatase.

RESIDUAL FUNCTIONAL CAPACITIES

The level of spinal cord injury has implications for the expected level of functioning in daily life (Table 20–2).

PATIENT EDUCATION

Major emphasis is placed on patient education throughout rehabilitation. The person with a spinal cord injury must learn to function with a substantially reduced physical capacity in a society that retains many physical and attitudinal barriers for persons with disability. The person with a spinal cord injury must learn to practice new preventive living habits and must learn to educate persons who come in contact with him or her as to proper care. The injured person must redevelop a positive self-image and learn to project in a constructive and self-assertive manner toward able-bodied persons who do not have experience in interacting with persons who have spinal cord injuries.[5]

DURATION OF INITIAL HOSPITALIZATION

A patient with mid- to low-level complete paraplegia may expect a 2- to 3-month initial hospital stay. A patient with tetraplegia may expect a 3- to 5-month stay if he or she has a relatively uncomplicated course.

TABLE 20–2 Functional Goals for Patients With Spinal Cord Injury, by Level

Goal	*Level of Injury**							
	C-4	*C-5*	*C-6*	*C-7*	*C-8 to T-1*	*T-2 to T-12*	*L-1 to L-3*	*L-4 to S-1*
Self-care								
Feeding	O	P	P	I	I	I	I	I
Dressing	O	D	D	P/I	I	I	I	I
Grooming	O	D/P	P	P/I	I	I	I	I
Bladder, bowel	O	D	D/P	I	I	I	I	I
Bathing	O	D	P	P	I	I	I	I
Wheelchair activity								
Special control, powered	I	I	I	I	I	I	I	I
Manual propulsion	O	P	P/I	I	I	I	I	I
Transfers to and from	O	D	P	I	I	I	I	I
Bed mobility	O	D	P	I	I	I	I	I
Communications								
Telephone	P	P	I	I	I	I	I	I
Writing	O	D/P	P	P	I	I	I	I
Typing	P	P	P	P	I	I	I	I
Ambulation	O	O	O	O	O	D	P	P
Orthoses	ECU	UEO	UEO	UEO		KAFO	KAFO	AFO
Transportation								
Driving with hand controls	O	D/P	P	I	I	I	I	I
Public (train, plane)	O	D	D	P/I	I	I	I	I
Public (bus without lift)	O	O	O	O	O	O	O	P

* AFO, ankle-foot orthosis; D, dependent, but can assist; ECU, environmental control unit; I, full independence; KAFO, knee-ankle-foot orthosis; O, not possible; P, partial or full independence with special equipment; UEO, upper extremity orthosis.

From Stover et al.[2] By permission of the publisher.

FOLLOW-UP

Because many of the acute-care concerns remain significant risks for the rest of a patient's life, and many of the social, emotional, and vocational goals are pursued after the initial hospitalization, regular, life-long follow-up visits are essential for redeveloping and maintaining health and maximal functional capacities.

A typical follow-up schedule includes a return visit at 1 and 4 months after dismissal and at yearly intervals thereafter for a complete review. Additional follow-up contacts are made as necessary (Table 20–3).

TABLE 20–3 Guidelines for Annual Follow-Up of Persons With Spinal Cord Injury

History and physical examination, with special emphasis on
1. the status of the spine, spinal cord, and brain
2. the function of the genitourinary, musculoskeletal, gastrointestinal, vascular, and respiratory systems and skin
3. nutritional, psychosocial, and vocational aspects of independent living and healthy living habits

Laboratory studies, to screen the overall state of health, including complete blood count, chemistry group, sedimentation rate, urinalysis, urine Gram stain, urine culture and susceptibilities, residual urine volume(s), iothalamate short renal clearance, roentgenograms of kidneys, ureters, and bladder, excretory urogram with 20-minute film (or diethylenetriamine pentaacetic acid short renal scan), cystometrogram-electromyogram with urethral pressure profile, cystoscopy, and spine roentgenograms as appropriate

Physical therapy review for mobility, transfers, range-of-motion exercises and stretching exercises, wheelchair and wheelchair mobility, braces, possible upper extremity reconstruction or tendon transfers

Occupational therapy review for activities of daily living, adaptive equipment, driving, possible upper extremity reconstruction

As appropriate, review by social services, psychologist, recreational therapist, orthopedist, neurologist or neurosurgeon, urologist, internist

In general,
1. patients with uncomplicated courses who have paraplegia or low tetraplegia (C-6 to C-8 lesions) may be reviewed on an outpatient basis
2. patients with mid- to high-level tetraplegia (weak C-5 and above) are better served in the hospital

REFERENCES

1. Ruskin AP, ed. Spinal cord injury. In: Current therapy in physiatry: physical medicine and rehabilitation. Philadelphia: WB Saunders, 1984:379–456.
2. Stover SL, Donovan WH, Freed MM, et al. Rehabilitation in spinal cord disorders. In: Self-directed medical knowledge program in physical medicine and rehabilitation—syllabus. 2nd ed. Chicago: American Academy of Physical Medicine and Rehabilitation, 1985:K1–22.
3. Standards for neurological classification of spinal injury patients. Chicago: American Spinal Injury Association, October 1982.
4. Mayo Clinic Interdisciplinary Spinal Cord Injury Committee. Spinal cord injury preventive care guidelines. Rochester, Minnesota: Mayo Foundation, 1985.
5. SCI patient manual. Department of Physical Medicine and Rehabilitation, Mayo Clinic and Nursing Service, Rehabilitation Nursing, Saint Marys Hospital, Rochester, Minnesota, 1979.

21 BLADDER RETRAINING

Joachim L. Opitz, M.D.
Mark M. Mitros, M.D.

Bladder retraining has become an integral part of the rehabilitation of patients with spinal cord injury, [1–8] in selected brain-injured patients, and in patients who have atonic myogenic detrusor insufficiency associated with habit contraction of the external urethral sphincter.[9] Bladder retraining has been made efficient through the use of an organized training program[4] as assisted by modern urodynamic diagnostic procedures, biofeedback, neuropharmacology, and specific urologic surgical procedures.[3,5] The purpose of this chapter is to discuss the indications, contraindications, procedural guidelines, and results of bladder retraining.

GOALS

The goals of bladder retraining are (1) to ensure free flow of urine from the kidneys without overloading the ureteral work capacity, (2) to empty the bladder regularly (generally every 3 hours) and adequately (consistently less than 100 ml of residual urine volume) for the maintenance of abacteriuria without causing bladder hypertrophy of a degree that threatens the competence of the ureteral vesical junction, and (3) to reestablish urinary continence.

INDICATIONS

Patients must be motivated to spend between 20 and 60 days (average, 30 days) specifically learning the motor skills that are necessary to reachieve efficient, catheter-free voiding (within normal voiding pressures) while permanently maintaining a regular voiding and drinking schedule. Bladder retraining is indicated in patients who have neurogenic hyperreflexic bladder dysfunction with or without external sphincter dyssynergia, neurogenic hyporeflexic or areflexic bladder dysfunctions with or without dyssynergia, or atonic myogenic detrusor insufficiency. At times, patients with uninhibited bladder dysfunction due to brain injury may also profit from parts of the bladder retraining program.

CONTRAINDICATIONS

Bladder retraining is contraindicated in patients who have substantially decompensating renal function and in those with incompetent vesicoureteral junctions with impending or actual reflux and its sequelae for the upper urinary tract. It is also contraindicated in patients with severe cystitis, bladder calculi, or major structural changes of either the bladder or the urethra; in patients who cannot adhere to the necessary training procedures and record keeping; in the very young; in debilitated elderly patients; in unmotivated or undisciplined patients; and in patients who are unable to do the necessary manipulations for voiding, such as transferring to and from the toilet and dressing and undressing.

TEAM APPROACH

A team approach is necessary because bladder retraining requires (1) regular intermittent catheterization, (2) urodynamic testing and retesting, (3) acquisition of much new knowledge, (4) learning of new psychomotor skills and living habits by the patient, and (5) at times, neurourologic surgical procedures.

The team is headed by the physiatrist and includes the patient, the neurourologist, the physical therapist, the primary rehabilitation nurse, and members of the intermittent catheterization team.

The team is also supported by physicians specializing in infectious disease and nephrology, an epidemiology nurse, microbiologic laboratory support personnel, and data collection and program evaluation personnel.

Indispensable for successful bladder retraining is the participation of a knowledgeable primary physician (not infrequently a physiatrist) who has the proper understanding of (1) the urodynamics of the various bladder and urethral dysfunctions, (2) control of infection of the impaired urinary tract, (3) the effects of neurourologic medications, and (4) the indications for neurourologic procedures.

The physician must analyze the voiding data with the patient and associated staff daily in order to suggest optimal actions for bladder retraining, such as voiding technique, drug therapy, and urologic surgical procedures.

THE WORKUP

Because the success of bladder retraining depends on the correct urodynamic diagnosis, the psychosocial evaluation, and the exclusion of contraindications, bladder retraining should not be started until a stable neurourologic condition has developed, the workup has been completed, the lower urinary tract has become free of foreign bodies and infection, and intermittent catheterization yields acceptable volumes of retained urine (less than 400 to 500 ml).

Excretory urography (intravenous pyelography), [^{125}I]iothalamate short renal clearance test of renal function, and urine culture and sensitivity studies may be performed when the patient is still using an indwelling catheter. A complete blood count, serum electrolyte levels, serum creatinine value, and blood urea nitrogen value should also be determined. After the patient has been receiving specific antibiotics for 24 to 48 hours for any existing bacteriuria and fluid output has been reduced to less than 1,400 ml per 24 hours, intermittent catheterization may be started.

With intermittent catheterization, concomitant bacteriostatic medications should be used, such as trimethoprim-sulfamethoxazole (Septra or Bactrim, 1 single-strength tablet orally at bedtime) or methenamine salts (Mandelamine, 1 g four times a day, or Hiprex, 1 g twice a day). The patient is monitored with weekly urine cultures while in the hospital. In 85% of patients, the lower urinary tract can be kept free of infection during hospitalization. With weekly monitoring, recurrent asymptomatic bacteriuria can be treated promptly and specifically. Further, intermittent catheterization rids both the bladder and the urethra of the ongoing irritation of an indwelling catheter, which is especially detrimental in patients who have spastic spinal paralysis. After several days of intermittent catheterization, the bladder becomes less irritated.

If abacteriuria is demonstrated by a negative Gram stain on the day of the planned studies, a urodynamic evaluation is done with cystometrography/sphincter electromyography (CMG/EMG) and a urethral pressure profile (UPP). Cystoscopy, when indicated, may be performed thereafter. If bladder stones are suspected, cystoscopy may have to precede urodynamic studies.

CMG/EMG may be done with the patient in the lithotomy or sitting position. An indwelling Foley catheter is placed in the bladder and two EMG recording leads are placed at the 2 and 10 o'clock positions perianally to record the electrical activity of the pelvic floor musculature. The muscles of the pelvic floor in this area receive innervation from the same sacral root levels as does the external urethral sphincter. Therefore, increased electrical activity in these muscles is used as an indirect measure of the electrical activity of the external urethral sphincter—the greater the electrical activity, the tighter the sphincter closes about the urethra to obstruct urine flow.

Initially, the absence or presence of voluntary control of the pelvic floor musculature is documented. Then the presence or absence of the bulbocavernosus reflex mediated by the S2–4 nerve root is determined by tugging on the indwelling catheter and observing a momentary reflex increase in the activity of the pelvic floor musculature. Subsequently, carbon dioxide or normal saline is introduced into the bladder through the catheter at a rate of 100 ml per minute. The intravesicular (within the bladder) pressure is monitored during filling. The presence or absence of a sensation of fullness and of a need to void is monitored. Then, the quality, degree, control, or absence of a detrusor (bladder muscle) contraction is determined by observing the intravesicular pressure changes over time. The various voiding techniques (such as tapping, Credé maneuver, straining, massage, or perineal stimulation) are evaluated by observing the resulting pressure changes. It is important to observe whether the normal quieting of electrical activity in the pelvic floor musculature occurs with the contractions of the detrusor during attempted voiding. Incoordination may exist between the expulsive pressure (detrusor) and retentive pressure (external sphincter) when the detrusor and pelvic floor muscles co-contract. Such incoordination is called "detrusor-sphincter dyssynergia."

Finally, the catheter is slowly and smoothly pulled from the bladder, and the pressures along the urethra are recorded (UPP) while carbon dioxide is escaping from the catheter tip at 150 ml per minute. The catheter movement through the urethra is thought to serve as a stimulus for maximal contraction of the external urethral sphincter, and the peak pressure recorded is generally thought to be the maximal (retentive) pressure that can be elicited within the urethra by the external urethral sphincter and the bladder neck (internal urethral sphincter).

The internal urethral sphincter is actually the base of the bladder that normally forms a funnel shape when voiding is attempted. In certain types of bladder dysfunction, this funneling may not occur, and this results in an inability to empty the bladder properly without the use of a catheter. The function of this funneling can best be tested with the use of a modified CMG/EMG technique called cinecystourethrography, or "video CMG/EMG." For this test, a radiopaque liquid is used instead of carbon dioxide or normal saline, and real-time fluoroscopy can be used to visualize the anatomic function of the bladder neck (simultaneously, all the previously described factors are also recorded).

CMG/EMG may be difficult for various reasons. Patients may be unable to void while they are on the table or in the highly unfamiliar and populated diagnostic operating room.

Routinely, after the initial excretory urogram has been obtained, colleagues in neurourology are asked to evaluate the urologic data that have been obtained and to participate in and continue the urologic workup and surgical interventions needed during the ensuing bladder retraining. At the Mayo Clinic, the initial "diagnostic" CMG/EMG is performed immediately before cystoscopy in the operating room. Subsequent CMG/EMG studies, known as "therapeutic" CMG/EMG, are performed in a special procedures room of the rehabilitation unit.

THE TRAINING PROGRAM

Once the team members and the patient decide to pursue bladder retraining, the patient is instructed by a physical therapist or rehabilitation nurse with special experience and training in the basic anatomy involved, normal and specific abnormal urodynamic factors, the specific recording of data required of the patient, the purposes and technique of therapeutic CMG/EMG, and the rationale of specific retraining procedures as they relate to the specific bladder dysfunction that is present.

Because the team members can do no more than assist the patient in his or her own efforts at bladder retraining, the patient is made fully responsible for adhering to a previously agreed on drinking, voiding, and catheterization schedule. Until voiding has become efficient, the drinking schedule usually consists of a well-timed fluid intake of 1,800 ml per 24 hours (400 ml at meal times and 200 ml at 10 A.M., 2 P.M., and 4 P.M.). Attempts at voiding, by use of the specific techniques that gave the best response during CMG/EMG, should be made and promptly recorded by the patient at least every 3 hours during the day and preferably once during the night. The schedule of intermittent catheterization (every 6 hours) allows four determinations of residual urine volume to be made each day.

The patient is responsible for recording the following data as soon as they become available: intake, intentional voiding (amount in milliliters), unintentional voiding (in relative degrees), and the amount of residual urine volume obtained every 6 hours, after attempted voiding, by intermittent catheterization. The values for residual urine volume are particularly helpful for determining the efficiency of voiding. The patient records the data on a daily record sheet (Fig. 21–1), which is kept on a clipboard at the bedside. Bacteriostatic medications should be taken at bedtime (such as trimethoprim-sulfamethoxazole) or during the day (such as methenamine).

For an overview of the many data that accumulate day by day, the patient also records the values of the 24-hour fluid volumes of the preceding day in the form of a graph, which indicates an increase, a leveling off, or a decrease in the efficiency of voiding (Fig. 21–2). This graph sheet is also kept on a clipboard at the bedside. Initially, the 24-hour volumes of urine intentionally voided are much lower than the 24-hour volumes of residual urine. As success in bladder retraining evolves, a crossover occurs between the volumes of intentionally voided urine and those of residual urine, but the 24-hour fluid intake remains unchanged at about 1,800 ml. The graphic representation of the efficiency of voiding is a strong motivating factor for the patient. It also serves as an important instrument for quick orientation of the members of the rehabilitation team.

RECORD OF BLADDER RETRAINING

Date ________________ Name ________________________ MC No. ________

	FLUID INTAKE	FLUID OUTPUT			
		INTENTIONAL		UNINTENTIONAL	CATHETERIZATION
TIME	All beverages, also include soup, ice cream, jello, fruit	VOLITIONAL (*NOT* triggered, strained or manually expressed)	TRIGGERED, STRAINED or MANUALLY EXPRESSED	INCONTINENCE— or SPONTANEOUS voidings	RESIDUAL CHECKS or RETENTIONS SELF - TEAM
1:00 AM					
2:00					
3:00					
4:00					
5:00					
6:00					
7:00					
8:00					
9:00					
10:00					
11:00					
12:00 N					
1:00 PM					
2:00					
3:00					
4:00					
5:00					
6:00					
7:00					
8:00					
9:00					
10:00					
11:00					
12:00 MN					
SUBTOTAL					
TOTAL IN:		TOTAL OUT:			

Figure 21–1 Daily record sheet on which patients receiving bladder retraining record time and volumes of fluid intake, intentional and unintentional voidings, and residual urine volumes. (From Opitz.[9] By permission of the publisher.)

GUIDELINES TO RETRAINING FOR SPECIFIC BLADDER AND URETHRAL DYSFUNCTIONS

Uninhibited Neurogenic Bladder Dysfunction

Patients with brain injury in which a lesion exists between the cerebral cortex and the pontine micturition center have uninhibited neurogenic bladder dysfunction. Because the pontine micturition center, which is intact, is responsible for the coordinated function of the spinal micturition center (S–2 to S–4), the normal kinesiology of micturition is undisturbed. However, inasmuch as the patient lacks awareness of the urge to void and does not adequately suppress the pontine-spinal loops of micturition, incontinence by reflex voiding occurs and is usually frequent and complete.

Patients with brain injury (cerebrovascular accident, trauma, or tumor) in whom either urinary retention or incontinence persists after removal of the catheter need to have a detailed urologic

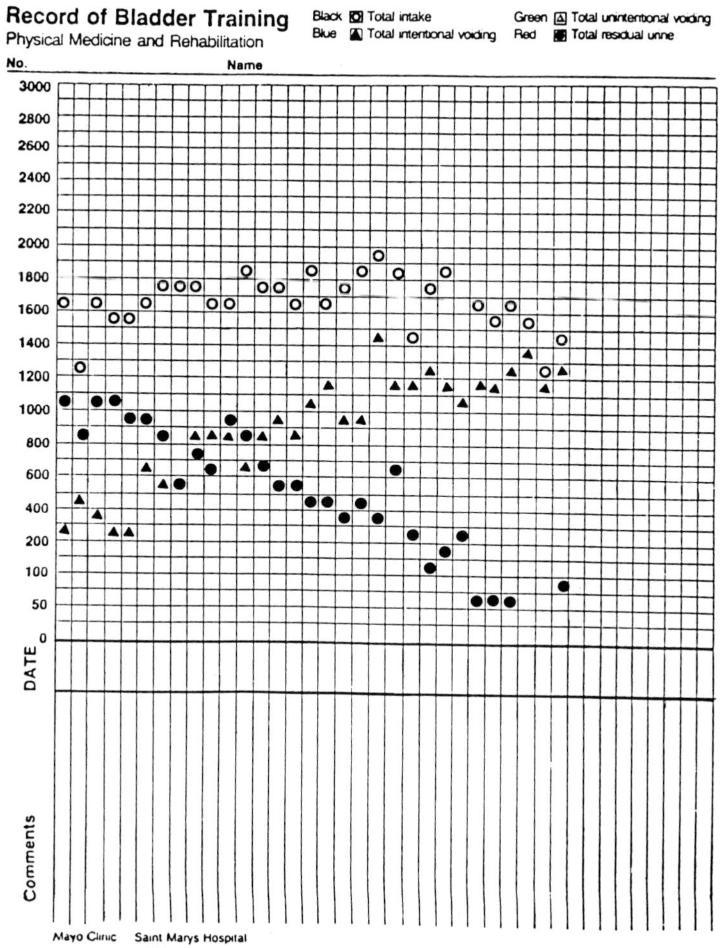

Figure 21–2 Data from woman with complete flaccid detrusor and external urethral sphincter paralysis after central disk compression of sacral cord. (From Opitz.[9] By permission of the publisher.)

workup (as previously described) to determine whether the cause is structural or functional or both.

If the lower urinary tract is normal, bladder retraining consists of regular attempts at voiding, concentrating on the patient's early, conscious awareness of bladder fullness. Such regular attempts at voiding should be coordinated with a regular balanced intake of liquids (that is, the fluid schedule outlined previously). Light suprapubic tapping or pulling of pubic hair may be helpful as an initial sensory cue; such a stimulus is consciously perceived and can be associated with the sensation of a full bladder and with the urge to void. Appropriate suppression of the urge to void then follows as the patient is able to focus attention on bladder function and suppress the micturition centers adequately until a time when it is socially acceptable to void.

Occasionally, the use of low-dose anticholinergic medications, such as propantheline bromide (Pro-Banthine) or oxybutynin (Ditropan), may lessen the resting tone of the bladder and, secondarily, the voiding reflex. Because these medications lessen the expulsive force of the detrusor, their use may result in urinary retention—especially in elderly men.

Hyperreflexic, Dyssynergic (Upper Motor Neuron) Bladder Dysfunction

A person with a neurologic lesion between the pontine and the sacral micturition center, which renders the center dyssynergic to varying degrees, experiences hyperreflexic, dyssynergic (upper motor neuron) dysfunction of the bladder and urethra. Emphasis in bladder retraining has to be placed on developing a spinal micturition reflex that favors detrusor contraction of adequate strength with minimal external sphincter co-contraction (dyssynergia).

Usually, the reflex is best developed by the use of rapid, yet light, suprapubic tapping (Fig. 21–3) at a place where the highest degree of reflex response is obtained. Performing heavy and slow suprapubic tapping—on the basis that if a little works, more is better—is a misconception to which uninformed staff and patients alike not infrequently succumb. Heavy tapping usually leads to in-

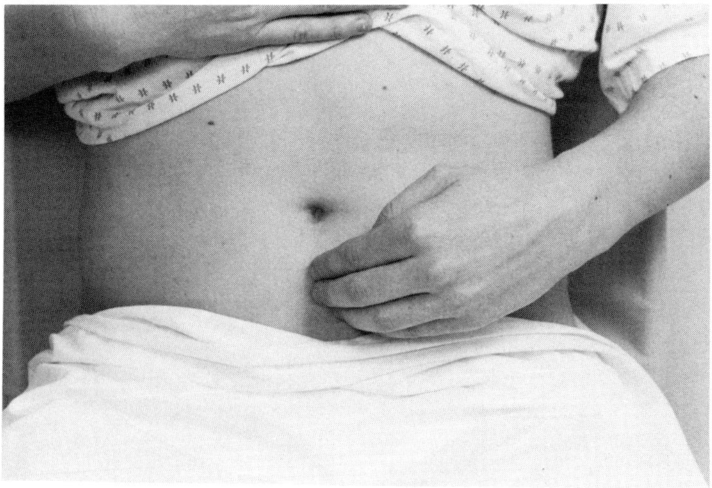

Figure 21–3 Method of catheter-free voiding for upper motor neuron bladder dysfunction: light tapping.

creasing degrees of dyssynergia, which give rise to a vicious cycle of associated increasing dyssynergia, increasing detrusor contractions, increasing residual urine volumes, increasing incidence of bladder infection, and further increases of dyssynergia with progressive bladder hypertrophy; eventually, vesicoureteral reflux and upper tract complications result.

Anticholinergic medications such as propantheline or oxybutynin are often useful for the management of upper motor neuron bladder dysfunction by decreasing detrusor reflexivity and force of contraction. Occasionally, an α-sympathetic blocking agent such as phenoxybenzamine can be helpful by decreasing the tone of the bladder neck and proximal urethral smooth muscle. To a lesser degree, the spasticity of the striated muscle of the external urethral sphincter may be relaxed by antispasticity medications such as baclofen, diazepam (Valium), or dantrolene (Dantrium).

At times, all of these methods fail and a surgical procedure may be beneficial. A limited external sphincterotomy or bladder neck resection or both (depending, of course, on the particular area of major dysfunction) may be required before the urethral resistance to urine flow is reduced.

Areflexic Detrusor and External Sphincter (Lower Motor Neuron) Bladder Dysfunction

A neurologic lesion involving either the sacral micturition center or its connections to the bladder and pelvic floor muscles gives rise to an areflexic detrusor and external sphincter (lower motor neuron) type of bladder dysfunction. Because the bladder lacks expulsive force, such force needs to be supplied by straining (Valsalva maneuver) (Fig. 21–4) or by the open-hand or closed-hand

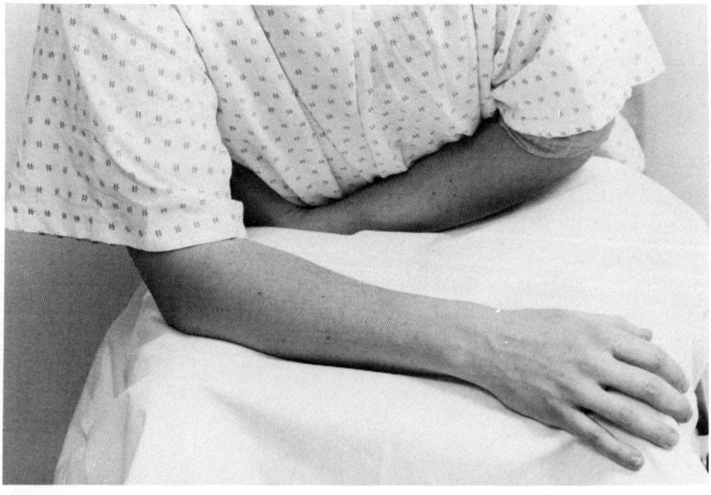

Figure 21–4 Method of catheter-free voiding for lower motor neuron bladder dysfunction: straining (Valsalva maneuver).

Credé maneuver (manual compression of the bladder (Fig. 21–5) so that the bladder neck is adequately pulled open for efficient emptying.

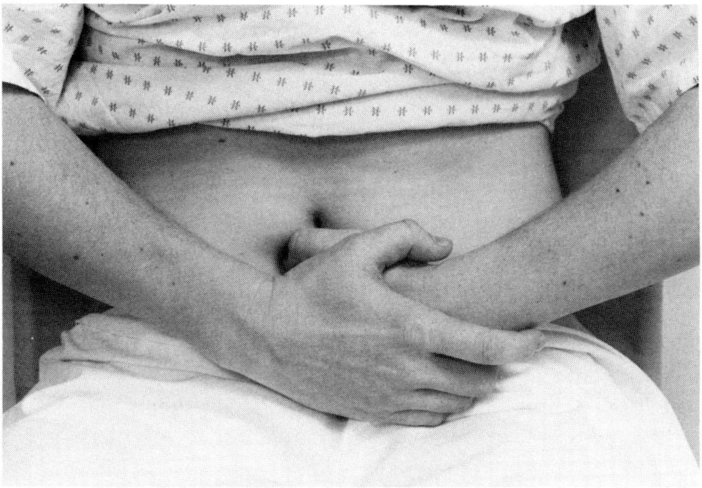

Figure 21–5 Method of catheter-free voiding for lower motor neuron bladder dysfunction: Credé maneuver.

Initial use of an α-sympathetic blocking agent such as phenoxybenzamine (10 to 20 mg daily) reduces the resistance to opening of the bladder neck as the intrabladder pressure is increased by either straining or the Credé maneuver. Once the tissue resistance of the bladder neck has decreased with frequently practiced voiding, use of phenoxybenzamine can usually be discontinued before the patient is dismissed.

The technique of straining (Valsalva maneuver) involves sitting and resting the abdomen forward on the thighs in both men and women. During straining in this position, hugging of the knees and legs may prevent any bulging of the abdomen. In this manner, all of the increase in intra-abdominal pressure may be put on the bladder and the pelvic floor.

The technique of voiding by the open-hand Credé method involves placing the thumb of each hand over the area of the left and right anterosuperior iliac spine and the digits over the suprapubic area with slight overlapping of the tips. The slightly overlapped digits are then pressed into the abdomen. When they have gotten well behind the symphysis, the pressure is directed downward to compress the fundus of the bladder. Both hands are then pressed as deeply as possible downward into the pelvic cavity. At times, the bladder can be compressed more efficiently by using the fist of one hand (closed-hand method) (Fig. 21–5) or a rolled-up towel.

Administering the cholinergic medication bethanechol 45 minutes before voiding may be helpful in association with mechanical stimulation of the detrusor by massage through the wall of the abdomen. Usually, this causes increased muscle tone of the bladder. Often, the previously entirely flaccid bladder can then be palpated suprapubically as a round organ with a definite tone. When it is then compressed with one of the Credé maneuvers, a higher transmural pressure can be generated and transmitted to the bladder neck for more efficient opening of the proximal urethra.

Straining (Valsalva maneuver) at the time the Credé maneuver is applied should be avoided because it increases the intra-abdominal pressure and causes bulging of the abdominal wall, which then tends to lift the compressing hands off the fundus of the bladder. Therefore, patients are asked to attempt voiding by one method first and then, after a period of relaxation, by the other method to determine whether it causes further voiding. In this way, both methods are tried alternately and the more efficient method for the patient can be determined. In our experience, the duration of bladder retraining is about the same in patients with spastic and in those with flaccid neurogenic dysfunction of the bladder.

Others

The management of mixed neurogenic bladder dysfunctions (types A and B) and areflexic myogenic detrusor insufficiency (end-organ failure) is beyond the scope of this chapter. A detailed description of them, the optimal voiding techniques, and helpful neurologic medications has been published.[9]

RESULTS

Data from nine studies comprising 737 patients who underwent bladder retraining between 1967 and 1978 (Table 21–1) indicated that the average acceptable residual urine volume after catheter-free voiding at the end of bladder retraining (mean duration, 39 days) was 102 ml. The success rate of bladder retraining was 72%. An average of 73% of 265 patients were free of catheter and urinary tract infection ($\leq 10^5$ colonies/ml) at dismissal.

Gjone and Ween[10] reported the follow-up data from 71 of their 116 patients (average duration of follow-up, 4½ years). Of these 71 patients, 63% had residual urine volumes of 150 ml or less at their follow-up visits. Episodes of recurrent bacteriuria occurred after dismissal in 42% of these patients. Positive findings on excretory urography were noted in 14% of the patients initially and in 11% at dismissal.

Viera et al.[11] analyzed the follow-up data from 99 patients. Of these 99 patients, 56 had their last follow-up examination more than 15 months after bladder retraining. The residual urine volume was 100 ml or less in 58%. The overall incidence of bacteriuria was 24% (colony count, $\leq 10^4$/ml).

TABLE 21–1 Success Rate of Bladder Retraining in Patients With Spinal Cord Injury

Reference	No. of Patients	Residual Urine, ml*	Mean Time of Training, Days	Retraining Successful, %	Abacteriuric Patients, %†
Bors[1]	36	–	–	78	–
Comarr[2]	109	Balanced bladder‡	–	87	–
Stover et al.[8]	33	150	21	57	32
Opitz[4]	120	65	62	78	91
Gjone and Ween[10]	116	150	59	80	65
Merritt and Ilstrup (unpublished data)	58	100	–	69	91
Sperling[6]	41	100	17	46	84
Perkash[5]	104	100	–	56	–
Fam et al.[3]	120	50	35	98	–
Total or average	737	102	39	72	73

* Acceptable maximal volume for catheter-free voiding.
† Colony counts were $\leq 10^5$/ml.
‡ Residual urine volume was usually $\leq$100 ml.
Modified from Opitz.[9]

SUMMARY

With the use of modern urodynamic evaluations (which may include exploration of the optimal features of voiding technique for an individual patient), neurourologically active medications, a well-structured program of bladder retraining, and carefully selected urologic operations, the success rate of bladder retraining has been increasing. With the normalization of voiding pressures during catheter-free voiding, careful eradication of bacteriuria, regular and careful voiding habits, and regular follow-up surveillance of persons with neurogenic bladder dysfunction after successful bladder retraining, the incidence of serious complications of the urinary tract can be expected to decrease further. A need exists for carefully conducted, prospective follow-up studies.

REFERENCES

1. Bors E. Intermittent catheterization in paraplegic patients. Urol Int 1967; 22:236–249.
2. Comarr AE. Follow-up on intermittent catheterization among spinal cord injury patients. Proc Vet Admin Spinal Cord Injury Conf 1969; 17:133–139.
3. Fam BA, Rossier AB, Blunt K, et al. Experience in the urologic management of 120 early spinal cord injury patients. J Urol 1978; 119:485–487.
4. Opitz JL. Bladder retraining: an organized program. Mayo Clin Proc 1976; 51:367–372.

5. Perkash I. Intermittent catheterization failure and an approach to bladder rehabilitation in spinal cord injury patients. Arch Phys Med Rehabil 1978; 59:9–17.
6. Sperling KB. Intermittent catheterization to obtain catheter-free bladder function in spinal cord injury. Arch Phys Med Rehabil 1978; 59:4–8.
7. Stolov WC. Rehabilitation of the bladder in injuries of the spinal cord. Arch Phys Med Rehabil 1959; 40:467–474.
8. Stover SL, Miller JM III, Nepomuceno CS. Intermittent catheterization in patients previously on indwelling catheter drainage. Arch Phys Med Rehabil 1973; 54:25–30.
9. Opitz JL. Treatment of voiding dysfunction in spinal-cord-injured patients: bladder retraining. In: Barrett DM, Wein AJ, eds. Controversies in neuro-urology. New York: Churchill Livingstone, 1984:437–451.
10. Gjone RN, Ween E. Results of bladder training 1966–1974. Paraplegia 1977–1978; 15:47–54.
11. Viera A, Merritt JL, Erickson RP. Renal function in spinal cord injury: a preliminary report. Arch Phys Med Rehabil 1986; 67:257–259.

22 EXAMINATION AND TREATMENT OF PATIENTS WITH BACK AND NECK PAIN

Robert R. Sawtell, M.D.

Neck and back problems are extremely common. Nearly every physician is apt to become involved in caring for patients with these complaints. Some cases are complex and difficult to manage, but most can be understood well enough to develop a reasonable plan of action. Backaches can often be understood if they are revisualized by taking a proper history. The physical examination also helps one to revisualize the precipitating event, especially if the pain can be duplicated by certain maneuvers. The diagnosis is then validated and reinforced by appropriate radiographic and laboratory data.

LUMBAR DISK PROBLEMS

The use of the history, physical examination, and laboratory findings for diagnosis will be illustrated within the context of disk problems and sciatica. Fortunately, disk problems are not as common as one may be led to believe, but the drama of the event aids the revisualization exercise. When obtaining the history, one usually first develops the central theme and talks about the present episode of back pain. Both the physician and the patient are interested in the location of the pain, its severity, its type, and whether it spreads or radiates. One needs to ask when and how the precipitating event happened, whether the event took place at work or at home, and other specifics, such as how the patient was standing, how much weight was being lifted, and how high the object was off the floor. Patients often like to demonstrate how it happened, but one must take care that they do not reinjure themselves in their effort to reenact the event.

After the central theme has been developed, one needs to sketch in the background material. One important question to ask is whether similar events have occurred in the past and, if so, how they occurred and how long they lasted. Most disk problems are characterized by distinct episodes (one or two times a year) that last from 7 to 10 days. Often, patients are vulnerable to an attack because of fatigue from overwork or a recent illness. Questions regarding general health are important so the physician can be aware of whether the patient has, for example, a heart problem or diabetes or has recently had an operation. Back problems may not be a truly inherited disease but, nevertheless, it is helpful to ask about the incidence of back pain in near relatives.

One should ask the patient whether anything gives some degree of relief. Patients with disk problems often state that lying flat on the floor with the feet elevated and knees bent or lying on a side with the knees flexed is of some help. Also, most patients find some degree of relief with heat or aspirin. Some patients resort to narcotics, an action that may indicate the severity of the pain. Many patients have consulted a chiropractor but are reluctant to admit so to their physician; however, one needs to know what avenues have been explored in an attempt to find relief. Other helpful information is whether the pain is worse with movements such as coughing and straining, jolting of any kind, riding in a car, lifting, or twisting the back. The results of previous radiographic and laboratory studies, such as electromyography, computed tomography, routine roentgenography, and bone scanning, should be reviewed. The patient should be asked about any previous treatment, such as physical therapy, surgery, or chymopapain injections. All of these questions are helpful for designing a therapy program.

The first part of any physical examination is observation. Observation should start while the history is being taken. Pain behavior and whether the patient is comfortable sitting or moving should be noted. One of the first things to be determined is the presence of an antalgic list, which is leaning to one side or the other to avoid pain. Sometimes a patient will lean away from the pain to open up the foramina and allow more space for the nerve root, or a patient may lean toward the pain because of muscle spasm around that area. Often, lumbar lordosis is flattened because of increased muscle tone and splinting from the pain. The patient can be asked to point to the pain, and the physician should note whether the patient uses just the fingertip or the whole palm of the hand. The patient can also point out the pathway that the pain takes as it spreads up the back or down the leg. Disk pain usually has a very narrow, distinct route.

Keeping the knees straight, the patient should try to touch his or her toes with the fingertips. The distance between the fingertips and the floor can be measured for some objective evidence, but more important is observing the lower back and determining whether the spine actually flexes. Many people can touch their toes by flexing at the hips while maintaining a stiff back. Slowly and with a great deal of caution, the patient should extend the back.

When the back is extended, the spines are encroaching on each other, the muscles are shortening, and the foramina are becoming smaller and the patient is thus in jeopardy of pain. When the patient bends laterally, one should note whether the pain is contralateral, which would indicate muscular distress, or ipsilateral, which would likely indicate foraminal narrowing and nerve root encroachment. A helpful maneuver is to have the patient come up on the toes and then drop suddenly down on the heels. This jolt will often cause pain at the vertebral interspace where the disk is not acting as a shock absorber.

While the patient is walking away from the examiner, one can observe whether the rhythmic contractions of the paraspinal muscles are normal. With pain, the paraspinal muscles often are tense, splinting the back and not allowing the normal lordotic curve and pelvic sway. Also, the patient should walk away from the examiner on his or her toes so the presence of weakness of the gastrocnemius-soleus muscle group can be determined. These muscles are innervated chiefly by the first sacral nerve root. One can imagine that the Achilles tendon is a big number "1" on the back of the leg to refresh the memory. When the patient turns to walk back toward the examiner, he or she should try to walk on the heels so the strength of the anterior tibial muscle, which is innervated by L–5, can be checked. Weakness may have been noted earlier by listening to the sound of the foot slap when the patient walked into the office.

The back, buttocks, and thigh area can be easily examined by having the patient drape himself or herself over the examining table with the face down, the abdomen on a pillow, and the feet lightly touching the floor. In this position, the hips and knees are slightly flexed. The pressure on the abdomen often relieves some of the pain in the back; thus, if any muscle tension is noted in this position, it is chiefly due to residual pain and not to resistance to gravity. The spines and the spaces between them can be firmly palpated and the areas of pain can be marked with a pen. The paraspinal muscles can be easily palpated in this position to note pain or muscle tension. A disk syndrome often involves a relatively narrow track of spasm and occasionally some edema in the overlying skin. The sacroiliac joint, the greater trochanter, and the sciatic nerve should also be palpated while the patient is in this position. After examination of all of these areas, a helpful step is to repalpate the spines to determine whether the patient will accurately report the same painful areas that were previously marked with the pen.

The patient should then be asked to sit on the edge of the examining table, and the knee jerk and ankle jerk are checked. The strength of the hip flexor and of the quadriceps muscle can be checked with the patient in this position. One must remember that the quadriceps mechanism of the knee jerk is supplied by L–3 and L–4, which are nerve roots that do not go through the sciatic nerve but rather through the femoral nerve. This nerve is not stretched with the straight leg raising test but rather is stretched with hyperextension of the hip. Checking the quadriceps muscle results in a modified straight leg raising test, and if any degree of sciatica is present the patient will complain of pain and will lean backward and prop himself or herself up with the hands.

The examiner should closely observe how the patient lies down on his or her back. A patient who is having considerable pain will move slowly and will lower himself or herself with the hands to the side and then tuck the legs up on the table and roll over onto the back with the hips and knees flexed. While the patient is lying on the back, the straight leg raising maneuver can be performed to compare one extremity with the other.

A helpful modification of this test is to allow the knee to be flexed about 15° to 20° and then flex the hip until there is some degree of stretch along the back of the leg. With the patient in this position, the examiner can press firmly on the popliteal nerve that is spanning the popliteal space and determine whether there is any excruciating pain in the buttocks, posterior aspect of the thigh, calf, or back. This maneuver is sometimes called the "bowstring sign." Pressing on the nerve causes the nerve root to be irritated in the foramina. Further pain often results when the patient lifts the head because flexing the neck causes the spinal cord to shift cephalad, and if the sciatic nerve is being held down firmly at the knee the nerve root will tighten over the protruding disk.

The strength of the abdominal muscles is important and can be checked while the patient is supine. With the hips and knees flexed and the examiner holding the feet down firmly, the patient is asked to elevate the head and shoulders (Fig. 22–1). The examiner can check the comfort of the patient while on the back in the knee-chest position (Fig. 22–2) and also determine whether the patient can do a pelvic tilt. The pelvic tilt maneuver (Fig. 22–3) is basically rotating the pelvis so that the pubic area moves up and the spines go down against the table. Flexion of the lumbar spine would open the foramina and also stretch the paraspinal muscles.

MECHANICAL LOW BACK PAIN

The described technique of taking a history and performing a physical examination can be applied to most patients with back problems. Usually, as the picture develops, it will become apparent that the backache is not sciatica but rather "mechanical low back pain." This is a backache that results from stress to the muscles, tendons, ligaments, and bones, and the pain is not due to impingement of a nerve root. The history usually reveals a chronic day-after-day type of ache that is more severe in the afternoon and evening. It is often characterized by stiffness in the morning that is relieved by a hot shower or aspirin. Sometimes it involves pain extending down the leg, but the pain seldom goes below the knee and the pattern of pain is a wide pathway. The use of heat frequently

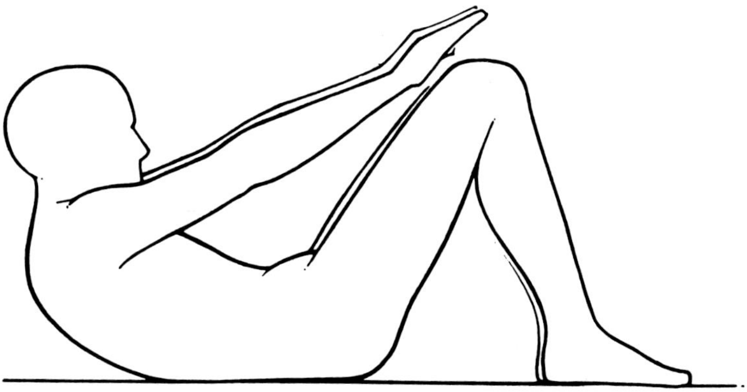

Figure 22–1 Maneuver used to check strength of abdominal muscles. Patient lies on back with knees bent and feet flat. With arms outstretched, patient raises head and shoulders, reaches hands toward knees, and returns to resting position. (From Mayo Clinic and Mayo Foundation, Department of Physical Medicine and Rehabilitation and Pain Management Center: Living With Low Back Pain. Rochester, Minnesota, Mayo Foundation, 1984. By permission of the publisher.)

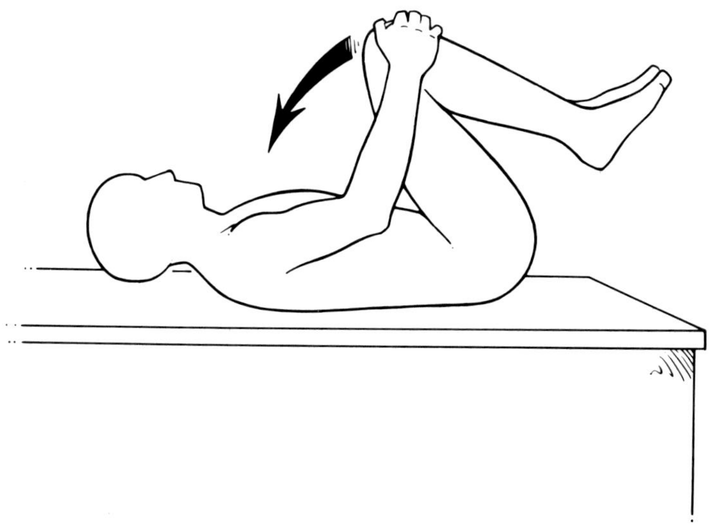

Figure 22–2 Knee-chest position is used to stretch lower part of back and open foramina. Patient lies on back and pulls both knees toward chest and slightly out toward flanks and then grasps knees with hands and pulls. (From Mayo Clinic and Mayo Foundation, Department of Physical Medicine and Rehabilitation and Pain Management Center: Living With Low Back Pain. Rochester, Minnesota, Mayo Foundation, 1984. By permission of the publisher.)

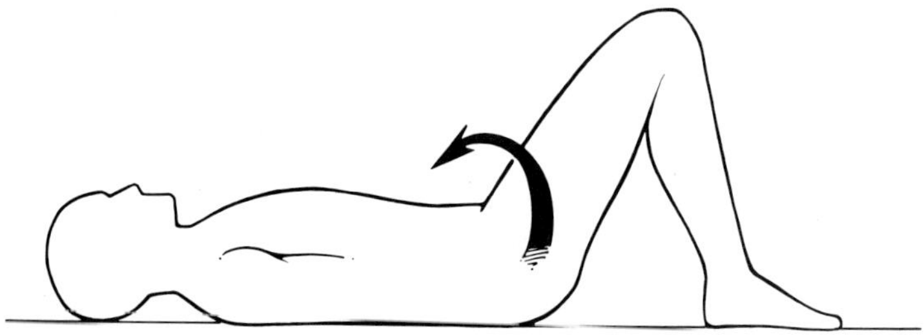

Figure 22–3 Pelvic tilt maneuver. Patient lies on back with knees bent and feet flat. Patient tightens abdominal muscles to roll pelvis up and back, thus flattening back against surface. (From Mayo Clinic and Mayo Foundation, Department of Physical Medicine and Rehabilitation and Pain Management Center: Living With Low Back Pain. Rochester, Minnesota, Mayo Foundation, 1984. By permission of the publisher.)

relieves the pain, and generally the aching is aggravated by continued hard use of the back. The physical examination reveals few, if any, neurologic findings but rather tender muscles with some increased tone and duplication of pain by stretching the muscle.

EMOTIONAL FACTORS

During the process of taking the history and performing the physical examination, one must be alert to emotional and psychologic factors. The meaning of pain and the fear of losing a job, compensation, sexual ability, or recreational pursuits will certainly color the picture. These elements are often frustrating to the physician, but they add to the challenge of treating the whole person rather than just the back.

FACET SYNDROME

Facet pain can often be suspected by the fact that the pain is localized over a facet. Often the pain can be duplicated by extension and lateral bending to the involved side. Occasionally, facet pain also radiates down the buttocks and thigh, but it seldom goes below the knee.

REST AND BACK PAIN

Noting the response of pain to rest is helpful. Usually, the patient with mechanical low back pain finds relief with rest but awakens in the morning with stiffness that lasts a short time. The patient with sciatica finds relief with prolonged rest after the muscles relax and no longer compact the vertebrae. When a patient seems to have increased pain during rest at night, one should be alerted to the possibility of metastasis to bone from a breast or prostatic tumor. Severe sacroiliac pain in the morning after sleep may be due to ankylosing spondylitis. Ankylosing spondylitis usually starts in the third or fourth decade of life and is more common in men, especially if their tissue type is HLA-B27.

NECK PAIN

Neck pain is similar in many ways to back pain, with a few unique features. Seldom is there a soft disk protrusion in the neck, but rather the nerve root is irritated by a "hard disk," which is an osteophyte. The most common nerve root to be involved is C–7, which innervates the triceps and wrist extensors. Usually, there is pain radiating down the arm to the thumb and forefinger when the head is tipped backward and laterally. Often the grip is weak. The finger flexors usually have adequate strength, but the grip power is decreased because of weak wrist extensors.

The most common neck pain is due to muscle tension. Muscle tension in the neck occurs for multiple reasons, including emotional stress and strain, job pressures, prolonged improper posturing of the neck, headaches, and injuries. These factors often become apparent as the patient describes the problem.

TREATMENT

Heat is an ancient way to treat neck and back pain. Heat will usually decrease the pain and also relax the muscles and allow greater freedom of movement. Various forms of heat can be used, but those most accessible at home are hot tub baths, heat lamps, and hot packs. Some heating pads have "hot spots" that can cause burns; nevertheless, patients frequently use them. Massage is helpful for gaining relaxation but is not an extremely important therapy. Certain flexing and stretching movements can be taught to the patients to ease neck and back pain. These maneuvers should be done slowly and gently and be followed by a few moments of relaxation. Some benefit can be gained by strengthening muscles such as the abdominal muscles and the anterior neck muscles. Abdominal strength is necessary to generate high hydraulic pressure in the abdominal cavity to support and protect the back. Occasionally, traction is used to treat the back, but it is more frequently used for the cervical region. Traction may distract the vertebrae to some extent, but its chief advantage is that it stretches the muscles and causes some relaxation.

Various cognitive relaxation techniques are helpful, especially for treating tension myalgia in the cervical region.

To avoid unnecessary stress to the neck and back, patients should be taught proper posture and lifting techniques. Energy-efficient methods of doing work can be taught by an occupational therapist.

CONCLUSION

Reconstructing and revisualizing the event or events that have triggered neck and back pain by obtaining a complete history and performing a physical examination and laboratory studies usually allow the examiner to determine the cause of neck and back pain. The examination should lead to a rational and reasonable treatment program. Frequently, the work environment needs to be altered so patients are better able to cope with their pain.

23 SPINAL OSTEOPOROSIS

Mehrsheed Sinaki, M.D.

Osteoporosis is the most common metabolic bone disease in the United States. It is an absolute reduction in bone mass. In a normal person, bone resorption is equal to bone formation, but in persons with osteoporosis, resorption is greater than formation. Osteoporosis involves a greater loss of trabecular bone than compact bone, a feature that accounts for the primary features of the disease (that is, crush fractures of vertebrae, fractures of the neck of the femur, and fractures of the distal end of the radius).

Osteoporosis is more common in women than men. About 25% of women older than 60 years demonstrate radiographic findings of osteoporosis.[1] It is more common in Caucasians and Orientals than in Blacks. Bone mass declines by about 10% per decade in women after menopause and by about 5% per decade in men after age 55 years.

ETIOLOGY

Several factors can cause osteoporosis: (1) a decrease in calcium absorption, which can be caused by aging or by drugs such as antacids and tetracycline; (2) hormonal factors, such as estrogen deficiency after surgical or natural menopause, an increased parathyroid hormone concentration, or decreased growth hormone or testosterone concentration; (3) drugs such as heparin, phenytoin, steroids, and methotrexate; (4) dietary factors, such as an insufficient calcium content, excessive phosphate content, vitamin D deficiency, or vitamin C deficiency; (5) altered vitamin D metabolism, which can result from a lack of or excessive vitamin D in the diet, decreased exposure to sunlight, excessive use of laxatives, malabsorption, decreased synthesis of 1,25-dihydroxycholecalciferol, use of cholestyramine or anticonvulsants, glucocorticoid excess (both exogenous and endogenous Cushing's disease), and chronic renal failure; and (6) physical inactivity (either generalized or localized) as a result of application of casts, severe weakness or paralysis, or rheumatoid arthritis. In some epidemiologic investigations, alcohol and smoking have also been implicated as risk factors. Another factor that may be important is body weight. Plasma-free estrogen levels are higher in overweight women. This could be the result of conversion of adrenal androgens to estrogens in adipose tissue.[1]

Hormonal and nutritional factors are well known to affect the process of bone loss. Furthermore, lack of physical activity or physical overactivity could be an important factor in osteoporosis.

Although the effect of inactivity on bones has been recognized for years, attention was only recently drawn to the role of inactivity on postmenopausal osteoporosis. The common causes of osteoporosis are listed in Table 23–1.

TABLE 23–1 Some Common Causes of Osteoporosis

Hereditary, congenital (osteogenesis imperfecta; neurologic disturbances: myotonia congenita, Werdnig-Hoffmann disease; gonadal dysgenesis)

Acquired

1. Generalized
    - Postmenopausal
    - Idiopathic
    - Malnutrition
    - Vitamin deficiency (C or D)
    - Vitamin overuse (D or A)
    - Calcium deficiency
    - Liver disease
    - Nephropathies
    - Chronic obstructive pulmonary disease
    - Malignancy (multiple myeloma)
    - Immobility
    - Senility
    - Endocrine disorders
        - Acromegaly
        - Hyperthyroidism
        - Cushing's syndrome (iatrogenic or endogenous)
        - Hyperparathyroidism
        - Diabetes
        - Hypogonadism
2. Localized
    - Inflammatory arthritis
    - Fractures and immobilization in cast
    - Limb dystrophies
    - Muscular paralysis

THE ROLE OF IMMOBILIZATION IN BONE LOSS

Patients lose calcium if confined to bed, and this loss does not subside until they become ambulatory.

In normal healthy volunteers[2] confined to bed in plaster fixation, calcium output increases for about 5 to 6 weeks and then maintains a consistently high level. In association with this increased output is nitrogen loss, an indication that both calcium and protein are being lost more rapidly than under normal conditions.

The phenomenon of atrophy and loss of bone density in association with motor paralysis is common in paraplegia, in which, with time, the bones below the level of the lesion undergo a greater degree of decalcification.

Weight bearing is much less effective than muscle contraction for limiting disuse osteoporosis.[3] Muscle action is the most effective stress on bone for prevention of disuse osteoporosis.

THE EFFECTS OF PHYSICAL ACTIVITY ON BONE

Physical activity has been recognized as one of the determinants of bone gain before maturity. The effect of exercise on the prevention of involutional bone loss has been studied.[4] The findings support the hypothesis that exercise can decrease involutional bone loss.

Muscle contraction leads to production of tension in the bone, which contributes to bone formation. It has been proposed that the weight of a muscle reflects the forces that it exerts on bones to which it is attached and that muscle weight is an important determinant of bone mass.[5] A significant correlation also has been demonstrated between the bone mineral density of the vertebral bodies and the strength of the back extensor muscles.[6]

The available literature indicates that a high level of physical activity throughout, and especially early in, life can provide a higher skeletal mass during the third to fourth decades of life. This high reservoir of bone mass at midlife may delay the clinical manifestations of involutional osteoporosis in later life.

Recently, attention has been drawn to the potential adverse consequences of prolonged and excessive physical activity on bone density, as observed in female marathon runners who were amenorrheic.[7]

SYMPTOMS

Back pain is usually a patient's main complaint. Vertebral compression fractures often occur in the low thoracic and upper lumbar bones, followed in order of frequency by the middle thoracic and lower lumbar bones. The cervical and upper thoracic vertebrae are rarely, if ever, involved. The compression fractures are manifested by pain in the involved level of the spine. The pain related to compression fractures may develop gradually or occur suddenly after a heavy object has been lifted or after strenuous activity. Back pain secondary to the compression fracture is self-limiting and usually resolves after 4 to 6 weeks. Persistent back pain necessitates further evaluation to rule out conditions such as multiple myeloma or other bone malignancies.

PHYSICAL THERAPY MEASURES

Acute Pain

The following measures can be used to relieve acute pain: (1) bed rest, (2) analgesics, (3) prevention of constipation, (4) proper posture principles (to avoid undue strain on the spine), and (5) physical therapy, such as mild heat and stroking massage.

Acute pain, which is usually due to a recent compression fracture, can be diminished by bed rest for 1 to 2 weeks on a hard mattress with a soft covering such as synthetic sheepskin. Prolonged bed rest can cause bone loss, but bone loss is not likely to be significantly aggravated by 1 week of bed rest. The patient should be in the supine position with a thin pillow under the head and a pillow of regular thickness under the knees to avoid undue strain on the spine. Some patients may have less pain if they lie on the side rather than the back and so should be allowed to do so. A small pillow should be used to fill the hollow of the flank when present. In this position, patients usually feel more comfortable with the hips and knees somewhat flexed. Placing a small pillow between the knees decreases the strain on the lower back caused by the adduction of the upper hip. At this stage, analgesics and an infrared heating lamp to decrease the pain and mild, stroking massage for relaxation of the paraspinal muscles are helpful. If pain persists despite the trial of bed rest, use of a back support for ambulatory activities should be considered (Fig. 23–1).

A properly fitted back support is appreciated more than any other measure by most affected patients. Fully supporting and rigid braces are preferred and usually give the best relief. Unfortunately, however, some patients, usually older persons, do not tolerate rigid back braces. In these instances, a semirigid thoracolumbar support with shoulder straps is a good alternative. The shoulder straps help remind the patient with kyphotic posture to avoid stooping (Fig. 23–1 *C*). Rigid back braces, which are usually better tolerated by younger patients, provide a stronger support for the osteoporotic spine. For small-framed patients who are less than 5 feet tall, the back support should be well fitted, preferably custom fitted, rather than obtained off the shelf or by mail order. If the patient has primarily unilateral low back pain referred to the buttock and hip areas, the use of a cane in the hand opposite to the painful side is helpful for decreasing the pain related to weight bearing (Table 23–2).

Chronic Pain

Chronic pain may be a result of compression fractures and kyphotic or scoliotic changes in the spine with inappropriate stretch of ligaments. Sometimes pressure of the lower rib cage over the pelvic rim in patients with severe kyphosis causes significant pain and tenderness in the loin area. Measures that improve a patient's

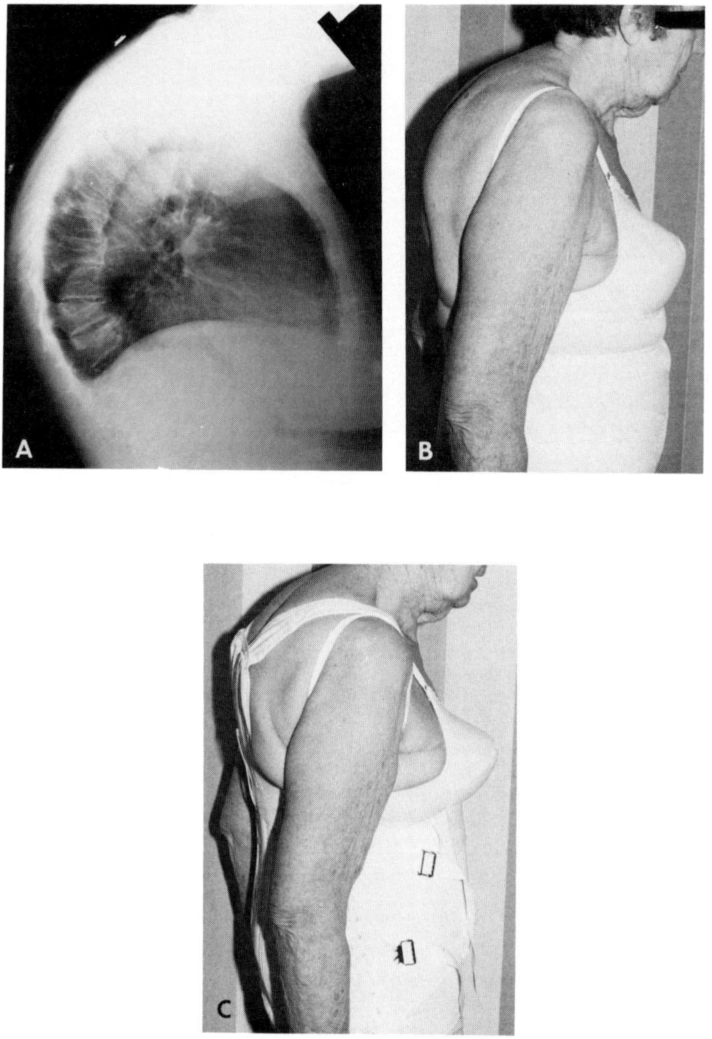

Figure 23–1 Patient with spinal osteoporosis. *A*, Lateral roentgenogram of thoracic spine demonstrates osteoporosis and compression fractures of several mid and lower thoracic vertebral bodies. *B*, Kyphotic posture resulting from osteoporosis and compression fractures. *C*, Patient fitted with thoracolumbar semirigid support with shoulder straps, which decreased back pain significantly. Stays in support are semirigid; if they are replaced with rigid stays, support is transformed into rigid back support.

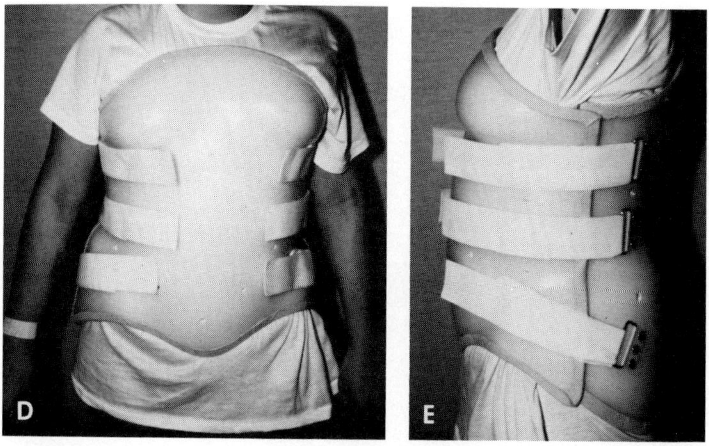

Figure 23–1 (continued) *D* and *E*, Anterior (*D*) and lateral (*E*) views of rigid back support or bivalved body jacket. This brace, made of polypropylene, is custom fitted. (From Sinaki.[8] By permission of Mayo Foundation.)

TABLE 23–2 Management of Acute Pain in Patients With Osteoporosis

Bed rest (less than 2 weeks)
Analgesics
Avoidance of constipation
Avoidance of exertional exercises. Significant aggravation of bone loss is not likely to occur during 1 to 2 weeks of bed rest
Proper positioning principles to avoid undue strain on spine
Physical therapy: mild heat and stroking massage

posture are needed. These measures include the use of a back support and proper back extension exercises. Semirigid or rigid back supports are used, depending on the severity of spinal osteoporosis and the patient's tolerance. We recommend extension exercises [8,9] (Fig. 23–2 *B* through *E*). Flexion exercises (Fig. 23–2 *A*) are not recommended; these can increase the vertical compression forces on the body of vertebral bones and may increase the possibility of compression fractures and further increase the kyphosis (Table 23–3).

TABLE 23–3 Management of Chronic Pain in Patients With Osteoporosis

Improve faulty posture, if possible
If beyond correction, apply a back support to decrease inappropriate stretch of ligaments
Avoid physical activities that increase vertical compression forces on body of vertebral bones
Prescribe a sound therapeutic exercise program
Start appropriate medical treatment, as indicated

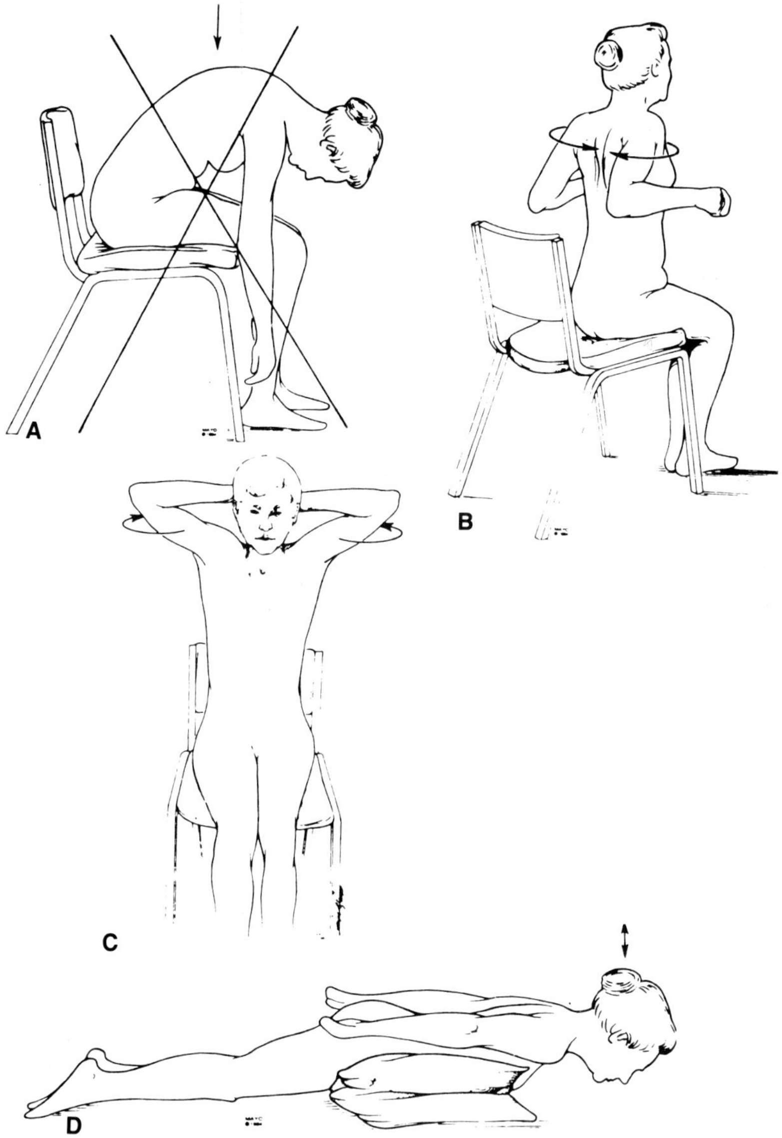

Figure 23–2 *A*, Lumbar flexion exercise that could contribute to kyphotic posture and cause more compression of osteoporotic vertebrae (to be avoided). *B*, Back extension exercise performed in sitting position. *C*, Deep-breathing exercises combined with pectoral stretching and back extension exercises. *D*, Back extension exercise performed in prone position. In patients with severe osteoporosis, pain can be avoided or minimized by having patient perform extension exercise in sitting position (*B*).

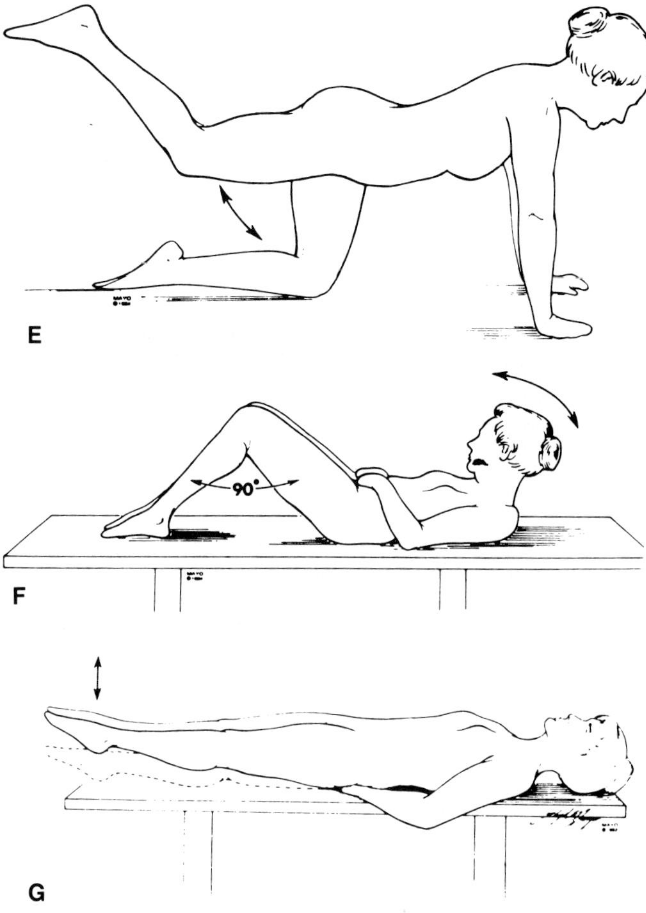

Figure 23–2 (continued) *E*, Exercise for improving strength in lumbar extensors and gluteus maximus muscles. *F* and *G*, Two techniques for strengthening abdominal muscles isometrically. (Redrawn from Sinaki.[8] By permission of Mayo Foundation.)

Complications of Severe Kyphotic Posture

Complications other than pain need to be given consideration. Attempts should be made to improve chest expansion. Stretching exercises of the pectoral muscles and other respiratory muscles such as the intercostals are recommended. Figure 23–2 *C* demonstrates deep-breathing exercises combined with pectoral stretching and thoracic spine extension.

Patients should be instructed to avoid stooping during ambulatory daily activities. The patient's desk and chair may need to be adjusted and a thin pillow used against the backrest of the chair for better support of the lower back. A hard mattress with a covering of synthetic sheepskin provides a soft contact over the spinous processes and decreases the possibility of developing pressure sores.

MEDICAL TREATMENT

Medical therapy should include a dietary evaluation and determination of the need for calcium and estrogen. A daily intake of 400 IU of dietary or supplementary vitamin D is recommended. Treatment with calcitonin has special indications. Sodium fluoride stimulates osteoblasts and has been recommended to be used in conjunction with calcium and vitamin D for some patients.[10] However, sodium fluoride is still under investigation. If sodium fluoride is used, the serum level of fluoride should be checked and controlled. At the Mayo Clinic, the therapeutic level is less than 15 μmol/ liter (Table 23–4). In patients who are receiving estrogen, initial and periodic gynecologic evaluations for cancer of the uterus and breast are needed.

TABLE 23–4 Medical Treatment for Patients With Osteoporosis

Dietary supplement
- Elemental calcium and vitamin D as required

Estrogen replacement: the usual effective dose after menopause is 0.625 mg/day; estrogen and progesterone are used cyclically in the presence of uterus

Prevention of immobilization

Fluoride and calcium together—the fluoride stimulates osteoblastic activity

PREVENTIVE MEASURES

Patients should be instructed to avoid heavy lifting and bending. Use of a cane provides better balance, reduces the possibility of falls, and decreases the low back pain resulting from weight bearing.

Patients should be instructed to try pectoral stretching, deep-breathing, and back extension exercises and to avoid stooping. They should be encouraged to try swimming or bicycling as a means of keeping fit rather than exercises or recreational activities that could predispose them to vertebral compression. Weight-bearing exercises are more effective than swimming for improving the bone mineral density.[11] However, swimming is recommended when general conditioning and fitness are desired. Osteoporotic patients have to avoid flexion exercises because they seem to predispose the spine to compression fractures. Also, a balanced diet is important and should contain 1 g of elemental calcium daily, which is contained in three glasses of whole or skim milk or its equivalent in ice cream or cheese (1 g before menopause and 1.5 to 1.8 g after menopause). The beneficial effects of a high-calcium intake on age-related bone loss are debated extensively.[12]

REFERENCES

1. Wilson JD, Foster DW. Williams textbook of endocrinology. 7th ed. Philadelphia: WB Saunders, 1985.
2. Deitrick JE, Whedon GD, Shorr E. Effects of immobilization upon various metabolic and physiologic functions of normal men. Am J Med 1948; 4:3–36.
3. Abramson AS, Delagi EF. Influence of weight-bearing and muscle contraction on disuse osteoporosis. Arch Phys Med Rehabil 1961; 42:147–151.
4. Aloia JF. Exercise and skeletal health. J Am Geriatr Soc 1981; 29:104–107.
5. Doyle F, Brown J, Lachance C. Relation between bone mass and muscle weight. Lancet 1970; 1:391–393.
6. Sinaki M, McPhee MC, Hodgson SF, Merritt JM, Offord KP. Relationship between bone mineral density of spine and strength of back extensors in healthy postmenopausal women. Mayo Clin Proc 1986; 61:116–122.
7. Drinkwater BL, Nilson K, Chesnut CH III, Bremner WJ, Shainholtz S, Southworth MB. Bone mineral content of amenorrheic and eumenorrheic athletes. N Engl J Med 1984; 311:277–281.
8. Sinaki M. Postmenopausal spinal osteoporosis: physical therapy and rehabilitation principles. Mayo Clin Proc 1982; 57:699–703.
9. Sinaki M, Mikkelsen BA. Postmenopausal spinal osteoporosis: flexion versus extension exercises. Arch Phys Med Rehabil 1984; 65:593–596.
10. Riggs BL, Seeman E, Hodgson SF, Taves DR, O'Fallon WM. Effect of fluoride/calcium regimen on vertebral fracture occurrence in postmenopausal osteoporosis: comparison with conventional therapy. N Engl J Med 1982; 306:446–450.
11. Nilsson BE, Westlin NE. Bone density in athletes. Clin Orthop 1971; 77:179–182.
12. Heaney RP, Gallagher JC, Johnston CC, Neer R, Parfitt AM, Whedon GD. Calcium nutrition and bone health in the elderly. Am J Clin Nutr 1982; 36:986–1013.

24 ARTHRITIS

John L. Merritt, M.D., F.A.C.P.

Arthritis refers to a categorization of diseases and conditions that affect primarily joints. Arthritis may, however, also have profound effects on associated musculoskeletal and other organ systems. Arthritis comprises several dozen types, but the most common are (1) degenerative joint disease (osteoarthritis), (2) rheumatoid arthritis and its variants, (3) B27 arthropathies (for example, ankylosing spondylitis), (4) scleroderma, (5) lupus erythematosus, and (6) other mixed connective tissue diseases. Although arthritis, by definition, is associated with joint inflammation, osteoarthritis (or degenerative joint disease), the most common type, is primarily degenerative. The joint effects of scleroderma are secondary to noninflammatory changes in overlying and surrounding soft tissues. Rheumatoid arthritis and its variants, mixed connective tissue diseases, lupus erythematosus, and B27 arthropathies are all associated with significant and readily detectable joint inflammation.

Joint evaluation, discussed in Chapter 5, is essential for diagnosis and for establishing an effective management program. The intent of this chapter is not to discuss in detail the differential diagnosis or even the medical management, because excellent references are readily available for those purposes; instead, this chapter is intended to provide guidelines for formulating rational physical and rehabilitation management of two exemplary forms of arthritis. The physical management of arthritis, although generally recognized to be important, is much less discussed in the literature.[1–4]

RHEUMATOID ARTHRITIS

Rheumatoid arthritis is a disease of unknown cause for which no curative treatment is known. Effective treatment is, therefore, limited to controlling the disease and minimizing its effects. Rheumatoid arthritis is the epitome of an inflammatory disease of multiple joints. Therefore, management exemplifies the principles of controlling joint inflammation. Successful management of inflammatory arthropathies primarily depends on controlling and reducing joint inflammation.

The early effects of joint inflammation (synovitis) are joint swelling, pain, stiffness, limitation of motion, and consequential loss of function. These are at first a result of intra-articular effusions and swelling of inflamed synovia. Both effusion and synovial swelling distend and stretch joint capsules and the surrounding soft tissues. As the disease progresses, the swollen hypertrophic synovium develops into an aggressively invasive tissue that erodes joint cartilage, subchondral bone, and adjacent tendons, bursae, and capsules. The results are further limitations of motion, with consequential development of joint contractures, muscle atrophy, and weakened capsules, tendons, and ligaments. This loss of joint and tendon motion, in association with muscular weakness and incoordination, pain and stiffness, and finally joint deformities, results in progressive functional deterioration. Declining mobility and the psychologic and social consequences contribute further to the generally decreasing functional independence.

The goals of management of rheumatoid arthritis, therefore, are to reduce joint inflammation if possible and, if not, to prevent the consequences of progressive joint dysfunction.[3,4] Several medications reduce inflammation, but none are entirely effective alone. Salicylates remain the initial drug of choice, but other nonsteroidal anti-inflammatory drugs may be equally effective. Other second-line drugs include penicillamine, gold salts, and antimalarials. Steroids and cytotoxic medications are reserved for refractory and rapidly progressive synovitis. If inflamed joints are not protected physically, however, medications alone will inevitably be inadequate to control inflammation and its consequences. In addition, no medication can restore range of motion or increase strength, coordination, and endurance without physical adjuvants. Physical measures are, therefore, essential to the comprehensive and effective management of arthritis.

Physical measures include rest, exercise, heat, cold, joint protection techniques, patient education, splinting, and assistive devices (Fig. 24–1).

Rest

Rest is a powerful anti-inflammatory instrument. Before corticosteroids and nonsteroidal anti-inflammatory drugs were available, rest was the only effective anti-inflammatory prescription. Although rest still has strong advocates, it has taken a back seat to drug therapy.

Effective drugs and constraints on hospitalization or rest at home often result in neglecting rest as a therapeutic tool for arthri-

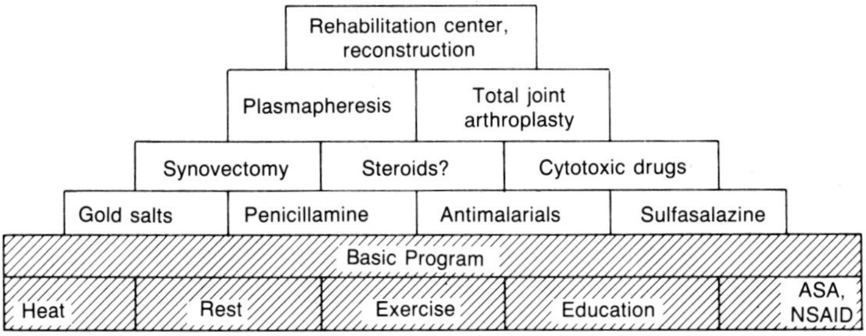

Figure 24–1 Management of rheumatoid arthritis. Items in lowest level, the basic program, are for all affected patients. Those who do not respond to this management are then treated with items in second level, in addition to items in first level. Note that four of the five first-level methods are physical, nonpharmacologic methods. ASA, acetylsalicylic acid; NSAID, nonsteroidal anti-inflammatory drug.

tis. However, the effectiveness of rest as a primary or adjuvant therapy for inflammatory joint disease was well described by Smith and Polley,[5] Partridge and Duthie,[6] and Gault and Spyker.[7] Gault and Spyker showed a reduction in the indices of inflammation after local joint rest (splinting). Smith and Polley long advocated an additional systemic benefit from general body rest. In a controlled trial, Partridge and Duthie reported a benefit from both general rest and joint splinting. Further study of joint rest is needed.

Most rheumatologists and physiatrists continue to agree that too much joint stress will increase joint inflammation and that rest should be a part of the management prescription for rheumatoid arthritis.[3–5] How much rest is needed and in what manner it is achieved, however, still need refinement. The main principle is that the more inflammation that is present on examination, the more rest that is needed. Thus, the quantity of rest should be increased or decreased according to symptoms and signs.

A frequent general guideline for moderate, early rheumatoid arthritis is 8 hours of rest at night, 1 hour of rest at noon, and 1 hour of rest before dinner. With this recommendation, many patients can continue employment or productive lives. Of course, heavy labor and strenuous or frequent repetitions of one motion should be avoided. Task modification, adaptive devices, and improved body and hand mechanics may further allow a productive life within a framework of joint protection and joint rest. Resting wrist-hand splints (see Fig. 25–1) can enhance rest for the hand and wrist joints at night and during general rest periods during the day. [8] These splints may also help reduce deforming stresses by maintaining proper joint alignment, but this theory is unproved. A wrist splint (the "cock-up" splint) can keep the wrist in a functional position during daily activities while allowing the hand and fingers freedom of movement. Maintaining the wrist or other joints in a middle range or functional position will also help keep intra-articular pressures low and thus reduce joint pain when synovial swelling or effusion is present.

Too much rest can, however, have detrimental effects on joints (contractures); bones (osteoporosis); muscles, tendons, ligaments, and capsules (weakness and atrophy); the brain and spinal reflexes (neuromuscular incoordination); and the respiratory and cardiovascular systems (loss of endurance and aerobic capacity). Rest must then be coupled with a concomitant exercise program.

Exercise

An exercise prescription requires as much care and specification as a drug prescription, especially for inflammatory arthritis. Exercises may include (1) range of motion (active, active-assisted, or passive), (2) stretching (active or passive), (3) strengthening (isotonic, isometric, or isokinetic), (4) reeducation, (5) coordination, and (6) endurance and conditioning (aerobic). Each type may be useful in some patients but may be useless, inappropriate, or even contraindicated in others.

Range-of-motion exercises are the mainstay of an exercise program for arthritis. Active, low-repetition (5 to 10 repetitions) exercises are usually preferable to passive range-of-motion exercises, but passive ones may be needed to achieve full range for joints in which the patient cannot perform full arcs of motion. Before a range-of-motion exercise program is prescribed, however, the reason that loss of motion is present or expected should be carefully considered for each joint (Table 24–1).

TABLE 24–1 Causes of Limitation of Joint Motion

- Contracture
  - Tendon
  - Muscle
  - Joint capsule
- Capsular distention
  - Effusion
  - Synovial proliferation
- Intra-articular free bodies
  - Foreign body
  - Meniscus tear
  - Villonodular synovitis
  - Synovial plica
- Joint surface incongruity

Joint contractures can limit motion. Such a limitation is most commonly due to contractures of joint capsules. Joint capsules readily develop contractures because of the anatomy of their braid-like intersecting fibers. These intersecting fibers automatically tighten to form a more closely knit network if the whole capsule is not stretched frequently (daily). All joint capsules have large "redundancies" that allow the joint to move through a full arc without tightening the capsule until the full arc for that motion is achieved. If these capsular redundancies are reduced by contractures, the capsule will tighten before the full natural arc of motion is achieved, effectively limiting the motion of the joint (Fig. 24–2). This type of capsular contractor is readily recognized by the skilled examiner by the type of resistance encountered at the end of an arc of passive motion (a "soft-end" feel).

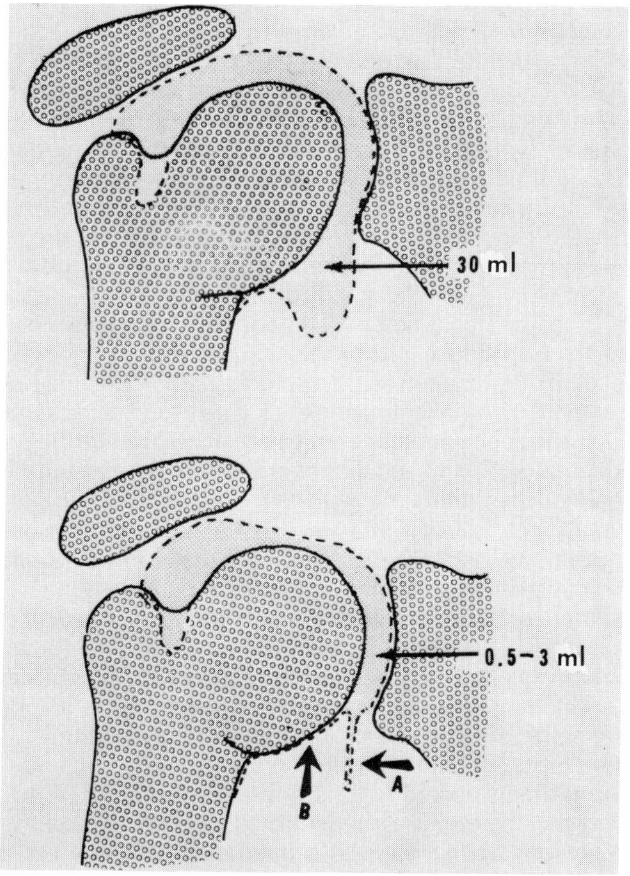

Figure 24–2 *Upper*, Normal shoulder capsule. *Lower*, Adhesive capsulitis, with contracted, adhered capsule (*A* and *B*); capsule volume is reduced markedly. Joint capsular "redundancies" allow joint motion. A contracted capsule limits range of motion, as does a distended capsule. (From Cailliet R. Shoulder pain. 2nd ed. Philadelphia: FA Davis, 1981. By permission of the publisher.)

Tendons, unlike joint capsules, usually are not readily shortened. Most supposed tendon tightness (for example, "heel cord contractures") has, in fact, been shown to be contractures of the respective muscles. Once a contracture has developed, whether of a capsule or of a muscle, range-of-motion exercises are inadequate to reverse the contracture. Appropriate stretching exercises are then indicated to restore motion. Range-of-motion exercises are appropriate primarily to maintain a given arc of motion and to help prevent joint contractures.

In the early stages of inflammatory arthritis, loss of motion is first and foremost due to joint capsular distention. As mentioned above, if capsular redundancies are reduced by contracture, the capsule will tighten before the full potential arc of motion is achieved. If, however, the capsular redundancies are filled with fluid from an effusion or with proliferative synovium, the redundancies are already "stretched" at middle range and further motion is not possible without further stress on painful capsular fibers. Joint motion is then limited by the capsular distention from effusion or proliferative synovium or both. In such cases, range-of-motion exercises will be ineffective to improve range of motion or even to prevent limitation of motion unless the effusion or synovial proliferation can be controlled or reduced. Likewise, stretching exercises will be painful and ineffective and may even result in capsular disruption. Aggressive medical anti-inflammatory measures are indicated instead. These will, of course, include rest (local or systemic) to help reduce inflammation (that is, effusion and synovial proliferation). Rest may, in fact, be part of a prescription to improve range of motion.[5] As inflammation ebbs, careful and painless range-of-motion and gentle stretching exercises can help restore the potential motion of each joint and thus help to prevent contractures from developing during this critical stage.

Loss of motion from intra-articular bodies or from joint surface incongruity (end-stage cartilage erosions) can be effectively resolved only with surgical intervention. Joint resurfacing (total joint arthroplasty) is the most effective procedure for joint surface incongruity.

In each patient, of course, different degrees and combinations of factors limiting joint motion are present. Thus, range-of-motion and stretching exercises, rest, anti-inflammatory measures, and operation may, and frequently are, combined and changed as the situation warrants according to the principles outlined here.

Strengthening exercises are indicated, in general, when weakness is present, when weakness is interfering with function, and when strengthening is possible and will not worsen the disease or cause damage. Weakness is common in patients with rheumatoid arthritis, due in part to a general decline in activities as well as a reduction in the intensity of activities. Generalized vasoconstriction, especially to major muscles, has also been implicated but not proved. Weakness of two major muscle groups, the hip and knee extensors (the glutei and quadriceps femoris), has particular functional significance (Fig. 24–3). Weakness in these two groups results in increasing difficulty getting out of chairs and climbing or safely descending stairs.

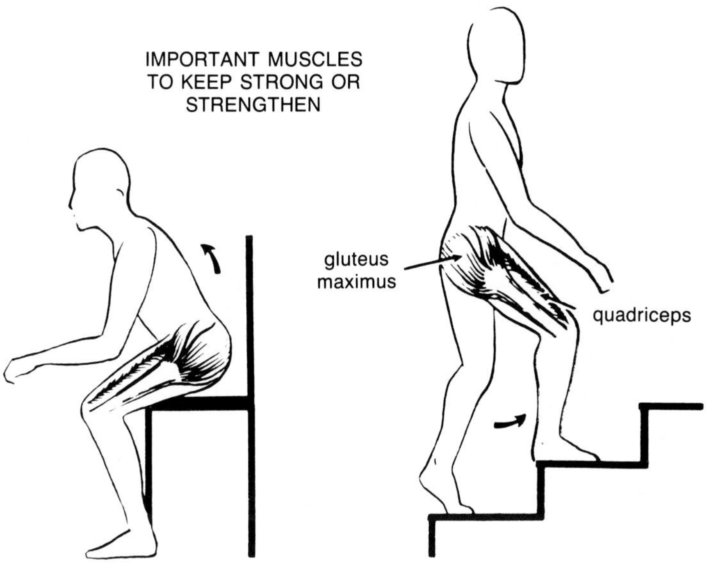

Figure 24–3 Hip and knee extensor muscles are important functionally.

Strengthening exercises can be performed in patients with arthritis, but not with traditional isotonic, weight-lifting methods. Isometric exercises can strengthen muscles as effectively as isotonic exercises. Isometric exercises (weight holding) allow significant resistance to the muscle with minimal effects on joint inflammation. Clinical experience and animal studies have concluded that isometric exercises cause the least adverse effects on inflammation.[9] However, allowing the slightest joint movement during a vigorous muscle contraction may increase joint inflammation. Thus, careful attention to correct technique is necessary to achieve selective muscle strengthening in rheumatoid arthritis. The Magnus belt exercise technique is one simple and effective method of accomplishing this (Fig. 24–4 *A*). Isometric strengthening of the quadriceps femoris with sandbags has an advantage in that quantification is possible, progression can be monitored, and patient feedback is present (Fig. 24–4 *B*).

Isometric exercises may, however, be painful during the muscle contraction and for a few moments afterward because of an increase in intra-articular pressure during the muscular contraction. Increased intra-articular pressure is present with isotonic and isometric contractions as well as, although to a lesser extent, with passive motion. This transient increase is not, however, apparently a stimulus for increased inflammation, at least with isometric exercises. A general rule of exercise is that pain may be allowed if it is transient, does not last for more than 1 hour, and is not associated with detectable increases in joint swelling, warmth, or

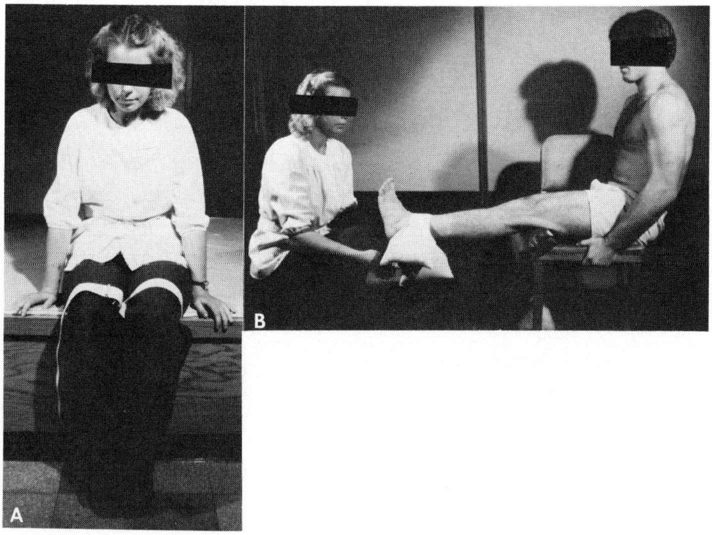

Figure 24–4 Two methods of isometric strengthening of hip and knee extensors. *A*, Magnus belt exercise. *B*, Progressive resistance exercise with sandbags.

tenderness. If these occur, the exercise should be modified or temporarily discontinued. A common problem is a change to an *isotonic* technique at home, even when instructions have stressed an *isometric* technique. We have frequently encountered this, even in bright, well-motivated patients. On a recheck examination, the patient should always be asked to demonstrate the exercise he or she has or had been doing to identify this common error.

Stiff joints and pain inevitably lead to muscle contraction and incoordination. Muscle reeducation is warranted for this frequent situation.

Patients who have been immobile for increasing durations often need general neuromuscular coordination and endurance training as disease, mobility, and strength permit. Individualized programs are necessary.

Exercises for the rheumatoid hand need special attention. The same principles for the prevention of loss of motion, for reduction of joint inflammation, and for restoration of function apply to hand joints. However, the goals for maintaining hand function and preventing deformities require some special rules.

Rheumatoid hand deformities include digital ulnar deviation, "intrinsic plus" (or "seal flap") hands, boutonniere and swan-neck finger deformities, and various thumb deformities. Several factors contribute to ulnar deviation (Fig. 24–5): (1) the shape of the metacarpal head that tilts radially, (2) a relatively weaker metacarpal radial collateral ligament compared with the ulnar ligament, (3) the ulnar pull of the finger flexor tendons during power grip, (4) metacarpal subluxation, which is inevitably volar and radial, (5) radial and volar subluxation of the wrist, which adds to the ulnar pull of finger flexors, and (6) functional lengthening of the finger flexors when bony absorption of the carpal bones causes shortening of the wrist. Many of these factors relate to forces transmitted through finger flexors.[10] As a consequence, strengthening of finger flexors is undesirable in the rheumatoid hand because strong flexors increase ulnar deviating forces. Power grip is also discouraged. Squeezing a rubber ball is to be avoided. Motion and dexterity are instead emphasized. A general rule is to perform only low stress exercises and activities for the upper extremities.

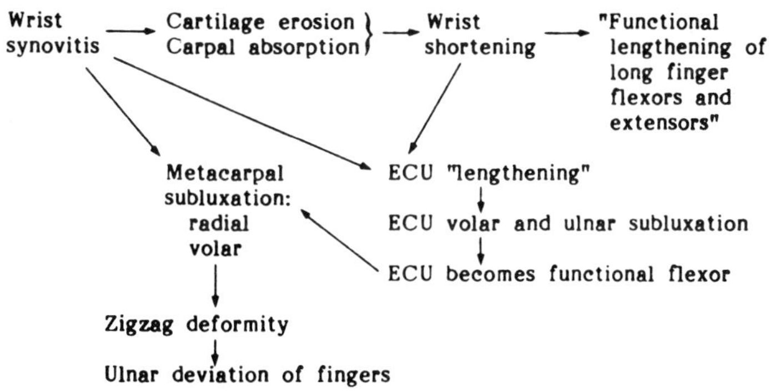

Figure 24–5 The role of the wrist in promoting ulnar deviation of fingers in rheumatoid arthritis. ECU, extensor carpi ulnaris.

Opening doors, jars, and other containers with counterclockwise resistance, if done with the right hand, as is most common, stretches the radial collateral ligaments and promotes ulnar deformity. Jar and door openers can help with these tasks and thus spare the radial ligaments. Alternatively, one could open containers (counterclockwise forces) with the left hand and close them (clockwise forces) with the right hand. The use of such assistive devices and joint protection procedures can potentially reduce subsequent hand deformities and help preserve function.

The "intrinsic plus" hand is due to a gradual tightening of the intrinsic muscles, secondary to pain and persistent spasm of these groups. Methods to reduce pain should thus be a part of a daily routine, as should stretching exercises for the intrinsic muscles. Intrinsic stretches are performed by actively flexing the proximal interphalangeal joints while the metacarpophalangeal joints are held in extension. These can often be performed simultaneously with warm soaks or during contrast baths.

Deformities of the wrist are reflected in "zigzag" deformities in the more distal aspect of the hand and fingers. Therefore, stabilization and early correction of volar and radial subluxation of the wrist with wrist splints are indicated.

Physical Methods

Heat, cold, massage, vibration, transcutaneous electrical nerve stimulation, and hydrotherapy are frequently prescribed for patients with rheumatoid arthritis. Each of these methods has unique physical properties, indications, and rationales.

Heat is the most frequently prescribed physical treatment for rheumatoid arthritis. The local and systemic effects of heat are well known and described, but most of these effects are undesirable in inflamed joints. Heating of human tissue increases local blood flow, local metabolism, capillary pressure, and intracellular edema. Increased blood flow results in increases in local oxygen and nutrients and also leukocyte and antibody concentrations and increases the activity of collagenases. With this in mind, the application of cold packs to inflamed joints has been advocated. However, as has been well demonstrated, neither hot packs nor cold packs actually change the temperature of underlying large joints (shoulders, hips, or knees). Only ultrasound therapy can effectively heat deep joints (Fig. 24–6).

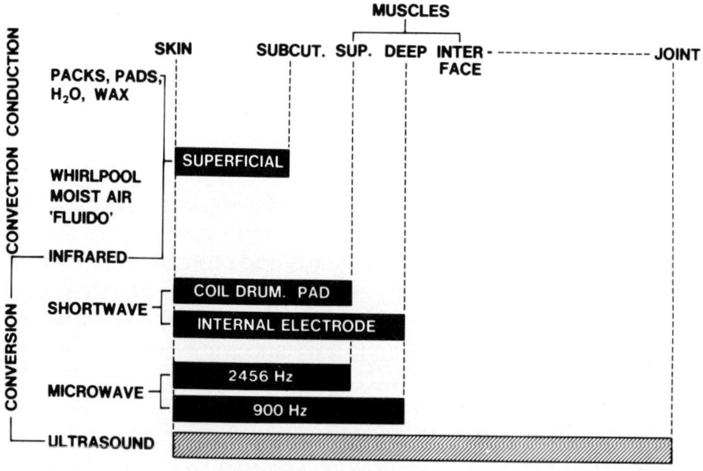

Figure 24–6 Methods of tissue heating and depth of heating. Note that only ultrasound therapy can effectively heat deep joints. Subcut., subcutaneous; Sup., superficial.

Heat and cold, as well as transcutaneous electrical nerve stimulation, vibration, massage, and a host of other physical methods, do relieve pain even though they do not directly heat or cool the joint. This nonspecific analgesia is apparently mediated through a neuromechanism (the "gate control" pain modulation theory). Pain relief may thus be achieved by local superficial heat, and adverse intra-articular heating effects are avoided. Even though cold packs can also relieve pain, they are not tolerated as well in patients with generalized vasoconstriction, such as those with active rheumatoid arthritis, and patients generally prefer heat for pain relief.

Warm water baths, showers, or soaks remain favorite and effective methods to reduce pain and stiffness and thus to allow a more effective exercise program or increased function. Warm soaks can, however, cause hand or foot edema. An empiric system that combines the vasodilatation of warm water and the vasoconstriction of cool water was developed to minimize edema formation. This contrast bath consists of alternating warm (110°F) and cool (60° to 65°F) water soaks (Fig. 24–7). This is a popular and convenient method to reduce pain and stiffness in hands and feet without edema formation.

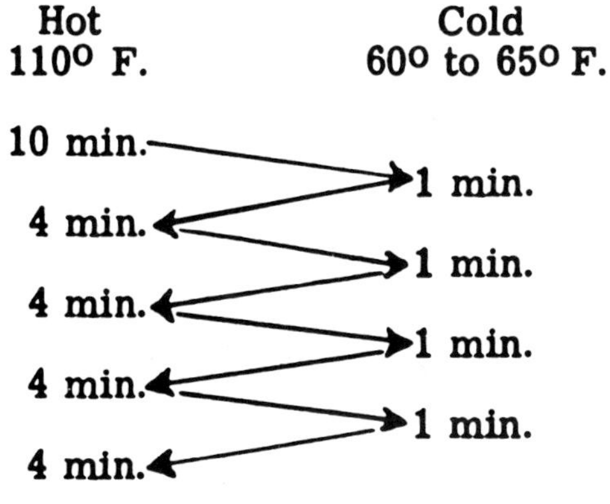

Figure 24–7 Program for contrast baths. Start and finish in warm water. Temperatures can be modified as needed and tolerated. (From Martin GM. Physical therapy in the general practitioner's office. Minn Med 1959; 42:235–239. By permission of the Minnesota Medical Association.)

Education

Patients with rheumatoid arthritis, like those with other chronic diseases, need a thorough base of knowledge about the disease, its effects, and its chronicity. They need to know that the cause of the disease is unknown, that there is no known cure, and that treatment is designed to prevent the effects of the incurable disease. They need thorough instruction in home therapy programs, in general health care, in hand care, and in joint protection measures. They need to be aware of possible adaptations to the home, for a hobby, and to their environment (Fig. 24–8 and 24–9). A knowledge of organizations such as social services, public health nursing programs, and therapy and vocational rehabilitation services can be valuable. Families are affected by the disease and may participate in its treatment; therefore, they also need to be included in the educational process. Finally, patients with rheumatoid arthri-

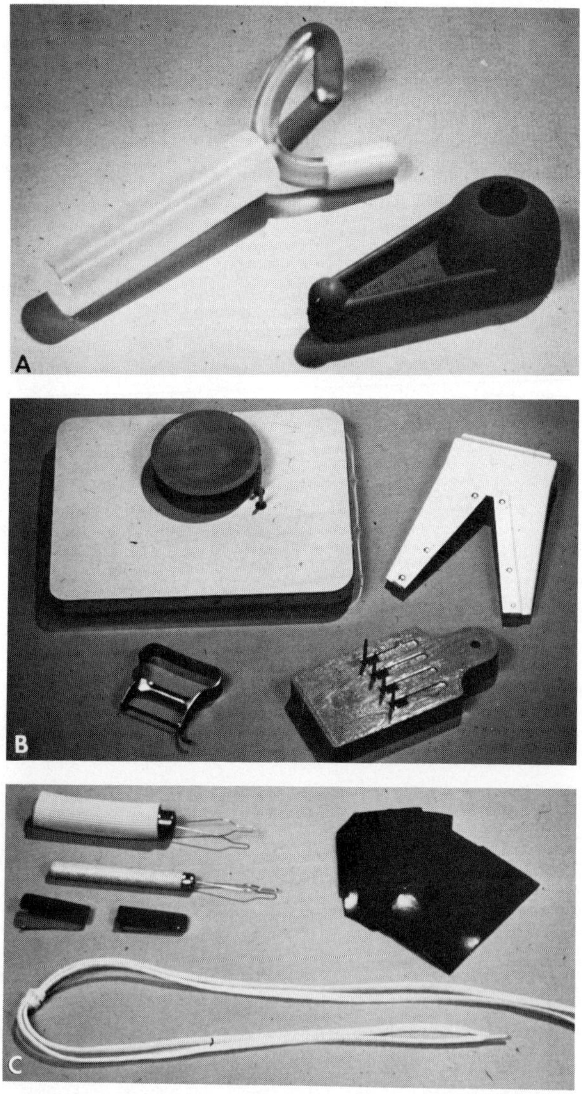

Figure 24–8 Assistive devices commonly used by patients with rheumatoid arthritis. *A*, Car door opener (left) and door knob turner (right). *B*, Jar openers and holders. *C*, Buttonhooks (left), friction rubber gripper (right), elastic shoe strings (bottom).

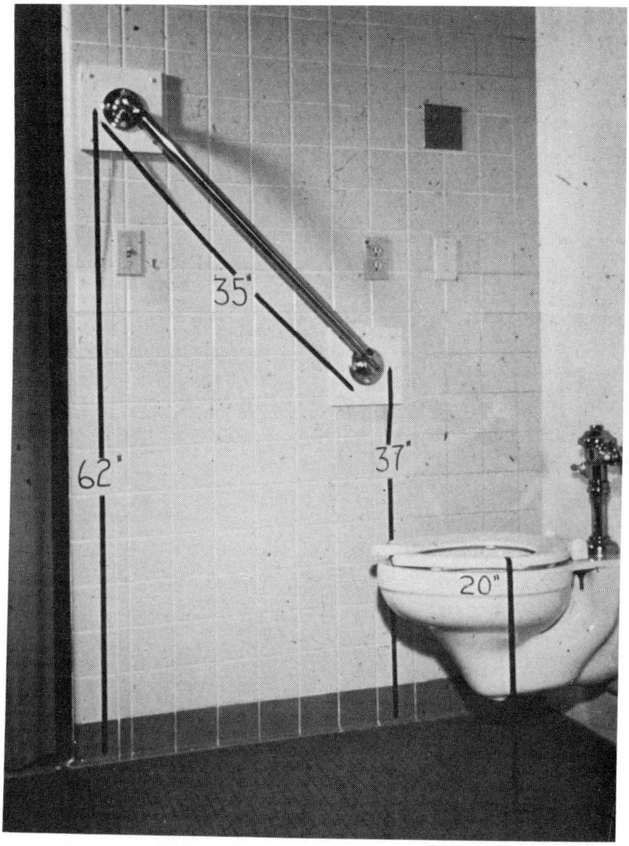

Figure 24–9 Dimensions for toilet and grab bar placement. If these cannot be remembered accurately, the patient should be sent to an occupational therapist who can provide this detailed information. (From Ellwood PM Jr. Transfers—methods, equipment, and preparation. In: Kattke FJ, Stillwell, GK, Lehmann JK, eds. Krusen's handbook of physical medicine and rehabilitation Philadelphia: WB Saunders, 1982: 473–491. By permission of the publisher.)

tis, like those with cancer, need to be aware that quackery is widespread and aimed specifically at people with diseases such as theirs. Peer-oriented organizations such as the Arthritis Foundation can provide assistance and valuable advice.

Mobility

Various mobility aids are available to reduce lower extremity stress and to improve mobility in the later stages of progressive arthritis. Canes, crutches, and walkers may be prescribed to reduce stress on inflamed hips, knees, ankles, or feet; however, this change simply transfers that stress to the upper extremities, including the wrist and hand. One way to avoid this stress on the hand and wrist is to add platforms to the gait aids (see Fig. 8–1 and 8–3). These devices, although still shifting stress to the upper extremities, eliminate weight-bearing stresses on the wrists and hands. Stair gliders enable one to ascend or descend stairs despite inflamed joints or weak muscles. Wheelchairs can provide an energy-efficient method for mobility, but propelling a wheelchair is not less stressful on the upper extremities than is walking on the lower extremities. If a wheelchair is needed for mobility, consideration should include an electric wheelchair. Vans with hydraulic lifts may allow improved mobility for wheelchair-dependent patients.

ANKYLOSING SPONDYLITIS

Ankylosing spondylitis is a unique disorder. The synovitis associated with it is predominantly localized to the posterior joints of the spine, including the spinal facet joints, the costovertebral joints, and the sacroiliac joints. Loss of motion of the cervical, thoracic, and lumbar spine and loss of chest wall motion result. Not only is ankylosis of the spine the final result, but characteristic ankylosis in a flexed, stooped posture causes severe functional impairment (Fig. 24–10).

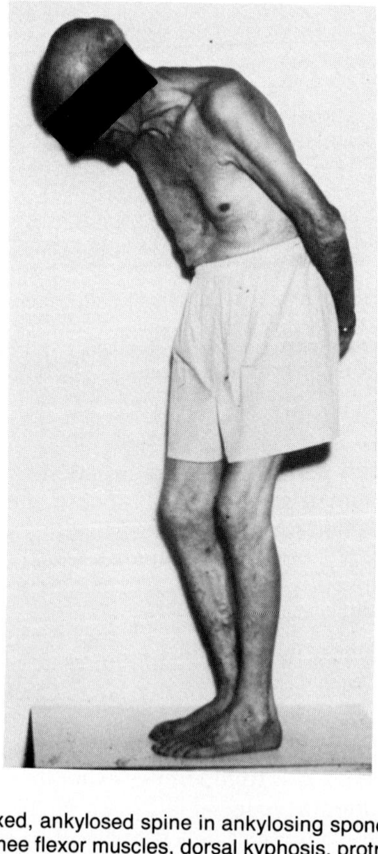

Figure 24–10 Flexed, ankylosed spine in ankylosing spondylitis. Note tight pectoral, hip, and knee flexor muscles, dorsal kyphosis, protracted shoulders, loss of cervical lordosis, and proximity of rib cage to iliac crest.

If spinal fusion occurs in this flexed position, balance, ambulation, and respiration can be severely impaired. Although no cure is available and no treatment can necessarily prevent spinal ankylosis, efforts to prevent fusion in a flexed position should be made. It is necessary to understand that such a flexed posture is a result of one's attempt to reduce pain by flexing the spine, therefore unloading the inflamed facet joints. Exercises that stretch the chest flexors (pectoral stretches) and strengthen the spinal extensors are provided (see Fig. 23–2), as are range-of-motion exercises for the neck and shoulders, deep-breathing exercises, and posture principles. But these principles must be accompanied by pain relief, including heat, massage, and nonsteroidal anti-inflammatory medications. Regular physical examinations should include measurements of height, chest expansion, and the C-7 to S-1 spinal flexion (in centimeters).

REFERENCES

1. Rossky E. Joint conservation and protection. In: Ehrlich GE, ed. Rehabilitation management of rheumatic conditions. Baltimore: Williams & Wilkins, 1980:234–242.
2. Neubauer P. The role of the physiotherapist in a multidisciplinary arthritis program. In: Ehrlich GE, ed. Rehabilitation management of rheumatic conditions. Baltimore: Williams & Wilkins, 1980:252–257.
3. Hollander JL, McCarty DJ, eds. Arthritis and allied conditions, a textbook of rheumatology. 8th ed. Philadelphia: Lea & Febiger, 1972:541–698.
4. Swezey RL. Arthritis: rational therapy and rehabilitation. Philadelphia: WB Saunders, 1978:1–192.
5. Smith RD, Polley HF. Rest therapy for rheumatoid arthritis. Mayo Clin Proc 1978; 53:141–145.
6. Partridge REH, Duthie JJR. Controlled trial of the effect of complete immobilization of the joints in rheumatoid arthritis. Ann Rheum Dis 1963; 22:91–98.
7. Gault SJ, Spyker JM. Beneficial effect of immobilization of joints in rheumatoid and related arthritides: a splint study using sequential analysis. Arthritis Rheum 1969; 12:34–44.
8. Gruen H. Splinting in the rheumatic diseases. In: Ehrlich GE, ed. Rehabilitation management of rheumatic conditions. Baltimore: Williams & Wilkins, 1980:243–251.
9. Merritt JL, Hunder GG. Passive range of motion, not isometric exercises, amplifies acute urate synovitis. Arch Phys Med Rehabil 1983; 64:130–131.
10. Gramse RR. The rheumatoid hand, mechanism of deformity, and the rationale for using splints. Semin Phys Med Rehabil, Mayo Clinic October 1977; 25.

25 HAND DISABILITIES

Jane L. Reiman, M.D.

Injury to one or both hands can be serious or devastating to the person who is injured. For someone whose vocation depends on his or her hands, even a small injury can be disabling. Even if it is still possible to perform one's vocation after a hand injury, the effect can be disabling if a favorite hobby has to be abandoned. Most of our activities of daily living such as grooming and hygiene depend on complete use of the hands. The purpose of hand rehabilitation is to restore the most complete function possible to the injured, operated, or diseased hand.

Patients may be referred for hand therapy for various reasons. For example, any number of possible injuries can occur to the hand. Some of the most common are fractures, tendon injuries, crush injuries, amputations, or a combination of these. Hand rehabilitation services may also be needed for patients with arthritis. Many postoperative conditions, such as release of the carpal tunnel in median neuropathy of the wrist, require hand rehabilitation. A patient is most often evaluated in the department of physical medicine and rehabilitation after the hand surgeon has completed the initial operation, treatment, and casting. Even though a patient's hand may be in a cast or dressing, therapy can be initiated.

COMPLICATIONS AND TREATMENT

Certain complications can be prevented or diminished by early evaluation and treatment. Some of the complications are edema, pain, loss of range of motion, loss of strength, adhesions, hypersensitivity, misuse of the extremity, disuse of the extremity, and, occasionally, overuse of the extremity (Table 25–1).

Edema is common after injury or operation. In part, it is due to immobilization of the hand and subsequent loss of the muscle

TABLE 25–1 Complications of Hand Injury and Some Recommended Therapeutic Measures

Complications	*Treatment*
Edema	Early active range of motion Elevation Decongestive massage Elastic wrap or glove
Pain	Cold, immediately postoperatively Heat methods (avoid swelling) Sedative massage Transcutaneous electrical nerve stimulation
Loss of range of motion	Control edema Range-of-motion exercises Joint mobilization techniques Splinting
Loss of strength	Progressive resistance exercises, isometric or isotonic
Adhesions	Friction massage Ultrasound, usually in water
Hypersensitivity	Desensitization massage
Misuse Disuse Overuse	Neuromuscular reeducation

"pump" in moving lymph from the hand. Also, the delicate lymph channels on the dorsum of the hand may be overwhelmed by rapid return of circulation after release of the tourniquet used during operation. Early active range of motion helps prevent edema and should be started in whichever joints can be moved. Even a small amount of motion can be helpful. Patients are instructed to keep the hand elevated whenever possible when swelling is a problem or a potential problem. They are instructed in decongestive massage, which is a distal-to-proximal massage to push the edema fluid out of the fingers or hand. They also learn to use elastic wrap (Coban) or string to wrap the fingers temporarily to decrease edema. Some patients wear elastic gloves to control swelling. If edema persists, soft tissue fibrosis may develop, which can result in loss of motion of joints and tendons.

Pain is also common after injury or for a short time postoperatively. Various types of hand therapy are used for relief. A whirlpool at moderate temperatures, fluidotherapy, contrast baths, light or deep sedative massage, paraffin baths, ultrasound, and transcutaneous electrical stimulation are some examples. It is important not to increase edema by overuse of heat, especially when the hand is in the dependent position, such as in the whirlpool. If there is a danger of swelling, whirlpool temperatures should be kept lower than the temperature of the limb, that is, lower than 35.5° or 36°C. Severe, persistent pain unrelieved by these treatments requires further investigation and therapy.

Loss of range of motion is another complication of hand trauma or operation. Often, such loss can be prevented by early use of appropriate hand therapy. Several mechanisms contribute to loss of range of motion. One is edema interfering mechanically with the function of the finger joints. The areas of edema may become fibrosed, causing swelling and stiffness to be persistent or permanent. Another cause for loss of range of motion is capsular and ligamentous tightness after immobilization of joints. Sometimes joints must be immobilized to allow for healing of bones or structures that have been repaired. Any joints that are not immobilized should have range of motion started immediately to help prevent loss. This includes the shoulder and elbow as well as the wrist and finger joints. The shoulder especially has a tendency to become stiff and painful when the patient is unable to use the hand. The purpose of the shoulder is to place the hand where it is needed. If the hand is not used normally, the shoulder will not be used normally, and specific range-of-motion exercises will help the patient use the shoulder and maintain the range of motion.

Although active exercises are most commonly used to maintain and increase range of motion, other forms of maintaining or increasing range of motion are used. Passive range of motion, in which an external force produces the motion, may be used. This does not imply stretching. Such exercises are done within the available range of motion. Active-assisted range of motion involves the patient actively moving the part as far as possible, and an external force completes the movement through the available range without stretching. This external force may be the therapist's hand or the patient's other hand. Gentle prolonged stretch, if desired, must be specified in the therapy prescription. Initially, the patient may tolerate only a few minutes of stretch, but the time ideally is increased gradually to 20 minutes, four times a day. It requires the cooperation of the patient, but the prolonged gentle stretch often achieves the goal of increasing the range of motion.

The addition of ultrasound to the gentle stretching program will enhance the effect of stretch alone. Stretching should be done simultaneously with the application of ultrasound and should be continued for several minutes thereafter while the tissues are cooling. This simultaneous heating and stretching enhances the flexibility of the tissues and makes them more amenable to stretch.

Heat methods other than ultrasound, such as a whirlpool or other superficial heat, during or before treatment may make movement easier.

Joint mobilization techniques, performed by the therapist, may be used to gain full "joint play" or capsular motion. They are not a home treatment, however.

Techniques other than therapeutic exercise can improve range of motion. If scar tissue or skin is tight over an area with loss of range of motion, friction massage will help. Dynamic splints may increase range of motion, and static splints maintain range of motion.

Splints (orthoses) are of many types, but the two basic are static and dynamic. Static splints have no movement built into them, and dynamic splints have movement (Fig. 25–1 and 25–2). Dynamic splints may be made with hinges or external joints and usually have a source of stored energy such as a rubber band or spring that provides movement.

Splints may be used to align, support, resist, assist, and simulate movement. All of these functions are used for hands at various times. Alignment and support are important in the resting splint for the arthritic patient. Static splints may resist abnormal or undesirable movements, such as a splint that prevents the patient from putting tension on a newly repaired tendon. Splints may assist movement dynamically, such as when rubber bands or springs assist movement of a weak muscle, or statically, such as in the wrist

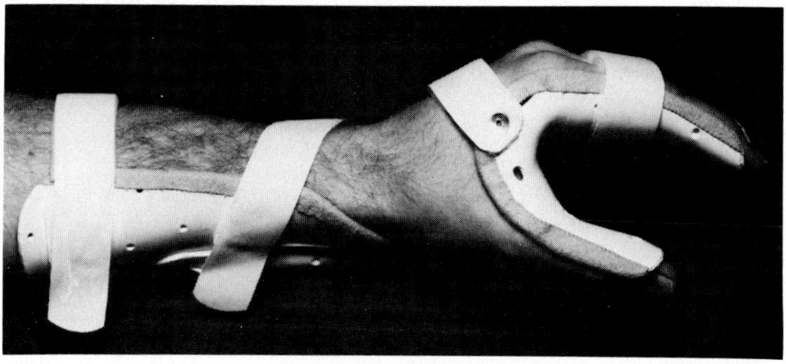

Figure 25–1 Static type of wrist-hand orthosis (splint). This type has no moving parts.

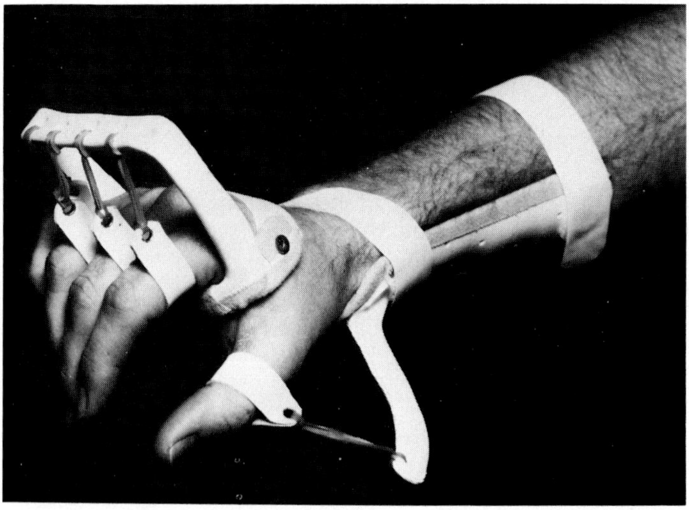

Figure 25–2 Dynamic type of wrist-hand orthosis (splint). The rubber bands assist extension of the metacarpophalangeal joints.

cock-up splint that supports the hand with weak or paralyzed wrist extensors. The simulation of function also involves movement built into the splint; also, these splints have a source of stored energy that can be activated by the patient's own muscles or by an external power source.

Splints can be made for individual joints, for the entire area of the elbow, hand, and wrist, or for portions of the extremity. Splints can be fabricated from special plastics that soften when heated, or occasionally they are made of metal or of canvas with metal supports; they can also be prefabricated, although a better fit is usually achieved with a custom-made hand splint.

The duration the splint is worn depends on the purpose. Sometimes splints must be worn constantly, such as when sound healing of a tendon or fracture is sought. Dynamic splints, which provide prolonged gentle stretch, are worn for a prescribed time, such as a half hour four times daily.

MUSCLE REEDUCATION

The hand therapist will often spend much time on muscle reeducation, regardless of whether tendon transfers have been performed. The classic method of reeducation, as described by Sister Kenny,[1] consists of progression from passive relaxed range of motion to active-assisted and to active range of motion followed by strengthening. The patient must concentrate and be aware of the desired action by feeling the muscle with the other hand and by observing muscle action. Electrical stimulation and electromyographic biofeedback can be used to enhance awareness of the desired action.

During the course of reeducation, the therapist and physician must be aware of and try to prevent misuse, disuse, or overuse of the affected muscles and other muscles of the extremity.

Misuse is using the extremity in the wrong fashion. This includes substitution, co-contraction, and guarding. Substitution is use of the wrong muscles for the desired movement. Co-contraction is contraction of the agonist and the antagonist at the same time while attempting a movement. If one tries to flex the elbow while simultaneously contracting the biceps and the triceps, elbow motion becomes difficult and uncomfortable because of fatigue of the muscles and extra forces on the joint. Misuse of the muscles of the extremity is inefficient and fatiguing. Co-contraction causes trembling and shaking. Guarding is tightening the muscles in a protective fashion.

Disuse is insufficient use of the extremity. Disuse may occur if the patient uses the extremity only for exercises and not for functional activities. Instruction in functional activities is given as soon as the patient is able to do them.

Overuse is using the extremity too much. Too quick a return to normal activities can result in pain and edema. Progression of activities from ''light'' to ''moderate'' to ''heavy'' should be monitored in each patient.

Sensory reeducation is important when the hand has nerve damage. If there is hypersensitivity, desensitization techniques are used. If all or part of the hand is anesthetic, the patient must be instructed in measures to protect the insensate part to avoid injury. As sensation returns, first in very gross rather than fine form, the patient is instructed in activities to practice sensation, thereby making the fullest use of the neurons present and increasing awareness of the sensation that is present. The progression is from identifying textures to differentiating small objects, temperatures, and hard from soft. Small assembly tasks are the final stage.

Although the road to full rehabilitation of hand disabilities may be long, much can be accomplished by the hand physiatrist, the hand therapist (physical or occupational therapist), and other members of the rehabilitation team working with the hand surgeon. Delays in referral to physical medicine and rehabilitation can result in slow or suboptimal rehabilitation; thus, cooperation and communication between the hand surgeon and physiatrist is of extreme importance and is for the benefit of the patient.

REFERENCE

1. Knapp ME. The contribution of Sister Elizabeth Kenny to the treatment of poliomyelitis. Arch Phys Med Rehabil 1955; 36:510–517.

26 TENSION MYALGIA

Mehrsheed Sinaki, M.D.

The term "tension myalgia" has been used for years. "Tension" suggests a major characteristic—increased muscle tone, whether it is spasm or increased muscle tone related to other factors. One of these factors may be psychologic tension or stress. "Myalgia" refers to the most characteristic finding—muscle pain, including pain in the muscular attachment areas. Tension myalgia is also called fibromyalgia, fibrositis, fibromyositis, myofascitis, myofascial pain, and nonarticular rheumatism (muscular rheumatism). Its incidence is not known precisely, but it is considered common. After osteoarthritis, tension myalgia is the second most frequent rheumatologic diagnosis.

ETIOLOGY

Poor posture or spinal curvature may be involved by increasing mechanical stresses. Clinical evidence has shown that anxiety, tension, depression, poor sleep, overwork, or physical activity can be a factor in the pain process. It is also associated with a higher than expected incidence of peptic ulcer, colitis, and migraine headaches.

SYMPTOMS

The incidence of tension myalgia can only be estimated because no population studies have been done. Most patients are women,[1] and onset is before age 35 years in more than 70% of patients. Symptoms may include generalized aches and pains, tiredness or fatigue, stiffness, anxiety, depression, disturbed sleep patterns, headaches, irritable bowel symptoms, subjective sensation of joint swelling, and numbness. The most common sites of tender points are the nuchal and upper back muscular attachment areas, lateral epicondyle, pectoralis attachment areas, gluteal attachment areas, gastrocnemius attachment areas, and suboccipital attachment areas.

Cold or humid weather, fatigue (physical or mental), a sedentary state, overactivity, anxiety, and poor sleep aggravate tension myalgia. Relieving factors include warm or dry weather, a hot shower, local heat, massage, modest physical activity, general relaxation, vacation, and restful sleep. Tension myalgia sometimes may mimic lumbar disk protrusion or cervical radiculopathy.

SUGGESTED CRITERIA FOR DIAGNOSIS

The criteria essential for a diagnosis of tension myalgia include (1) the presence of aches and pains with or without prominent stiffness involving various anatomic sites; (2) the absence of secondary causes, for example, trauma, overuse, and infective, endocrine, or malignant disorders; and (3) normal results of roentgenograms and pertinent laboratory tests.

Other criteria that can be used for diagnosis include (1) the presence of typical and consistent trigger points, (2) modulation of symptoms by physical activity and changes in temperature and humidity ("weather factors"), (3) a poor sleep pattern, (4) general feelings of fatigue or tiredness, (5) anxiety, distress, or depression, (6) chronic headache, (7) irritable bowel syndrome, (8) a subjective sensation of swelling, and (9) numbness. Appropriate studies must be done to rule out the secondary causes mentioned above, and the patient also must be observed in case these conditions evolve. In tension myalgia, muscle stretch reflexes and muscle strength are normal. Electromyography fails to show evidence of myopathy or any neurogenic change. The serum creatine kinase value is normal.

The differential diagnoses include (1) bursitis, (2) tendinitis, (3) costochondritis, (4) posttraumatic fibrositis, (5) rheumatoid arthritis, (6) palindromic rheumatism, (7) psychogenic rheumatism, (8) systemic lupus erythematosus, (9) vasculitis, (10) osteoarthritis, (11) polymyositis, (12) dermatomyositis, (13) polymyalgia rheumatica, (14) hyperthyroidism or hypothyroidism, and (15) early parkinsonism.

PATHOPHYSIOLOGY

Tension myalgia is not associated with any specific laboratory or roentgenographic abnormalities. Pain probably results from mechanical and other local stresses that contribute to a state of hyperalgesia of pain-sensitive tissues. The pain may be referred and poorly localized. Pain can be accentuated by stress factors such as cold, anxiety, abuse or overuse of muscles, and lack of adequate rest. Likewise, soothing activities may improve the symptoms.

TREATMENT

The patient needs to be reassured that the disease is benign and that it is not imagined. Rest and relaxation on a periodic basis are important (including a vacation, day or night sleep or a restful period, and muscle relaxants). Physical therapy may consist of heat in the form of hydrotherapy or infrared heating lamp, massage, or stretching exercises; sometimes, transcutaneous nerve stimulation may be helpful. Proper posture during activities of daily living is imperative. In selected cases, psychotherapy to relieve the cause of stress and teaching self-relaxation with and without biofeedback techniques[2] are additional therapeutic approaches. Patients need to have insight into the relationship between personality and pain. Analgesic medications such as acetaminophen, acetylsalicylic acid, or other nonsteroidal anti-inflammatory drugs are often useful. Tricyclic antidepressants sometimes are of benefit. Injection of tender points with local analgesics can sometimes be helpful in well-selected cases.

PELVIC FLOOR TENSION MYALGIA

The syndrome of pelvic floor myalgia is a form of tension myalgia involving the musculature of the pelvic floor and causing pain in these muscles or in their areas of attachment such as the sacrum, coccyx, ischial tuberosity, and pubic rami. The symptoms associated with pelvic floor myalgia are often vague. They are frequently difficult for the patient to describe or localize accurately. Patients usually complain of an aching discomfort in the rectum, pelvis, or lower back. Indeed, many patients are initially treated fruitlessly for low back strain, lumbar disk syndrome, or degenerative joint disease of the lumbar spine. Various terms such as piriformis syndrome,[3] levator ani spasm syndrome, diaphragma pelvis spastica, and coccygodynia (without any traumatic cause) have appeared in the literature, all of them referring more or less to the same entity.

Initial Complaints

A study at the Mayo Clinic[4] demonstrated the major symptoms to be low back pain in 82% of patients, a heavy feeling in the pelvis in 64%, leg pain in 48%, pain with bowel movement in 33%, constipation in 26%, coccyx pain in 19%, dyspareunia in 13%, and urine retention or psychogenic bladder in a few percent.

Aggravating factors are sitting for extended periods, tension, physical activity, standing for a long time, and sexual intercourse.[4]

Alleviating factors are analgesics, muscle relaxants, and sedatives; being in a lying position; relaxing; and a hot tub bath.[4]

Diagnostic Findings

The diagnosis of pelvic floor tension myalgia can easily be missed if the examiner does not consider it in the differential diagnosis. The physical finding that most often leads to the diagnosis is tenderness of one or more pelvic floor muscles on rectal examination. For the examiner to reach the piriformis muscles during rectal examination, the patient should be positioned on the side with the lower limb that is on the top bent at the hip and at the knee. Other reported associated findings are poor posture in about a third of cases, deconditioned abdominal muscles in a third of patients, and generalized muscle tenderness.

Suggested Criteria for Diagnosis

In the absence of a pathologic process in the pelvis, the criteria for diagnosis are tenderness of the pelvic floor muscles on rectal examination, aggravation of pain while in the sitting position, and tenderness of pelvic muscular attachments.

Treatment

The physical therapeutic techniques vary from deep heat (coil diathermy or ultrasound) to hydrotherapy, stretching massage of the pelvic floor muscles via the rectum, relaxation exercises, abdominal and back muscle strengthening exercises, posture instructions, and biofeedback techniques for relaxation. During recent years, significant success has been achieved with superficial heat and relaxation exercises applied with biofeedback techniques[5]; ultrasound therapy and diathermy are used only in selected cases. One or more of these treatments can be used. The duration of the treatment program is usually 5 to 10 days.

Reeducation for Pelvic Floor Muscles.[5] To maintain the skill of keeping pelvic floor muscles relaxed, the patients are instructed to practice the following exercise four times a day: (1) place one's hand over the anal cleft and, to feel the pelvic floor tension, tighten these muscles gently (but do not pinch the buttocks together); (2) tighten the muscles gently and feel the anal cleft being drawn up and in; and (3) in order to relax these muscles, feel the anal cleft bulge against one's hand and keep this relaxed position. Patients should learn how these relaxed muscles feel in order to be able to maintain the relaxed state. When the patient feels confident about keeping the pelvic floor muscles relaxed, indoor and then outdoor activities should be gradually increased. Keeping these muscles relaxed will become easier as the pain and discomfort are diminished.

Treatment Goals. The goals of treatment are (1) to relieve pain by inducing muscle relaxation with deep or superficial heat or exercises with biofeedback measures; (2) to avoid provoking factors;

and (3) to teach conscious, frequent relaxation of the pelvic muscles.

Summary

Important points to remember are that (1) this syndrome is little known to some physicians; (2) the diagnosis is obscured by vague complaints in a patient who is often neurotic as a result of pain or a premorbid personality; (3) a diagnostic clue is severe tenderness of the pelvic diaphragm muscles on rectal examination, and the tenderness may be in the posterior or anterior part of the pelvic diaphragm or in the attachment areas of the pelvic floor muscles; and (4) a patient may have a past history of generalized tension myalgia, generalized deconditioning, poor posture, or previous orthopedic or gynecologic operation or pelvic operation.

REFERENCES

1. Yunus M, Masi AT, Calabro JJ, Shah IK. Primary fibromyalgia. Am Fam Physician 1982; 25:115–121.
2. Basmajian JV. Biofeedback in rehabilitation: a review of principles and practices. Arch Phys Med Rehabil 1981; 62:469–475.
3. Thiele GH. Coccygodynia: cause and treatment. Dis Colon Rectum 1963; 6:422–436.
4. Sinaki M, Merritt JL, Stillwell GK. Tension myalgia of the pelvic floor. Mayo Clin Proc 1977; 52:717–722.
5. Department of Physical Medicine and Rehabilitation. Home instructions for relief of pelvic-floor pain. Rochester, Minnesota: Mayo Clinic, 1983.

27 ATHLETIC REHABILITATION *

Steven G. Scott, D.O.

Recent growth in the field of physical medicine and rehabilitation has coincided with the growing interest in sports and sports medicine. There are more than 500 sports medicine clinics in the United States, and the upward trend in rehabilitation medicine has led to an increased interest in both rehabilitation and sports medicine. The specialty of physical medicine and rehabilitation offers a unique contribution to the treatment of athletes because of its coordinated team approach and its broad base of knowledge. Numerous sports exist in which persons can have injuries or medical problems. These sports involve all ages—from infants to elderly persons—and physically disabled as well as able-bodied persons. Innovations in physical methods, therapeutic exercises, measurements of fitness, and prevention of athletic injuries provide the basis for this chapter.

CAUSES OF SPORTS INJURIES

Sports injuries can result from various causes that can be grouped into two particular types. One is blunt trauma, which occurs, for example, when a football player tackles another player or a hockey player sustains a body check from an opposing player. Injuries can range from simple to catastrophic—from contusions to closed head injuries or spinal trauma. The second major type is overuse of the musculoskeletal system, or microtrauma. In this type, repetitive sports activities gradually cause repetitive overuse syndromes. This injury often occurs in long-distance running, swimming, and ice skating. Individual sports can predispose the ath-

* Major portions of this material appeared in the *Mayo Clinic Proceedings* 1984; 59:83–90. Used with permission of the Mayo Foundation.

lete to specific types of athletic injuries. Repetitive use of the incorrect backhand in tennis can lead to tennis elbow, or lateral epicondylitis. If a skier falls on a thumb while grasping a ski pole, the ulnar collateral ligament can sustain blunt trauma and injury. The specific causes of sports injuries can range from pure chance to inadequate rehabilitation or poor supervision.

SPORTS INJURIES

Head, Back, and Trunk Injuries (Table 27–1)

Among sports injuries to the head and face are concussions during sports such as boxing and dental injuries from being kicked in a sport such as soccer. Eye injuries are common in all sports, especially in racquet sports that use a high-velocity ball. Facial injuries mainly involve lacerations and nasal bleeding and fractures from direct trauma. Injuries to the cervical spine range from strains and sprains to spinal cord injuries. Likewise, injuries to the lumbar spine also vary from strains and sprains to traumatic spondylolysis in young athletes involved in sports that involve repetitive hyperextension of the spine (such as gymnastics).

Visceral injuries involving blunt trauma to the chest or abdominal regions can be serious. Splenic injuries can become life-threatening. They often need emergency medical attention and will always be of some concern to the sports medicine physician. Injuries to the kidneys or to the abdominal region can usually be prevented with proper protective padding.

TABLE 27–1 Sports Injuries to the Head, Back, and Trunk

Concussions
Dental problems
Eye injuries
Back strains and sprains
Spinal cord injuries
Spondylolysis
Abdominal visceral injuries

Upper Extremity Injuries (Table 27–2)

Shoulder injuries in sports consist of instability, impingement, muscle tears, and acromioclavicular strains. The shoulder can easily be subluxed or dislocated in sports that involve tackling or falling on an outreached hand. Repetitive overhead use of the arms in sports such as swimming or throwing can cause an impingement of the subacromion structures and irritation of the rotator cuff muscles and tendons. Also, the small muscles of the rotator cuff easily tear from repetitive overuse or physical trauma. Also, acromioclavicular strains can occur from a fall on an outreached hand or from direct trauma.

TABLE 27–2 Sports Injuries to the Upper Extremity

Shoulder instability
Shoulder impingement syndrome
Rotator cuff tear
Acromioclavicular strain
Lateral and medial epicondylitis
Olecranon bursitis
Forearm tenosynovitis
Wrist strains
Hand contusion
Finger strain
Mallet finger

Elbow injuries are usually caused by repetitive overuse of the forearm extensor origin muscles on the lateral epicondyle, as in tennis, or by overuse of the forearm flexor origin muscles on the medial epicondyle, as in golf. Throwing a javelin can cause hyperextension problems in the elbow and olecranon bursitis. Repetitive wrist and hand activities, such as in the sport of motocross, can cause tenosynovitis of the forearm. Wrist strains or injuries are common in sports such as weight lifting and rowing. The hand is also injured frequently. Contusions of the hands and strains of the fingers are common in football, as are dislocations of the fingers. Baseball players receive direct trauma to the tips of their fingers from a baseball and experience a mallet finger or the inability to extend the distal phalanx when the distal extensor tendon is involved.

Lower Extremity Injuries (Table 27–3)

Hip and pelvic injuries, although not common in sports, occur in sports such as dancing and ice skating. However, poor flexibility in hockey players may lead to frequent strains of the groin muscles from repetitive stress. The knee is the most severely injured joint in sports, and an injury can often compromise the ability of the athlete to participate in competitive sports. Severe injuries to the anterior or posterior cruciate ligaments can lead to major

TABLE 27–3 Sports Injuries to the Lower Extremity

Groin strain
Knee ligamentous injuries
Patellar tendinitis
Patellofemoral pain syndrome
Medial tibial stress syndrome
Ankle sprain
Planter fasciitis
"Turf" toe

surgery. Common knee injuries are patellar tendinitis from repetitive jumping activities and patellofemoral pain syndrome from structural malalignment of the lower extremities. Shin splints or medial tibial stress syndromes commonly result from excessive running. More specific diagnoses of this problem are tendinitis, periostitis, stress fractures, and compartmental syndromes.

Ankle sprain is the most common reason athletes are held from competition. The athlete often is afflicted by an inversion strain of the lateral ankle ligaments. Injuries to the foot also can easily prevent the athlete from participating in sports. Plantar fasciitis of the foot is often a disabling problem in running and can take up to 6 months to heal. Other running injuries, such as "turf" toe or hyperextension strains of the first metatarsal, can prevent participation.

COMPREHENSIVE REHABILITATION PROGRAM

Rehabilitation of the injured athlete involves (1) care and treatment of athletic injuries, (2) sports fitness, and (3) prevention of sports injuries. In the care and treatment of athletic injuries, initial measures provide comfort and continued efforts help regain and maintain motion, strength, endurance, and skill. Measurements of sports fitness provide objective criteria for exercise prescription and for a return to full participation in sports activities. Supervisory, educational, and follow-up activities of the physician for the prevention of athletic injuries round out the comprehensive rehabilitation program.

CARE AND TREATMENT OF ATHLETIC INJURIES

Provision of Comfort

Rehabilitation can be effective only when pain is reduced enough to allow comfortable, coordinated motion. Currently, physical methods, manual therapy, electrotherapy, and anti-inflammatory medications are used to relieve discomfort.

The use of physical methods to reduce pain, swelling, and inflammation has not changed substantially over the years. Initially, the treatment of an acute athletic injury consists of protection, rest, ice, compression, and elevation. Cold therapy is still used early after injury to raise the threshold of pain, act as a local vasoconstrictor, decrease muscle spasm, and limit the degree of injury. Cold therapy is usually continued until the hemorrhage, edema, and hyperthermia of the skin have subsided. If used too long after injuries, cold therapy can impair healing of the wound and tissue.

Protection and rest are facilitated by crutches, orthoses, and taping. The use of elastic supports to protect and support a muscle or tendon can allow early freedom of joint movement. Edema can be controlled with cold therapy, elevation of the edematous part, avoidance of heat, isometric exercise, and elastic compression wraps. An intermittent-pulse pneumatic compression pump (Fig. 27–1), or an air splint, reduces the swelling of a sprained ankle and thus often shortens the rehabilitation time.

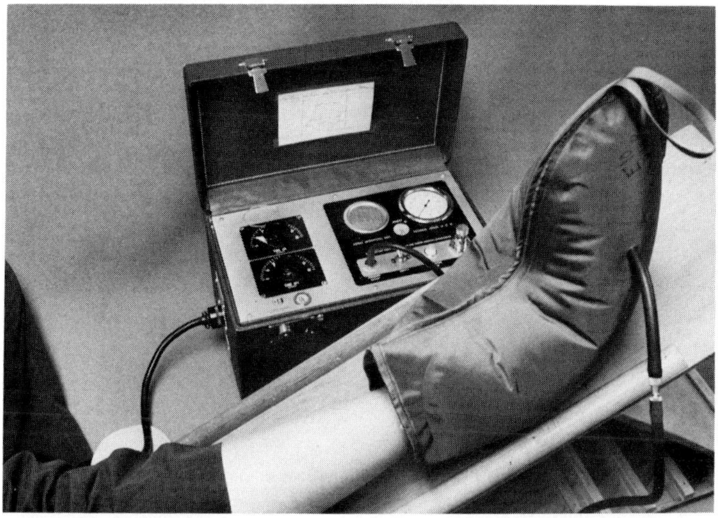

Figure 27–1 Intermittent-pulse pneumatic compression pump (Jobst Institute, Inc., Toledo, Ohio). (From Scott SG. Current concepts in the rehabilitation of the injured athlete. Mayo Clin Proc 1984; 59:83–90. By permission of Mayo Foundation.)

Contrast bath treatments (alternate applications of heat and cold) are currently in wide use to manage sports injuries when the benefits of cold therapy have decreased and when heat therapy alone seems inappropriate. The cold treatments minimize the buildup of edema caused by the heat therapy, and the heat provides a sedative effect. The distal aspects of the extremities can be bathed for a 30-minute period consisting of an initial 10 minutes in warm water and alternating periods of 1 minute in cold water and 4 minutes in warm water. Other intervals for the contrast therapy and different physical methods may be used.

After the first 24 to 48 hours from the time of injury, cold therapy is often replaced with heat unless bleeding is suspected (as in severe contusions or hematomas). Heat therapy decreases joint stiffness, raises the threshold of pain, relieves muscle spasm, and produces a sedative analgesic effect. Heat can be applied by conduction (hot packs), convection (hydrotherapy), radiation, or conversion (diathermy or ultrasound). The most common methods of heating used in sports injuries are whirlpools and moist heat packs for superficial heat and ultrasound for deep heat. The therapeutic temperature range for heat is narrow (43°C to 45°C), and the duration of application is from 3 to 30 minutes.[1]

Manual therapies, such as massage and mobilization of soft tissues, are used early after injury to reduce swelling and alleviate pain. Stroking, compression, and percussion are commonly used forms of massage. Mobilization of soft tissues, which involves palpatory skills and complex manual therapies, should be performed only by persons who are well instructed in its use.

Electrotherapy often is used in the subacute stages of care to relieve pain. Transcutaneous nerve stimulation, a Microdyne II stimulator (Fig. 27–2), and an interferential current are used at present.

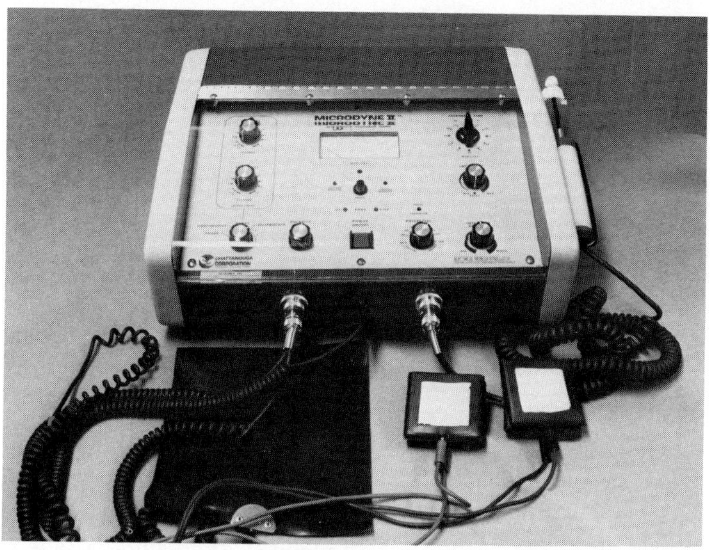

Figure 27–2 Microdyne II stimulator. (From Scott SG. Current concepts in the rehabilitation of the injured athlete. Mayo Clin Proc 1984; 59:83–90. By permission of Mayo Foundation.)

Anti-inflammatory medications are commonly prescribed early in the care of athletic injuries. Injections of corticosteroids can reduce the inflammation associated with injuries to the soft tissue, but serious weakening and rupture of tendons can occur if an inappropriate technique is used by inexperienced persons. If injections of local analgesics are given to relieve pain, pain-free motions can begin early in the rehabilitation program.

In summary, the athlete is first treated with ice, rest, anti-inflammatory medication, and protection. Contrast baths, heat, or manual therapies can be used next. Electrotherapy and injections are usually reserved for the subacute phases.

Restoration and Maintenance of Motion, Strength, and Endurance

Therapeutic exercises to maintain or increase mobility are begun early after injury—as soon as a reasonable degree of comfort has been obtained. Recent studies have shown that early joint movement aids in tendon and ligament healing and prevents contractures. Early passive or active range-of-motion exercises should be done in a pain-free range. Motor incoordination causing substitution movements or co-contractions of the antagonist muscles necessitates neuromuscular reeducation, preferably with electromyographic biofeedback.

The difficulty in estimating the tensile strength of tissue that is healing often leads to uncertainty in the prescription of safe stretching exercises. The amount of stretching needed to improve range of motion is related to the duration of stretch, the temperature of the tissues being stretched, and the forces applied. Gentle, prolonged, pain-free stretching at a moderate tension is more effective than the short intermittent or ballistic stretches that once were widely used. Elevation of tissue temperatures (45°C) with heat techniques in combination with gentle prolonged stretching promotes extensibility of tissue and increases range of motion (Fig. 27–3).[2] Thus, ultrasound therapy and prolonged stretching exercises are commonly used together to increase flexibility.

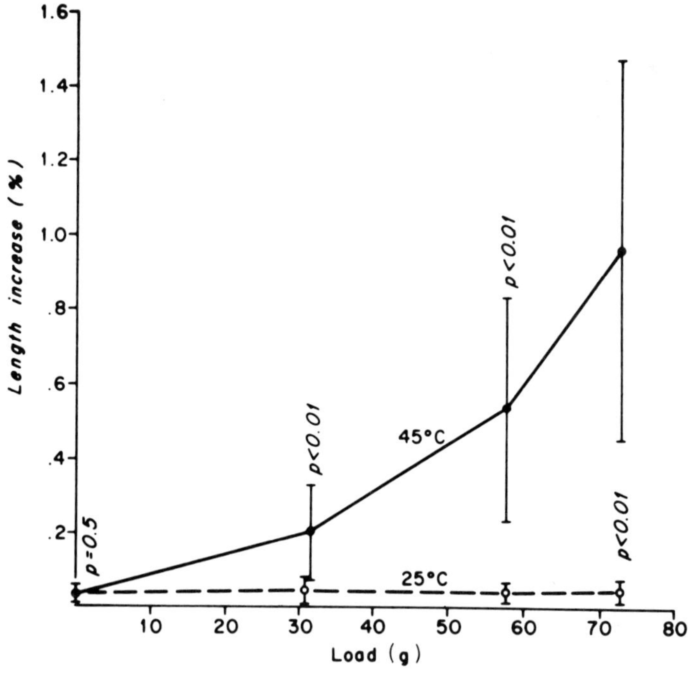

Figure 27–3 Percentage increase in tendon length at 45°C and 25°C. (From Scott SG. Current concepts in the rehabilitation of the injured athlete. Mayo Clin Proc 1984; 59:83–90. By permission of Mayo Foundation.)

Strengthening exercises usually are begun once comfort has been attained. The trend in the rehabilitation of injured athletes is to begin strengthening exercises soon after an injury. The important point to remember, however, is that pain and effusion in joints can inhibit and decrease strength. If the strengthening exercises are started too early and cause more pain or effusion, the patient will gain less strength and have more motor incoordination, and the course of rehabilitation will be prolonged. The gain in strength depends on the mode (type) and the rate of strengthening exercise, the resistance of the muscle contractions, and the number of repetitions. The best mode of strengthening exercise remains controversial.

Modes of strength training can be divided into two categories: static and dynamic. Static, or isometric, strengthening exercises, usually begun in the initial stages of rehabilitation, should be done in a way that produces no discomfort. Isometric strengthening can be used if the range-of-motion exercises cause pain and if joint movements need to be restricted. Limitations include poor compliance by patients and lack of carryover to specific motor skills. The added benefits of doing isometric exercises more frequently throughout the day, as is often prescribed in the rehabilitation of injured athletes, are unknown.

High-intensity electric stimulation with a current intensity of 60 mA and a modulated sine wave frequently is used in the early and intermediate stages of rehabilitation of injured athletes as a means of static isometric strengthening and reeducation of specific muscles (Fig. 27–4). The stimulation, which produces a maximal tetanic contraction within the athlete's tolerance of pain, usually is applied once daily for 10 to 15 minutes. Studies have shown that muscle atrophy is less during the period of joint immobilization and improvements in strength are greater with stimulation than with isometrics.[3] Other studies have not shown that electric stimulation achieves a considerable gain in strength.[4] The advantages of electric muscle stimulation over volitional isometrics are that stimulation can strengthen or reeducate specific muscles and seems to raise the patient's threshold of pain.

Once maximal static (isometric) contractions are done at multiple joint angles, or when 70% to 80% of the pain-free range of motion is achieved, dynamic strengthening exercises are usually begun. Dynamic strengthening exercises can be classified into three types: constant resistance, variable resistance, and accommodating resistance. Each of these exercises has its advantages and disadvantages in the rehabilitation of injured athletes.

Constant resistance (isotonic) exercises are the most frequently used strengthening mode in rehabilitation. Examples of isotonic strengthening modes are free weights and the universal gym. A disadvantage of this exercise mode is that the weight resistance is limited to the weakest angle in the arc of motion. Also, once inertia is overcome, little added work is needed to move the weight.

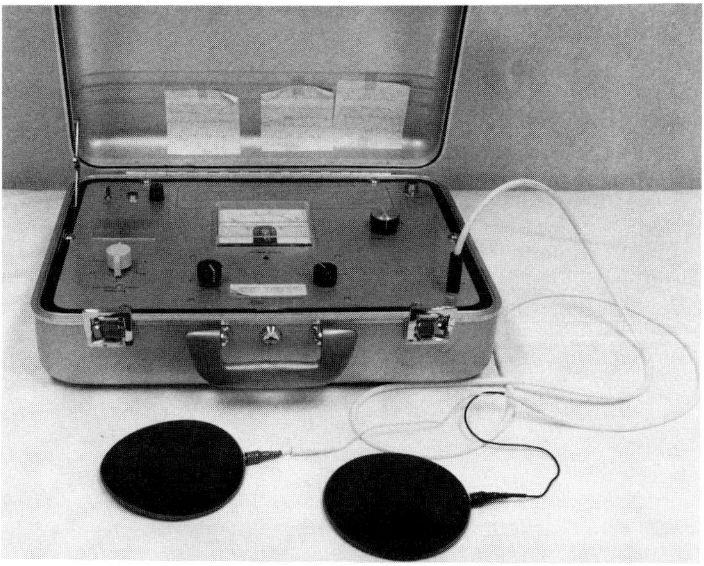

Figure 27–4 High-intensity muscle stimulator. (From Scott SG. Current concepts in the rehabilitation of the injured athlete. Mayo Clin Proc 1984; 59:83–90. By permission of Mayo Foundation.)

Another concept of strengthening in the rehabilitation of injured athletes is the variable resistance mode. Simpler forms of this mode are the use of elastic bands and manual resistance. Hydraulic or cam-shaped machines (for example, Nautilus, Sports Medical Industries, De Land, Florida) that provide varying resistance throughout the full range of motion are a more complex but increasingly more available form of variable resistance. The resistance on the cam-shaped exercise equipment attempts to match the angle-specific strength capacities of muscles. Limited studies have shown little difference in gains of strength between persons who use equipment that provides variable resistance modes and those who use constant resistance modes.[5] Advantages of the cam-shaped exercise machines are the ability to strengthen both eccentrically and concentrically and thus to improve flexibility and the capacity to work the muscles at a higher maximal rate than that attainable with the constant resistance modes.

Another type of exercise commonly used for the rehabilitation of injured athletes uses the accommodating resistance mode (isokinetics). Isokinetics involves exercising at a constant velocity of joint motion. The most common isokinetic equipment used is the Cybex machine (Cybex, Division of Lumex, Ronkonkoma, New York), which provides an isokinetic dynamometer to give a direct measurement of muscle torque, power, and endurance under reproducible velocities (Fig. 27-5). The advantage of the isokinetic

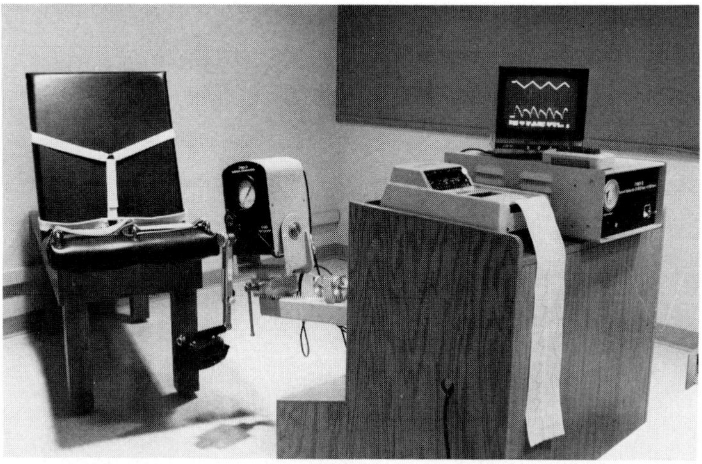

Figure 27–5 Cybex isokinetic machine. (From Scott SG. Current concepts in the rehabilitation of the injured athlete. Mayo Clin Proc 1984; 59:83–90. By permission of Mayo Foundation.)

mode is that the resistance matches a person's muscular exertion at a specific velocity. As the muscles become fatigued or limited in strength by discomfort, the torque output exerted by the muscles may decrease, and the Cybex machine accommodates this decrease with less resistance. Thus, it is safer to use this exercise mode early in rehabilitation. Another advantage of isokinetic equipment is its ability to train muscle contractions at high velocities that match speeds used in athletic skills. Most functional activities involve joint ranges of motion that exceed 90º per second, and many sports activities involve speeds that exceed a range of 240º per second. These speeds are much faster than those that can be attained with the other strengthening modes. Also, the muscle resistance is maximal throughout the full range of motion, a factor that allows more work to be performed with each repetition of exercises than can be done with the other modes.

A new advancement in strength training is the Kin-Com kinetic machine (Chattecx Corp., Chattanooga, Tennessee) (Fig. 27-6). Force, velocity, and range of motion can all be automatically controlled through a programmed computer. By means of robotics and computer technology, the machine can lead the patient through eccentric, concentric, passive, and static muscle contractions at different velocities, forces, and ranges. Television disk display and software programming make this strengthening machine versatile in sports medicine.

Once a degree of muscle strength has been achieved, the trend is to begin training in muscular endurance and power. Muscular endurance is the ability of a muscle to sustain continuous work at a moderate intensity. It results from increased frequency of repe-

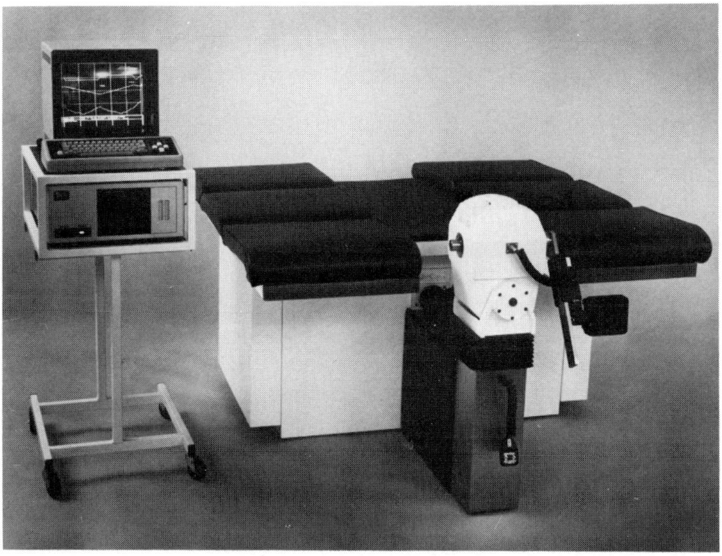

Figure 27–6 Kin-Com kinetic machine. (From Scott SG. Current concepts in the rehabilitation of the injured athlete. Mayo Clin Proc 1984; 59:83–90. By permission of Mayo Foundation.)

titions during light resistance in any of the dynamic strengthening modes. Muscular power, the rate at which a muscle can exert force through a specific distance, is gaining emphasis in the rehabilitation of the injured athlete. Muscular power in sports activities is derived from muscles that act in synergy or stabilize the body for balance. These muscles are most active in free-weight exercises, which continue to have a place in power development in the rehabilitation of the injured athlete.

In summary, the rehabilitation of patients for strength, muscular endurance, and power begins with isometric strengthening or high-intensity galvanic stimulation at multiple joint angles. Once a strong isometric contraction can be done at multiple angles, dynamic resistance exercises can be begun within the pain-free range of motion. The rate and resistance of weight training are gradually changed to improve muscular endurance and power. An important point to remember is that regardless of the cost of exercise equipment for strengthening muscles, motivation of the patient is the most important factor in strength training.

Maintenance of Cardiovascular Endurance

Exercises for cardiovascular endurance can also begin early in the rehabilitation program so that the aerobic fitness level can be maintained. Such exercises usually involve continuous muscle activity of large muscles. Examples are jogging, walking, swimming, jumping rope, bicycling, and rowing. Often in upper or lower extremity injuries, athletes can begin bicycling or swimming or other pool activities.

Refinement of Motor Skills

Restoration of skilled activities related to the sport is the next step in rehabilitation, and it can be done only after the athlete has achieved a proper amount of comfort, range of motion, and strength. During the return to the specific sport skills, activities that improve reaction time, speed, balance, and agility should be begun. The ability to move fast and react quickly is often lost after injury because of the failure of the mechanoreceptor feedback as a result of injury, operation, or immobilization. Activities that involve a series of exercises that emphasize regaining proper receptor coordination and muscle recruitment can be done. One example is the use of a tilt board or ankle disk to improve the reaction time of athletes with recurrent ankle injuries. The effectiveness of these methods has not been proved. Another skill that should be considered is balance. Balance activities could include the use of a beam, one-legged stands, and hopping. Also, speed activities that emphasize rapid movement of body parts, rate-of-acceleration running, and maximal running speed can be initiated in this phase of rehabilitation.

Jogging, plyometrics, and agility training are done during the refinement of motor skills. Jogging is usually allowed for athletes with lower extremity injuries who have achieved 80% of their strength in the uninjured leg as measured by Cybex isokinetic testing. Hopping and the use of medicine balls are forms of plyometric training. Plyometric training is based on the assumption that muscles can react more forcefully and quickly from a prestretched position than from a relaxed state. Agility, the ability of the body to change direction rapidly, is a combination of reaction time, speed of movement, coordination, strength, and power. In athletes with lower extremity injuries, agility training is usually begun when about 9% of strength in the injured extremity has been regained. Activities such as figures-of-eight, dodging, jumping rope, zigzags, and shuttle runs can be practiced.

In the final phase of rehabilitation, the athlete begins to perform specific sports activities at a low level and gradually increases their intensity. The athlete who has regained normal strength, endurance, and flexibility and is able to run, jump, and change directions without pain or weakness may return to the sport.

Provision of Psychologic Support

Although not discussed in depth in this chapter, treatment of the psychologic problems of the injured athlete is one of the most important considerations in rehabilitation. Depression is often present in an injured athlete and should be identified early so that the athlete can be counseled and, if necessary, referred for appropriate help. Also, malingerers should be identified and treated properly with psychologic instead of physical rehabilitation. Psychologic difficulties of the injured athlete can be widespread, involving learning, personal, developmental, and social problems. The psychologic preparation of an athlete to return to a sporting event is as important as the retraining of the physical skills.

SPORTS FITNESS

Another new concept in rehabilitation of the injured athlete is the evaluation of sports fitness. Specialists can determine many fitness profiles, including aerobic capacity, flexibility, strength, muscle and body composition, and agility. Measurement of fitness in rehabilitation necessitates establishing normal values in individual athletes, giving objective criteria for returning to sports after an injury, analyzing the physical potential of the athlete in a specific sport, offering guidance and advice on a particular physical weakness or strength, and helping to establish a more objective exercise prescription for the athlete. The accuracy and reliability of current techniques to measure these variables need further scientific investigation.

PREVENTION OF SPORTS INJURIES

Another major aspect in the complete rehabilitation program for an injured athlete is the prevention of sports injuries. Prevention includes correction of improper techniques, attempts to modify or change rules, proper supervision and coaching during preseason training and conditioning, correct training habits, safe equipment, and taping.

SUMMARY

Sports medicine is a rapidly growing area of interest in the field of physical medicine and rehabilitation. Multiple injuries requiring rehabilitation in a steplike manner occur in many sports. Rehabilitation of athletes includes not only the care and treatment of athletic injuries but also sports fitness and prevention of injuries.

REFERENCES

1. Kottke FJ, Stillwell GK, Lehmann JF, eds. Krusen's handbook of physical medicine and rehabilitation. 3rd ed. Philadelphia: WB Saunders, 1982.
2. Warren CG, Lehmann JF, Koblanski JN. Heat and stretch procedures: an evaluation using rat tail tendon. Arch Phys Med Rehabil 1976; 57:122–126.

3. Laughman RK, Youdas JW, Garrett TR, Chao EYS. Strength changes in the normal quadriceps femoris muscle as a result of electrical stimulation. Phys Ther 1983; 63:494–499.
4. Massey BH, Nelson RC, Sharkey BC, Comden T. Effects of high frequency electrical stimulation on the size and strength of skeletal muscle. J Sports Med 1965; 5:136–144.
5. Sanders MT. A comparison of two methods of training on the development of muscular strength and endurance. J Orthop Sports Phys Ther 1980; 1:210–213.

28 GERIATRIC REHABILITATION

Kevin P. Murphy, M.D.
Mehrsheed Sinaki, M.D.

According to US census statistics, the number of Americans older than 65 years has been growing at a rate 3 times faster than that of the general population. In 1950, 12 million people older than 65 years were living in the United States.[1] Currently, approximately 25 million people older than 65 years are living in the United States, and this number will rise to approximately 55 million by the year 2030.[1] This increase is expected because persons born during the baby boom (following the end of World War II) will reach this age by the year 2030. At present, about 5% (1.3 million) of the nation's elderly population resides in nursing homes; by the year 2000, this number is expected to increase by approximately 50%.[1]

As the elderly population increases in number, it will require an increasing proportion of medical care. At present, this group uses more medical services than any other age-group, being hospitalized twice as often and staying in the hospital twice as long.[1] Traditional medical care competently handles, in an increasingly professional manner, the life-and-death matters that contribute to the duration of life. It is a simple fact that sophisticated medical technology and profound medical knowledge have added years to the average human life span.

Rehabilitation medicine has been evolving rapidly since World War II and deals directly with the quality of life. To keep up with the estimated needs of the present and the future, the subspecialty of geriatric rehabilitation is beginning to define itself. Because little has been written about this topic from a physiatric and rehabilitation point of view, we hope this discussion will outline some basic considerations that have become apparent to us. Many of the basic physical medicine and rehabilitation principles for different disease states and for therapeutic exercise have been discussed in previous chapters or apply to patients of all ages and will not be discussed further here. Any rehabilitation plan must first establish the patient's overall general medical condition and subsequently optimize this condition toward obtaining maximal rehabilitation goals and potential.

MEDICAL CONSIDERATIONS

Certain *medical conditions* appear with high frequency in the elderly population and have a considerable effect on the outcomes of rehabilitation.[2] Anemia is prevalent in the elderly population and may explain why a patient is falling short of goals in mobility and therapeutic exercise. Other conditions that can contribute to suboptimal performance are myxedema, occult malignancy, cardiovascular disease, chronic infection, metabolic imbalance, and pulmonary dysfunction. With aging, maximal voluntary ventilation and vital capacity decrease, as do respiratory muscular strength and endurance. These effects contribute significantly to easy fatigue and lowered working capacity.

Nutritional deficits are of major concern also. The basic metabolic rate decreases about 2% per decade in adults, and the average protein requirement remains about 1 g/kg per day throughout life.[3] Calorie requirements remain essentially the same throughout adult life at approximately 1,800 to 2,000 calories per day.[4] Vitamin deficiency in elderly persons is relatively uncommon, probably because of the many over-the-counter supplements available and ample support by the media for increased vitamin intake.[5] Anorexia and subsequent cachexia are common, especially in the presence of chronic disease. Reasons for poor nutrition include restricted mobility and inconvenience for food preparation, loss of appetite, depression, decreased motivation, gastritis and gastroesophageal reflux, dysphagia, poor dentures, and excessive medications. *Polypharmacy* is a common problem in the elderly patient, and it is magnified when the patient does not have the cognitive ability to adhere to a therapeutic medication schedule. The side effects and toxicity of excessive medications are real, limiting, and, at times, deadly.

The effects of *immobility* need some basic consideration. About 3% of muscle strength can be lost per day during complete immobilization.[6] Therefore, an immobilized individual who has marginal mobility and self-care ability can quickly become totally dependent because of loss of muscle strength. Other effects of chronic immobility include contractures, osteoporosis, orthostatic hypotension, reduced cardiac performance and blood volume, negative nitrogen and calcium balance, electrolyte imbalance, urinary tract stones, deep venous thromboses and pulmonary emboli, skin pressure sores, and pulmonary hypoventilation syndromes.[7] No less disabling consequences are those that arise from severe sensory and emotional deprivation, which may lead to increased confusion, depression, and general disorientation.

Skin tolerance to pressure is decreased in the elderly population. This results from atrophy of subcutaneous adipose tissue and possible sensory motor neuropathies.[5] Peripheral edema and venous stasis syndromes also lead to decreased skin tolerance, and pressure sores may easily develop along the hindfoot and medial and lateral malleolar areas. Capillary closing pressure in adults is estimated to be 25 mm Hg and is of consideration when prescribing elastic support garments.[2] In general, over-the-counter elastic stockings provide approximately 10 mm Hg of pressure and, in this capacity, have an optimal effect on the control of peripheral edema only when the patient is supine. The energy expenditure for donning high-pressure elastic garments can be tremendous, and a high level of manual dexterity and eye-hand coordination is required.

Visual and auditory impairment can be tremendously disabling to the elderly patient and is often mistaken for depression, poor cooperation, cognitive dysfunction, hostility, and speech impairment. A cataract in a patient with severe loss of distal proprioception can be exceptionally disabling because visual feedback to correct for the loss of joint position is inadequate. In such a patient, removal of the cataract may allow independent living and a maximal quality of life. In an amputee who is visually impaired, a prosthetic lower extremity may provide more sensory-motor feedback, distal proprioception, and thus more self-independence than if a wheelchair were used. An observation that cannot be overemphasized is that a minor illness in elderly patients can, and often does, lead to much more serious complications. For example, an equinous deformity at the ankle can lead to metatarsalgia and antalgic gait and be compounded by inappropriate footwear, gait aids, and therapeutic exercise. A result from this can be a fall in which a hip is broken with subsequent death occurring from pulmonary embolism. Similar cases can result from all aspects of suboptimal medical and rehabilitation care.

NEUROMUSCULAR-SKELETAL CONSIDERATIONS

Therapeutic exercise in the elderly population has some special considerations. Both anaerobic and aerobic programs need assessment if the physical and cardiopulmonary limitations mentioned above are present. Stationary bicycling, swimming, and daily walking can be excellent aerobic and general mobility programs. An aerobic workout for 20 minutes three times a week that does not exceed 60% to 80% of the maximal heart rate, with appropriate warm-up and cool-down periods, may be optimal but certainly must be individualized carefully.[8] Isometric exercises, in contrast to an isotonic strengthening program, seem to demand more from the cardiovascular system because a steady equilibrium state is not achieved.[9] Deep-breathing exercises and postural drainage techniques may be especially important in a patient with chronic pulmonary disease. Appropriate shoe modification to allow comfort while walking may allow a patient to remain active and well conditioned. For less mobile, bedridden patients, bimanual activities can be used for both anaerobic and aerobic conditioning. The perceived scale of exertion can be helpful for discerning the limitations of the aerobic exercise program. According to Müller,[6] one 6-second isometric contraction per day per muscle group can be enough to ward off the daily 3% decline in muscle strength that results from complete immobilization.

Neuromuscular reeducation and relaxation techniques, including biofeedback, may be limited in elderly patients with mild-to-moderate cognitive dysfunction and senile dementia. Stretching exercises should be done with care because of a probable decrease in the tensile strength of the soft tissue masses. Daily range-of-motion exercises and stretching by simple techniques are especially important for preventing contracture formation and further limited mobility (Fig. 28-1 and 28-2). The simple knee or hip flexion-contracture can create a significant leg-length discrepancy or flexed

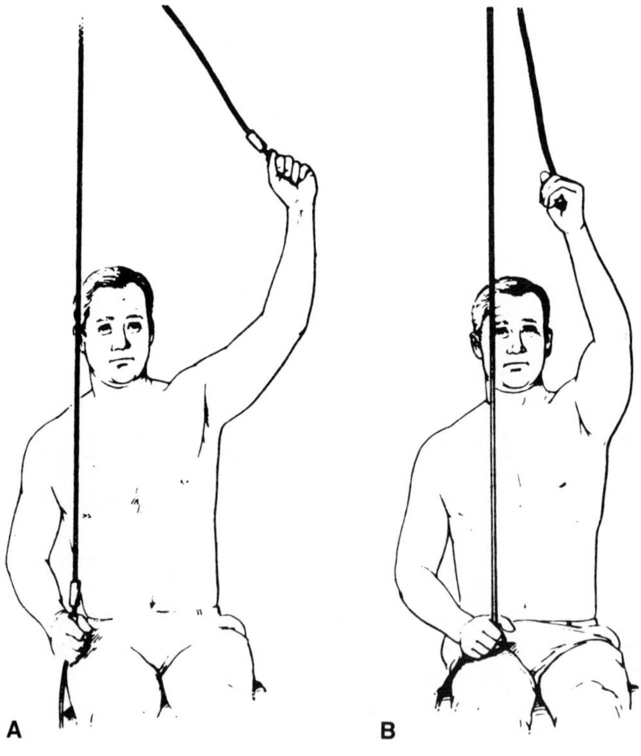

A B

Figure 28–1 Range-of-motion exercises for shoulders, with pulley. *A*, Abduction. *B*, Flexion.

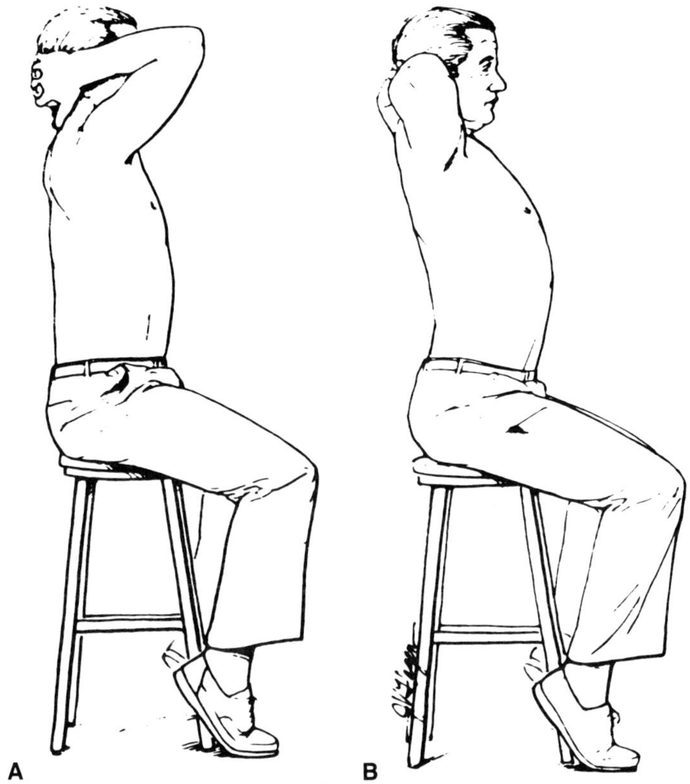

Figure 28–2 *A*, Shoulder abduction and external rotation combined with pectoral stretching. *B*, Deep-breathing combined with pectoral stretching to prevent stooped posture.

posture during the gait cycle. This may increase the energy consumption of walking above the physiologic tolerance of the patient and result in falling, cessation of gait, and the subsequent sequelae of trauma and immobilization. Simple techniques in the supine or upright posture for stretching hip and knee flexors and the pectoral muscles can be of great benefit for avoiding these problems (Fig. 28-3 through 28-5). In the presence of weakness and ataxia, stretching while in the supine position is preferred. In any therapeutic exercise program, especially in elderly patients, the work-rest cycle needs to be optimal.

Use of physical methods in the elderly population demands appropriate understanding of the contraindications. In general, microwave and shortwave methods are contraindicated in the presence of joint arthroplasties, cardiac pacemakers, insensate regions of the body, areas of poor arterial perfusion, and areas of malignancy.[10] Therapeutic electricity can also be contraindicated

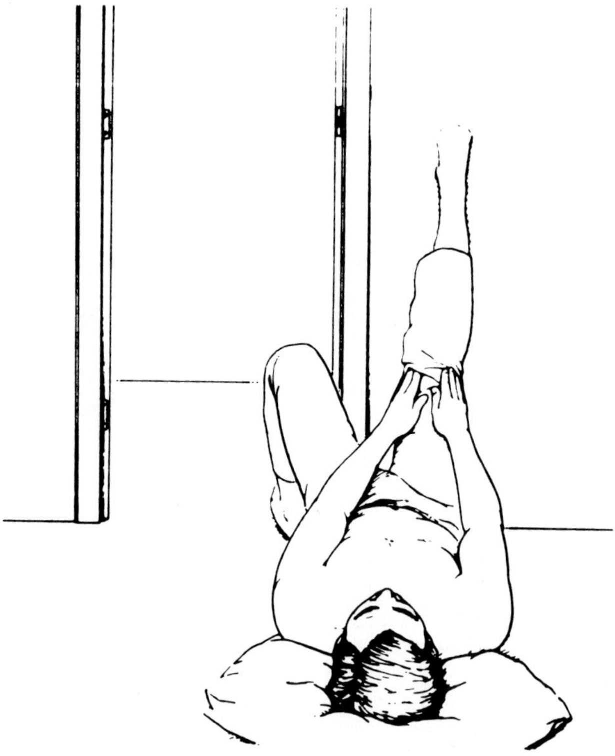

Figure 28–3 Stretching hamstrings while in supine (resting) position. This technique can be applied in the presence of ataxia and poor coordination.

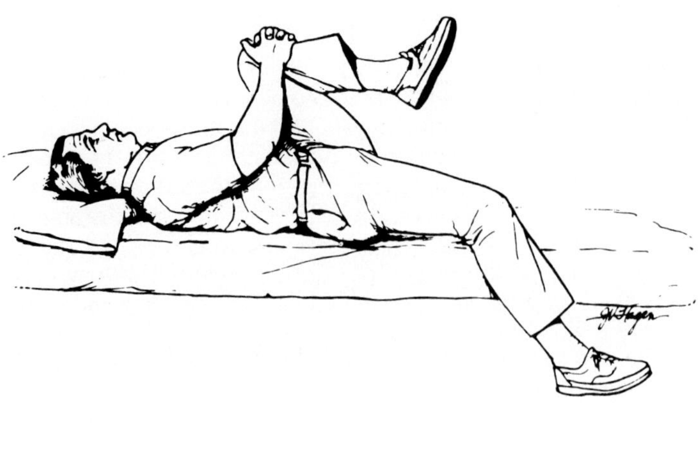

Figure 28–4 Simple technique for stretching hip flexors.

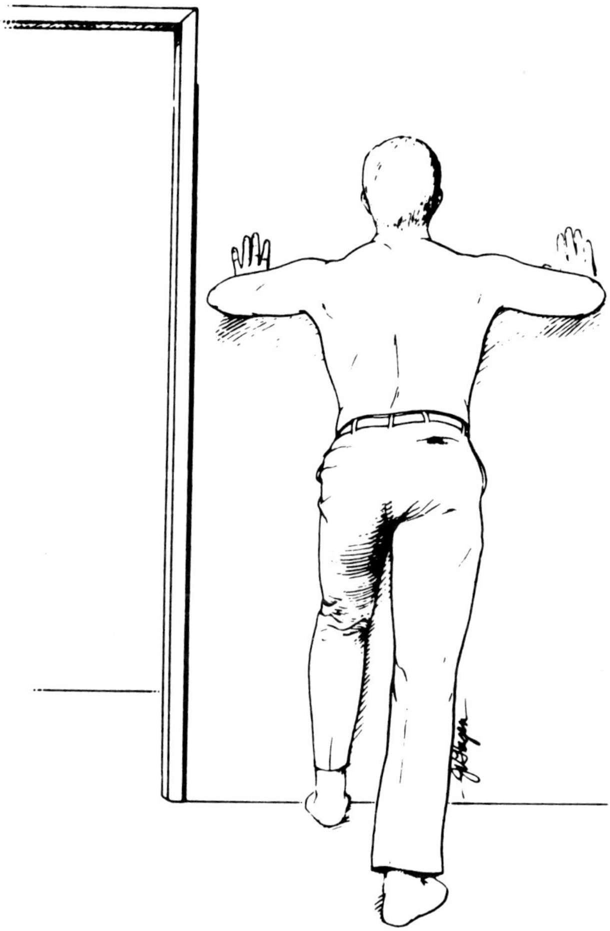

Figure 28–5 Method of stretching hamstring and pectoral muscles in ambulatory patients.

in patients with cardiac disorders or pacemakers.[10] Use of cold therapy can trigger Raynaud's phenomenon and cryoglobulinemia.[10]

Osteoporotic patients—particularly postmenopausal women—need special consideration for therapeutic exercise and protective spinal bracing. Vertebral compression fractures are common in osteoporosis and can be an extreme cause of limitation and chronic pain. Evidence suggests that spinal extension and isometric exercises are most appropriate for patients with postmenopausal osteoporosis to ward off vertebral compression fractures.[11] If osteoporosis is severe, bone mineral density should be ascertained and possible medical treatments should be evaluated. Degenerative joint disease and rheumatoid arthritis are discussed in Chapter 24.

MOBILITY

Mobility in the geriatric population varies from playing tennis and mountain climbing to being wheelchair-bound because of degenerative joint disease.

In general, approximately 70% of nursing home residents have some form of restricted mobility, which varies from needing a cane or a wheelchair to being bedridden.[1] Mobility is certainly one of the most important factors used to determine whether institutional care is needed for an elderly patient. A comprehensive rehabilitation program is probably the best way to assess and perpetuate functional mobility. An important part of this program is the therapeutic principles of exercise mentioned above, including contracture-free range of motion, strengthening, posture principles, coordination routines, appropriate footwear modification, gait-aid assessment, and a functional prescription for the amputee.

Significant consideration must be given to energy expenditure and the various forms of gait aids that are available. In general, crutch walking consumes about 70% more energy than the normal gait pattern.[12] According to most studies, wheelchair mobility on level ground increases the energy expenditure by only 7% to 10%.[12] Foremost in any consideration of mobility in the elderly population should be the idea of safety over function. This is of utmost importance to prevent trauma such as fractured hips and chronic subdural hematomas. Architectural barriers, such as stairs, curbs, carpet, and tile, need special consideration.

One basic and often forgotten consideration in all age-groups, especially the elderly, is the value of transfer ability. The ability to perform independent transfers or transfers with minimal assistance may allow the patient to be placed in a low- rather than high-nursing-skill unit with subsequent improvement in the quality of life. The ability to transfer into and out of a chair or onto or off a commode is basic and simple, yet it is commonly overlooked in a patient's overall care. The idea of achieving such small gains in ability with the help of a rehabilitation program, resulting in tremendous differences in degrees of independence, needs to be conveyed to the medical community as a whole. Safety, in regard to mobility, in patients receiving anticoagulants is often overlooked, and the result can be a life-threatening situation. Mobility may be limited in patients with normal neuromuscular function who have significant cognitive, visual, or perceptual dysfunctions.

ACTIVITIES OF DAILY LIVING

The activities of daily living are of prime importance in determining an independent living status in elderly patients. Dysphagia of multiple causes and a comprehensive swallowing evaluation with clear liquids and various food substances may be important considerations. For the evaluation of dressing ability, energy conservation techniques need attention, as do practical time limits for dressing and undressing. A metal razor blade may be too dangerous for shaving in some patients, especially those who have significant cognitive dysfunction or have been receiving anticoagulants for a long time. A detailed occupational assessment must include household duties, vocational and avocational interests, and safety and judgment evaluations. For example, a patient who leaves a burner ignited on a stove after finishing a meal has poor safety habits and judgment ability, as does a senile, visually impaired carpenter who continues to use power tools and electric saws. A patient's ability to gain access to an emergency care system must also be assessed. This assessment involves evaluating the ability to dial the "911" emergency telephone number or the telephone number of a hospital facility, neighbor, or friend.

Toileting ability is an important determinant of quality of life, regardless of age-group. A good bowel program with a high-fiber diet, psyllium hydrophilic mucilloid (Metamucil) (twice a day), adequate fluids, and every-other-day use of rectal suppositories may prevent unwanted intestinal ileus and provide for predictable bowel evacuation. Many nursing homes do not provide assistance with intermittent catheterization schedules; thus, long-term indwelling catheters are relatively common in nursing home residents. Antibiotic suppression is contraindicated in such cases because of the possibility for developing resistant urinary tract infections.[13] Most therapy plans recommend changing the catheter every 2 to 3 weeks in addition to urinalysis, Gram stain, and culture. If the urine becomes cloudy or fever, catheter leakage, unexplained leukocyte elevation, or dysuria develops, the catheter may need to be changed and the urine cultured.

PSYCHIATRIC CONSIDERATIONS

More than 50% of nursing home residents are estimated to have some form of senile dementia, mostly Alzheimer's type.[1] These persons need to be differentiated from delirious patients whose conditions may be secondary to medications or an abnormal metabolic state and usually follow a more acute to subacute time course. Depression can masquerade as several somatic complaints, including chronic pain, absentmindedness, anorexia with weight loss, and insomnia. Antidepressant medications may be of benefit in patients with strong vegetative symptoms, and their anticholinergic side effects need consideration. A patient with chronic pain behavior may respond better to an approach that involves controlled use of analgesics and measures of behavior modification. In a proper environment, one can decrease the use of analgesics in an organized fashion through substitution with other physical measures. Codeine should not be used as an analgesic in order to avoid the problem of constipation, which is common in elderly persons.

Communication disorders, including apraxias and dysphasias, can make it difficult to determine the degree of cognitive impairment that is present. Most psychometric evaluations demand some recognition of objects or the written or spoken word. General orientation to place and environment, carry-over from day to day of various activities, and following one- or two-step simple commands are probably the most basic abilities needed for an effective cognitive retraining program. The use of cognitive stimulation with both auditory and visual agents can be an effective way of maintaining arousal and improving psychomotor activity. Motivation, a quality that transcends psychiatric doctrines, is certainly a key element in achieving rehabilitation goals and potential. Many times there is an organic explanation for a poorly motivated patient, and a change in medication or the establishment of hormonal or electrolyte balance may provide the needed impetus for progressive rehabilitation gains. A patient with mental confusion who also has an ataxic gait and incontinence should be evaluated for the possibility of normal-pressure hydrocephalus or for cerebral mass lesions.

Elderly patients can be difficult to teach because they may think they are "too old to learn." Some of them may be resistant to change or have a significant fear of failure. The role of a rehabilitation psychologist as a member of the rehabilitation team cannot be overemphasized. Further considerations include discussions about death and dying and the practice of sexuality. Many older people are sexually active, and almost all need and want some form of companionship. More centers are beginning to realize this need for companionship in the long-term care of elderly persons and are allowing for quiet areas where married couples can spend time with each other.

SOCIAL CONSIDERATIONS

The degree of family support is probably the sole most important ingredient in determining whether an elderly patient can live safely outside of a nursing home.[14] Other factors in this decision process were mentioned above and have various degrees of importance. Community assistance and home health aids, including public health nurses, can be of major importance in providing a safe disposition for elderly patients. Numerous senior citizen living centers with a registered nurse on call 24 hours a day are providing a heightened quality of life for many elderly people throughout the United States. Further growth in these institutions is hoped for in order to accommodate the estimated needs of the 21st century.

Driving ability is of major importance when assessing the overall independence of an elderly patient, and it is often a most difficult area to discuss when the results of the evaluation are negative. Senior citizen bus passes, discount cab rates, and institutional shuttles can significantly relieve this transportation void. The feelings of loneliness, desperation, and isolation are heightened tremendously by the inability to operate a motor vehicle. Alternatively, the operation of a motor vehicle by an unsafe, cognitively impaired driver, regardless of age, is a major cause of morbidity and mortality throughout the world.

Disposition is a family decision in which the patient actively participates whenever reasonable cognitive capacity exists. Various forms of voluntary employment exist both within and outside institutional care homes and may fulfill a heightened need in some patients. Avocational considerations need to be addressed, and hobbies and various leisure activities need to be pursued for as long as is reasonably possible. At some point, modifications in past hobbies and leisure activities by a competent recreational therapist or concerned medical care provider can help patients find increased avocational satisfaction. Occasional trips outside the living environment and being part of the mainstream of society can be a most valuable therapeutic intervention. Variance in care, geographic location, and patient and family preference are important variables when choosing among various nursing home options.

CONCLUSION

The standard rehabilitation care is of benefit to the geriatric population when the patients to be treated show no significant degree of mental impairment. Such techniques are of unclear benefit to those with a mild degree of mental impairment and are without benefit to those with a severe degree of mental impairment.[15] Patients with significant dementia should be treated in programs specifically designed for them rather than in the usual rehabilitation programs. Other variables, as discussed above, must also be considered when deciding on a patient's rehabilitation potential and the optimal use of rehabilitation facilities and professionals. Almost all severely disabled persons can benefit in some small way from a comprehensive individualized rehabilitation program. Also, because of the limited time and resources available, selection of the most appropriate candidates for rehabilitation is a much needed and difficult area of decision making. As a part of this decision-making process, the trained medical professional must summate the "cumulative disability" of a patient in the hope of setting realistic goals and limitations. At the present time, the economic cost of chronic disability and dependence seems to be much higher than the monetary cost of a successful rehabilitation program.[16] Certainly of more importance than the monetary gains are the heightened levels of satisfaction and quality of life that come with independence in living.

REFERENCES

1. DDHS Publication No. (OHDS) 81-20704. "The need for long term care: a chartbook on the federal council on aging." Section I (numbers), and Section III (utilization).

2. Petersdorf RG, Adams RD, Braunwald E, Isselbacher KJ, Martin JB, Wilson JD. Harrison's principles of internal medicine. 10th ed. New York: McGraw-Hill, 1983.
3. Robinson CH, Lawler MR, Chenoweth WL, Garwick AE. Normal and therapeutic nutrition. 17th ed. New York: Macmillan Publishing, 1986.
4. Blackburn GL, Bistrian BR, Maini BS, Schlamm HT, Smith MF. Nutritional and metabolic assessment of the hospitalized patient. JPEN J Parenter Enteral Nutr 1977; 1:11-22.
5. Andres R, Bierman EL, Hazzard WR. Principles of geriatric medicine. New York: McGraw-Hill, 1985.
6. Müller EA. Influence of training and of inactivity on muscle strength. Arch Phys Med Rehabil 1970; 51:449–462.
7. Kottke FJ. The effects of limitation of activity upon the human body. JAMA 1966; 196:825-830.
8. American Heart Association. The Committee on Exercise. Kattus AA, Chairman. Exercise testing and training of individuals with heart disease or at high risk for its development: a handbook for physicians, 1975.
9. Fardy PS. Isometric exercise and the cardiovascular system. Physician Sportsmedicine Sept 1981; 9:43-56.
10. Kottke FJ, Stillwell GK, Lehmann JF. Krusen's handbook of physical medicine and rehabilitation. 3rd ed. Philadelphia: WB Saunders, 1982.
11. Sinaki M, Mikkelsen BA. Postmenopausal spinal osteoporosis: flexion versus extension exercises. Arch Phys Med Rehabil 1984; 65:593-596.
12. Fisher SV, Gullickson G Jr. Energy cost of ambulation in health and disability: a literature review. Arch Phys Med Rehabil 1978; 59:124-133.
13. Merritt JL. Urinary tract infections, causes and management, with particular reference to the patient with spinal cord injury: a review. Arch Phys Med Rehabil 1976; 57:365-373.
14. Lehmann JF, DeLateur BJ, Fowler RS Jr, et al. Stroke rehabilitation: outcome and prediction. Arch Phys Med Rehabil 1975; 56:383-389.
15. Schuman JE, Beattie EJ, Steed DA, Merry GM, Kraus AS. Geriatric patients with and without intellectual dysfunction: effectiveness of a standard rehabilitation program. Arch Phys Med Rehabil 1981; 62:612-618.
16. Lehmann JF, DeLateur BJ, Fowler RS Jr, et al. Stroke: does rehabilitation affect outcome? Arch Phys Med Rehabil 1975; 56:375-382.

INDEX

Note: Page numbers followed by (t) indicate tables; those followed by (f) indicate figures.

A

Abacteriuria, bladder retraining and, 196
Activities of daily living, 4
  elderly patients and, 272–273
Adjustment disorder, diagnostic criteria (DSM-III) for, 14–15t
Adjustment reaction, 16
Aerobic programs, for elderly population, 267
Age, as factor in brain injury outcome, 117
Agitation, causes of, 120
  after traumatic brain injury, 120
Alcohol abuse, 17–18
Alzheimer's type senile dementia, 273
Ambulation, assisting in, in primary muscle disease, 139
  in cerebral palsy, 129, 129f, 130f
  lower extremity in, 82–83, 82f
  upper extremity in, 83–84
Ambulatory activities, after stroke, 110, 110f
Ambulatory aids. *See* Gait aids
American Psychiatric Association, *Diagnostic and Statistical Manual of Mental Disorders*, 12, 14–15t
Amnesia, posttraumatic, as factor in brain injury outcome, 117
Amputation(s), above-elbow, prostheses for, 89, 89f
  above-knee, prostheses for, 86, 86f
  below-elbow, prostheses for, 88, 88f
  below-knee, prostheses for, 84–85, 85f
  in congenital limb deficiency, 81
  in disease, 80–81
  "major", definition of, 80
  management after, 92–94
  management before, 92
  in trauma, 81
  in tumor, 81
  vascular disease-associated, prevention of, 94
Amyotrophic lateral sclerosis, 153–163
  epidemiology and incidence of, 154
  exercise and rehabilitation programs in, 156t
  laboratory data in, 154–155
  symptomatic treatment in, 155–157, 157–162f, 163, 163t
  symptoms and signs of, 154
Analgesia, electrical stimulation for, 68–69
  local heating for, 63, 64f
Anemia, in elderly population, 266
Ankle, extension and flexion, 59f
  orthosis to support, 90, 111f
Ankle disk, 262
Ankylosing spondylitis, 238–239, 238f
  back pain in, 213
Anorexia, in elderly population, 266
Anosognosia, 16
  after stroke, 111
Antalgic list, in lumbar disk problems, 208
Anti-inflammatory drugs, in tension myalgia, 248
Antibiotics, in lymphedema, 98
Anticholinergic therapy, in multiple sclerosis, 179–180
Anticoagulation, in spinal cord injury, 186–187
Anticonvulsant medications, in thalamic pain of stroke, 109
Antidepressants, 19–20
  in tension myalgia, 248
Anxiety, in disability, 13
Aphasia, after stroke, 107
Apraxia, in elderly, 274
Architectural barriers, elderly population and, 272
Arthritis, 225–238
  rheumatoid. *See* Rheumatoid arthritis

types of, 225
Arthrograms, 33f
Aspiration pneumonia, in cerebral palsy, 128
Assessment, standardized, of psychologic functioning, 19
Assistive devices, in rheumatoid arthritis, 236f, 237f
Ataxia(s), 73
in multiple sclerosis, 178
Atelectasis, electrical stimulation in, 69
pulmonary, after stroke, 107
Athletic rehabilitation, 251–264
Autotopagnosia, 16

B

Back, sports injuries to, 252, 252t
Back pain, emotional factors in, 212
in facet syndrome, 212
low, mechanical, 210, 212
in lumbar disk problems, 207–210
in osteoporosis, 217–218 219f, 220, 220f, 220t, 221–222f
rest and, 212–213
Back support, in spinal osteoporosis, 218, 219–220f
Baclofen, in multiple sclerosis, 177
Balance, impaired, gait impairment in, 71, 72–73
Baths, contrast, in rheumatoid arthritis, 235, 235f
in sports injuries, 255
Beck's cognitive-behavioral therapy, in depression, 20
Behavior modification, in cerebral palsy, 134
for elderly, 273
Biofeedback, electromyographic, in athletic injuries, 257
in tension myalgia, 248, 249
training, in multiple sclerosis, 178
Bladder, dysfunction, areflexic detrusor and external sphincter, 202–204, 202f, 203f
hyperreflexic, dyssynergic, bladder retraining in, 201–202, 201f
uninhibited neurogenic, bladder retraining in, 199–201
function, in traumatic brain injury, 119
neurogenic, in stroke, 106t
problems, in multiple sclerosis, 179–180
psychogenic, in tension myalgia, 248
Bladder retraining, contraindications to, 195
goals of, 194
indications for, 194–195
program for, 198, 199f, 200f
results of, 204, 205t
in specific dysfunctions, 199–204, 201f, 202f, 203f
team approach in, 195
workup for, 195–198
Blood circulation, in tendinitis, 39f
Blunt trauma, in sports injuries, 251
Bobath digital spreader, in hemiplegia, 112
Bobath shoulder slings, 161f
Bobath sling, 112, 112f
Bobath therapy, in cerebral palsy, 132
Bone reconstructions, in cerebral palsy, 133
Bone, loss. *See* Osteoporosis
Bony landmarks, 61–62
Bony overgrowth, phantom pain in, 94
Bowel, care of, after stroke, 104, 106
dysfunction, in multiple sclerosis, 180
function, in traumatic brain injury, 119
in spinal cord injury, 188
Bowel program, for elderly population, 273
Brachial plexus injury, after stroke, 108
Bracing, in amyotrophic lateral sclerosis, 157f, 158f, 159f, 160f, 161f, 162f
in cerebral palsy, 132
in primary muscle disease, 139–140
in spinal osteoporosis, 218, 220f
Bradykinesia, in parkinsonism, 167, 167t, 171
Brain injury, bladder dysfunction in, 199–201
psychotic episodes after, 12
traumatic, 116–123
as silent epidemic, 116
complications of, 119
incidence of disability after, 116f
management in, 119–120
predicting outcome of, 117–118
prevention of, 117
Brainstem, involvement, in amyotrophic lateral sclerosis, 155
Brainstem reticular nuclei, activation of, 68
Breathing difficulty, in amyotrophic lateral sclerosis, 155, 157
Breech delivery, cerebral palsy in, 125

Bulbar palsy, progressive, 153
juvenile, of Fazio-Londe, 153
Bursitis, pain in, 37–39

C

Cachexia, in elderly population, 266
Calcium, absorption, osteoporosis and, 215
Cane(s), 74–75, 75f, 76f
Capsular distention, limitation of motion in, 32
Carbidopa-levodopa, in parkinsonism, 169–170
Cardiomyopathy, in acute polymyositis, 145
Carpal bones, as bony landmarks for goniometry, 61
Casting, in cerebral palsy, 132
Catheter(s), indwelling, for elderly, 273
in spinal cord injury, 187–188
Catheterization, intermittent, in spinal cord injury, 188
Cerebral palsy, 124–134
ataxic, 125, 126
atonic, 126
behavior modification in, 134
bracing in, 132
classification of, 125–128
defects in, 124
description of, 124
diagnosis of, 128
drug therapy in, 133
dyskinesis type, 125, 126
etiology of, 125, 127–128
examination in, 128
gait impairment in, 72
hyperkinesis type, 125, 126
incidence and prevalence of, 124
medical problems associated with, 128–129
mixed type, 125, 126
morbidity associated with, programs decreasing, 124
motion abnormalities in, 125
operative procedures in, 133
parents and therapy in, 133–134
persistent problems in, 132
pseudobulbar-type, 126
severity of involvement in, 127
sites of involvement in, 126
spastic, 125
splinting in, 132–133
symptoms of, 125–126
treatment of, 131–132
aims of, 129–130
Cervical collar, 161f, 162f
Cesarean section, cerebral palsy and, 125
Chemical dependency, 17–18
Circulation, in tendinitis, 39f
Clavicle, as bony landmark for goniometry, 61
Claw-hand deformity, splints in, 160f
Clinical evaluation, outline of, 5–9
CMG/EMG, bladder retraining and, 196–198
Co-contraction, in hand injury, 244
Cognitive and perceptual dysfunction, after traumatic brain injury, 121
Cognitive-behavioral therapy, in depression, 20
Cognitive impairment, 17
Cognitive rehabilitation, after traumatic brain injury, 120
Cold and heat, therapeutic, 63–66
Cold therapy. *See* Cooling, local
Coma, duration of, as factor in brain injury outcome, 117
Coma scale, Glasgow, 118, 118t
Communication, in cerebral palsy, 129, 131f
Compression pump, pneumatic, intermittent-phase, in athletic injuries, 255, 255f
Conditioning methods, inappropriate for elderly, 268, 269
Conductive cooling, 65–66
Conductive heating, 64
Constipation, in parkinsonism, 168
Contracture(s), capsular, 32
goniometry in, 41
intramuscular, 32
joint, in rheumatoid arthritis, 228–230, 229f
ligamentous, 32
limitation of motion in, 32
in neuropathic disease, 150
prevention of, in acute polymyositis, 146
in cerebral palsy, 130
orthoses for, 90
in primary muscle disease, 138
Contrast bath therapy, in athletic injuries, 255
Convective cooling, 66
Convective heating, 64–65
Conversion heating, 65
Cooling, local, in athletic injuries, 254
contraindications to, 65
indications for, 65
methods of, 65–66
in multiple sclerosis, 177
in neuropathic disease, 149–150
physiologic effects of, 65
in primary muscle disease, 137–138
Coordination, impaired, gait impairment in, 71, 72–73

Corticosteroids, in athletic injuries, 256
in multiple sclerosis, 180
Cranial nerves, examination of, 8
Credé maneuver, in bladder retraining, 202–204, 203f
in multiple sclerosis, 180
Crepitations, 34
Crutch gaits, for disorders involving one leg, 78
for two affected limbs, 78–79
Crutches, 75, 75f
Cybex isokinetic dynamometer, 259–260, 260f

D

Decubital ulcers, in multiple sclerosis, 179
Deltoid aid, after stroke, 109, 109f
Dementia, in parkinsonism, 169
senile, 273
Demyelination, in multiple sclerosis, 176
Denial, 16–17
Depression, 12–13
in amyotrophic lateral sclerosis, 163
as somatic complaint, in elderly, 273
in athletic injuries, 263
major, diagnostic criteria (DSM-III) for, 12–13, 14–15t
in multiple sclerosis, 178
in parkinsonism, 169
treatment of, 19–20
Dermatome(s), 182, 183f
Dermatomyositis, 144
Diagnosis(es), 9–11
Diagnostic criteria (DSM-III), for major depressive episodes, dysthymic disorder, and adjustment disorder, 12–13, 14–15t
Diazepam, in multiple sclerosis, 177
Dietary deficiencies, osteoporosis and, 215
Dietary therapy, in spinal osteoporosis, 223–224
Diplegia, in cerebral palsy, 126
Disability(ies), 240–245
anxiety in, 13–15
assessment of, 19
permanence of, minimizing of, 17
phobias in, 13
psychologic aspects of, 12–21
psychologic sequelae of, 12–19
sexuality and, 22–29
treatment of, 19–20
Type I, 24–25
Type II, 25
Type III, 25
Type IV, 25
Disk, "hard", neck pain in, 213
Disk pain, 208, 209
Disorientation, in elderly population, 266
Disuse, in hand injury, 244
Diuretics, in lymphedema, 98
Doppler studies, in spinal cord injury, 186
Dressing ability, of elderly population, assessment of, 272–273
Driving, by elderly, 274–275
Drooling, in cerebral palsy, 133
Drug(s), causing osteoporosis, 215
Dysarthria, after stroke, 106
in amyotropic lateral sclerosis, 154
in multiple sclerosis, 178
Dyskinesias, in cerebral palsy, 126
Dysphagia, in amyotrophic lateral sclerosis, 154
in elderly population, 272
in primary muscle disease, 142
Dysphonia, in amyotrophic lateral sclerosis, 157
Dyssynergia, detrusor-external sphincter, in multiple sclerosis, 180
Dysthymic disorder, diagnostic criteria (DSM-III) for, 12–13, 14–15t

E

Edema, in hand injury, 240–241
Education, in rheumatoid arthritis, 235–237
Elastic support, in lymphedema, 99, 100
Elbow, flexion and hyperextension, 43f
injuries, in sports, 253
Electrical stimulation, in athletic injuries, 256, 256f, 258f, 259f,
in hand injury, 244
Electricity, therapeutic, 67–70
in denervated muscle, 68
indications for, 67–68
in intact nerve supply, 67–68
Electroejaculations, 67
Electrolyte balance, establishing, in elderly, 274
Electromagnetic radiation, 65
Electromyographic biofeedback, in hand injury, 244
Electrotherapy, in athletic injuries, 256, 256f
Elevation, in lymphedema, 98
Emotional factors, in back pain, 212
Emotional lability, prevention of,

after stroke, 106
Endorphin system, activation of, 68, 69
Epicondylitis, lateral, 39
Equilibrium reactions, restoration of, after stroke, 107–108
Erections, psychogenic, in spinal cord injury, 26
reflexogenic, in spinal cord injury, 26
Estrogen deficiency, osteoporosis and, 215
Ethyl chloride, for local cooling, 66
Euphoria, in multiple sclerosis, 178
Evaluation, clinical, outline of, 5–9
history taking and, 4–11
Evaporation, as local cooling method, 66
Examination, physical, 7
Exercise(s), in acute polymyositis, 146–147
in amyotrophic lateral sclerosis, 156t
in ankylosing spondylitis, 221f–222f, 239
in athletic injuries, 257–261
in cerebral palsy, 130
for elderly population, 267–269, 271, 268f–271f
extension, in spinal osteoporosis, 220, 221f–222f
in hand injury, 242
in lymphedema, 99
mat, after stroke, 107–108
in multiple sclerosis, 177–178, 179
neck pain, 213
in neuropathic disease, 151
in osteoporosis, 271
in parkinsonism, 170–171, 170t
in primary muscle disease, 138
range-of-motion, after stroke, 104
rheumatoid arthritis, 228–234, 231f, 232f
in spinal osteoporosis, 223
Extroversion, 18–19

F

Facet syndrome, back pain in, 212
Family history, past, 6
Family reactions, after disability, 19
Fatigue, in multiple sclerosis, 177–178
Fecal impaction, prevention of, after stroke, 106
Femur, as bony landmark for goniometry, 61
[125I] Fibrinogen uptake scanning, in spinal cord injury, 186
Fibromyalgia. *See* Tension myalgia
Fibromyositis. *See* Tension myalgia
Fibrositis. *See* Tension myalgia
Fibula, as bony landmark for goniometry, 62
Finger(s), extension of, 51f
flexion of, 50f
Flail shoulder, prevention of overstretch of, after stroke, 103
Fluid intake, in spinal cord injury, 188
Foot, hind part of, motion of, 60f
orthosis to support, 90, 111f
Forearm, pronation and supination, 44f
Fracture, gait impairment in, 72
Functional abilities, assessment of, 5t

G

Gait, antalgic, 71, 73–74, 73t
assessment of, 10
impairment(s), conditions associated with, 71–73
Gait aids, 71–79
categories of, 74–77, 75f–77f
energy expenditure with, 272
evaluation of assets and impairment of patient for, 74
in neuropathic disease, 151
prescriptions for, 79, 79t
in rheumatoid arthritis, 237
selection of, 74–77
Gait cycle, human, 82–83, 82f
Gait training, after stroke, 110
in parkinsonism, 172
Galvanic stimulation, high-voltage, 69
Geriatric population, growth in, 265
Geriatric rehabilitation, 265–276
activities of daily living and, 272–273
medical considerations in, 266–267
mobility in, 272
neuromuscular considerations in, 267–271
social considerations in, 274–275
Glasgow coma scale, 118, 118t
Goniometer, 41, 42f
Goniometry, principles of, 40–41, 42f–60f
Grief, resolution of, 20
Grief reactions, 16
Guillain-Barré syndrome, 149, 151
treatment of, 151–152
Gutter splint, 113f

H

Hand, injury(ies), as devastating, 240
complications of, and treatment of, 240–244, 241t

muscle reeducation after, 244–245
in sports, 253
joints of, 45f
prosthetic, 87–88
rehabilitation, conditions needing, 240
rheumatoid, deformities of, 232–233, 233f
exercises for, 232
"intrinsic plus", 232, 233
Hand cone, in hemiplegia, 112
Hanging-arm syndrome, slings in, 161f
Head, sports injuries to, 252, 252t
trauma, cerebral palsy in, 127–128
Hearing, in elderly population, 267
Heat and cold, therapeutic, 63–66
Heating, local, contraindications to, 64
and deep, in athletic injuries, 255
in hand injury, 241
indications for, 64
methods of, 64–65
in neck pain, 213
in neuropathic disease, 149–150
physiologic effects of, 63, 64f
in primary muscle disease, 137–138
in rheumatoid arthritis, 234f, 234–235
in stroke, 108
Heating pad, electric, 64
Hemarthrosis, limitation of motion in, 32–33
Hemianopia, homonymous, after stroke, 111
Hemihook harness, 113f
Hemiplegia, in cerebral palsy, 126
Hemiplegic shoulder-hand syndrome, after stroke, 108
treatment of, 103f–104f, 108, 108f
Hemorrhage, in stroke, 101
Heparin, in acute polymyositis, 146
subcutaneous, after stroke, 107
Hip, abduction and adduction, 57f
disarticulation of, prostheses for, 87, 87f
extension, 55f
flexion, 54f
rotation, 56f
History, family, past, 6
medical, past, 6
History taking, assessment of functional abilities in, 5t
and evaluation, 4–11
Home health aids, for elderly, 274
Hooks, prosthetic, 87–88
Hopping, in athletic injuries, 262
Hot water bottle, 64
Humerus, as bony landmark for goniometry, 61
Hydrocephalus, mental confusion in, 274
Hydrotherapy, in acute polymyositis, 144
"Hyperextension", 41
Hyperkinesis, in cerebral palsy, 126
Hyperreflexia, in amyotrophic lateral sclerosis, 157
autonomic, in spinal cord injury, 188–189
Hypertension, stroke in, 101–102
Hypotension, orthostatic, in parkinsonism, 168
in spinal cord injury, 189–190

I

Ileus, electrical stimulation in, 69
Immobility, in elderly population, 266
in neuropathic disease, 150–151
Immobilization, osteoporosis and, 216–217
Immunologic abnormality, in multiple sclerosis, 175
Incontinence, electrical stimulation in, 67
Inflammatory diseases, gait impairment in, 72
Injections, in athletic injuries, 256
Interferential therapy, 69
Intimacy, 24
Isokinetics, in athletic injuries, 259
Isometric resistance, 31
Isotoner glove, in hemiplegia, 112

J

Jogging, in athletic injuries, 262
"Joint play", 34–35, 35f
Joint(s). *See also specific joints*
disease, degenerative, 33
evaluation, in arthritis, 225
examination of, 30–62
methodical, 30–31
recording chart for, 35–37, 36f
"right first rule" and, 31
inflammation, in rheumatoid arthritis, 225
mobilization, in hand injury, 242
motion. *See* Motion(s)

K

Kin-Com kinetic machine, 260, 261f
Knee, abduction and adduction, 59f
flexion and hyperextension, 58f
orthosis to support, 90

Kugelberg-Welander disease, 153
Kyphotic posture, complications of, 222–223

L

Language problems, after stroke, 107
Lapboard, 114,
Laplace, law of, 99
Levodopa, in parkinsonism, 169–170
Lhermitte's phenomenon, in multiple sclerosis, 176
Loebl measurements, 38f
Loose bodies, intra-articular, limitation of motion in, 32
Lumbar disk problems, back pain in, 207–210
Lungs, in spinal cord injury, 185–186
Lymph, production of, 96
 removal of, 97
Lymphedema, 96–100
 edema fluid in, control of, elastic support in, 99, 100
  measures to inhibit accumulation of, 99
  measures to move, 98–99
 physical treatment of, results of, 99–100
 postsurgical, 97–98
 treatment of, 98–99

M

Malingering, in athletic injuries, 263
Massage, in athletic injuries, 256
 in lymphedema, 98
 in neck pain, 213
 in neuropathic disease, 150
Masters and Johnson, 23
Medical history, past, 6
Meniscus, torn, 32
Mental retardation, in cerebral palsy, 128–129
Mental status, examination of, 7–8
Metacarpal bones, as bony landmarks for goniometry, 61
Metatarsals, as bony landmarks for goniometry, 62
Microdyne stimulation, 69, 256f
Micrographia, in parkinsonism, 167
Microwave diathermy, 65
Misuse, in hand injury, 244
Mobility, in elderly population, 272
Mobility aids, in rheumatoid arthritis, 237–238
Motion, abnormalities, in cerebral palsy, 125
 range of, loss of, in hand injury, 241–242
Motion(s), active and passive, 31
 active assisted, 31
 isometric resistance and, 31
 limitation(s) of, 32–34
  in rheumatoid arthritis, 226, 230
 major and minor, 35
 measurement of, 40–41, 42f–60f
 range of, maintenance of, in traumatic brain injury, 120
 spine, measurement of, 36–37, 37f, 38f
Motivation, for elderly, 274
Motor neuron disease(s), 153–164, 153t
Motor point block, in multiple sclerosis, 177
Motor power, decreased, in multiple sclerosis, 177
Motor skills, teaching of, in cerebral palsy, 131–132
Multiple sclerosis, ataxia in, 178
 course of, 176
 depression in, 178
 dysarthria in, 178
 etiology and epidemiology of, 175–176
 gait impairment in, 73
 manifestations of, 176
 outcome of, 180–181
 pathology of, 175
 positive predictive factors in, 180–181
 psychologic effects of, 178
 sensory deficits in, 178
 spasticity in, 176–177, 179
 weakness in, 177–178
"Muscle pump", lymph and, 97
Muscle strength, grading of, 8, 9t, 10
Muscle testing, manual, 8, 9t, 10
Muscle(s), abdominal, in lumbar disk problems, 210, 211f, 212f
 activation, electricity for, 67–68
 in cerebral palsy, 128
 denervated, electrical stimulation in, 68
 disease(s), primary, assistive devices for daily living in, 140, 141t, 142f
  considerations for rehabilitation in, 137
  genetic, 137
  irreversible, 137
  mobility training in, 139–140
  physical measures in, 137–138
  presentation of, 135–137
  therapeutic exercise in, 138
  types of, 136t
 reeducation, after hand injury, 244–245
  functional tasks to determine, 136t
  in neuropathic disease, 151

in pelvic floor tension myalgia, 249
in primary muscle disease, 138
of spinal cord, motor level classification of, 183t
tension, neck pain in, 213
weakness, in amyotrophic lateral sclerosis, 154
functional tasks to determine, 136t
in primary muscle disease, 135
Muscular atrophy, segmental spinal, of Sobue, 153
Musculoskeletal system, examination of, 8
Myalgia, in acute polymyositis, 144
tension. *See* Tension myalgia
Myofascitis. *See* Tension myalgia
Myopathy(ies), 135–143
Myotome, 182

N

Neck pain, causes of, 213
treatment of, 213
Nerve conduction studies, in amyotrophic lateral sclerosis, 154
Nerve stimulation, phrenic, 67
Nerve(s), cranial, examination of, 8
Neurectomies, in cerebral palsy, 133
Neuroma, painful, phantom pain in, 94
Neuromuscular reeducation, in athletic injuries, 257
for elderly, 268–269, 268f, 269f, 270f, 271f
electrical stimulation in, 67
Neuropathic disease, 149–152
motor involvement in, treatment of, 150–151
sensory involvement in, treatment of, 149–150
Neurosurgical procedures, in cerebral palsy, 133
Neurotoxin, causing parkinsonism, 165
Nursing, after traumatic brain injury, 122
in prosthetic prescription, 92
Nursing home care, factors determining need for, 274
factors influencing choice of, 275
Nutritional concerns, in traumatic brain injury, 119
Nutritional deficits, in elderly population, 266

O

Occupational therapy, after traumatic brain injury, 121
Orgasm, in spinal cord injury, 26
Orthosis(es), in adults with hemiplegia, 111–114, 111f, 112f, 113f, 114f, 157f
in amyotrophic lateral sclerosis, 157f, 158f, 159f, 160f, 161f, 162f
ankle-foot, 90, 111f
biomechanical principles for, 82–84
definition of, 80
electrophysiologic, 67
in hand injury, 242–243, 243f
indications for, 80–82
knee-ankle-foot, 90
materials for, 84
in neuropathic disease, 151
in primary muscle disease, 139–140
principles of, 90–91
upper extremity, 90–91, 243f
Orthostatism, in acute polymyositis, 145
Osmotic pressure, lymph production and, 97
Ossification, heterotopic, in spinal cord injury, 190–191
Osteoporosis, back pain in, 217, 218–220, 220t
exercise in, 271
and immobilization, 216–217
incidence and scope of, 215
in multiple sclerosis, 177
and physical activity, 217
spinal. *See* Spinal osteoporosis
Overuse, in hand injury, 244–245
Overuse injuries, in sports, 251

P

Pacemakers, electrical stimulation and, 69
Pain, back. *See* Back pain
chronic and acute, electrical stimulation in, 69
gait impairment in, 71–72
in Guillain-Barré syndrome, 152
in hand injury, 240–241
and inactivity, limitation of motion in, 33
myofascial. *See* Tension myalgia
in neck, causes of, 213
treatment of, 213
phantom, 92, 94
in tendinitis and bursitis, 37–39
thalamic, after stroke, 108–109
Palpation, in joint examination, 34
Paralysis, orthosis in, 81
Paraplegia, in cerebral palsy, 126
Parkinsonism, 165–174

clinical presentation of, 166–169
conditions exhibiting, 166t
occupational therapy in, 172–173, 173t
pathophysiology of, 165–166
pharmacologic treatment of, 169–170, 169t
physical therapy in, 170, 170t
speech therapy in, 173
Patient profile, 7
Pelvic tilt maneuver, in lumbar disk problems, 210, 212f
Pelvis, as bony landmark for goniometry, 61
floor of, tension myalgia of. *See* Tension myalgia, pelvic floor
Penile prosthesis, 26
in multiple sclerosis, 180
Peripheral vascular disease, amputations in, 80–81
Permanence of disability, minimizing of, 17
Personality disorder(s), long-standing, 18–19
premorbid, 17
Phalanges, as bony landmarks for goniometry, 61, 62
Phantom pain, 92, 94
Phantom sensation, 92
Phlebitis, after stroke, 107
Phobias, in disability, 13
Physical activity, osteoporosis and, 217
Physical examination, 7
Physical therapy, after traumatic brain injury, 121
in spinal osteoporosis, 218–223
Physician, role of, after traumatic brain injury, 122–123
in prosthetic prescription, 91
Plethysmography, in spinal cord injury, 186
PLISSIT model for sexual counseling, 26–28
Pneumonia, after stroke, 107
Polymyositis, acute, rehabilitation in, early acute phase, 144–146
middle phase, 146–147
remission phase, 147
side effects of, 147
Polypharmacy, in elderly population, 266
Positioning, in stroke, 103, 103f–104f, 105f
Postpolio weakness, 154
Postural adaptation, after stroke, 107
Postural adjustment, in cerebral palsy, 131
Postural drainage, after stroke, 107
Posture, kyphotic, complications of, 222–223
in parkinsonism, 167–168, 168f, 171
Prematurity, cerebral palsy in, 125, 127
Premorbid personality disturbance, 17
Pressure sores, prevention of, in acute polymyositis, 146
in stroke, 102–103
in spinal osteoporosis, 223
Prosody, in parkinsonism, 173
Prosthesis(es), above-elbow amputation sockets for, 89, 89f
above-knee amputation sockets for, 86, 86f
below-elbow amputation sockets for, 88, 88f
below-knee amputation sockets for, 84–85, 85f
biomechanical principles for, 82–84
complications of, 93–94
definition of, 80
elbow units of, 88
exoskeletal and endoskeletal systems, 89
fitting of, 93
foot and ankle mechanism for, 84, 85f
hand, 87–88
hemipelvectomy, 87, 87f
hip disarticulation, 87, 87f
indications for, 80–82
knee units for, 85–86
long-term management in use of, 93
materials for, 84
and orthoses, 80–95
prescription of, 93
principles of, 84–89
shoulder disarticulation and forequarter, 89
training in use of, 93
upper extremity, terminal devices for, 87–88
wrist units of, 88
Prosthetist, duties of, 91–92
Psychologic aspects of disability, 12–21
Psychologic disorders, acute, 18
Psychometric tests, after stroke, 114
Psychosis, 12
Psychotherapy, in tension myalgia, 248

R

Radial nerve palsy, orthosis in, 91
Radius, as bony landmark for

goniometry, 61
Rancho Los Amigos overhead suspension sling, 109f, 112–113
Recreation therapy, after traumatic brain injury, 122
Rectal examination, in tension myalgia, 249
Reflexes, in cerebral palsy, 128
examination of, 8
Rehabilitation, in amputation, process of, 92–94
definition of, 1–2
goal(s) of, 2, 11
in prosthetic prescription, 91
team, in prosthesis use, 91–92
in traumatic brain injury, 121–123
Rehabilitation medicine, definition of, 1
emphasis of, 2
history of, 2
team approach in, 2
Respiration, in traumatic brain injury, 120
Respirator(s), in acute polymyositis, 145
in amyotrophic lateral sclerosis, 155–157
Respiratory care, after stroke, 107
Respiratory failure, in primary muscle disease, 142
Rest, back pain and, 212–213
in rheumatoid arthritis, 226–228
in tension myalgia, 248
Rheumatism, muscular. *See* Tension myalgia
Rheumatoid arthritis, 225–238
joint inflammation in, 226
limitation of joint motion in, 228t
management of, goals of, 226
physical measures in, 226–238, 227f
orthosis in, 91, 243f
Righting reactions, restoration of, after stroke, 107
Rigid frame, in spinal cord injury, 185
Rigidity, gait disturbance in, 73
in parkinsonism, 167, 171
Rotator cuff injury, after stroke, 108
Rotator cuff repair, orthosis after, 91

S

Sacroiliac pain, 213
Salivation, excessive, in parkinsonism, 168
Scapula, as bony landmark for goniometry,61
Schober flexion test, modified, 37
Sclerosis, amyotrophic lateral. *See* Amyotrophic lateral sclerosis
multiple. *See* Multiple sclerosis
primary lateral, 153–154
"Sclerotic plaque", in multiple sclerosis, 175
Scoliosis, in cerebral palsy, 132
electrical stimulation in, 67
Seizure disorder, after stroke, 109
Senile dementia, 273
Sensation, examination of, 8
Sensory deficits, in multiple sclerosis, 178
Sensory reeducation, in hand injury, 245
Sex acts, 23–24
Sex drive, 23
Sexual Attitude Restructuring, 22
Sexual counseling, PLISSIT model for, 26–28
Sexual dysfunction, in disabled persons, 24
in multiple sclerosis, 180
Sexual function, impact on, types of disability and, 24–25
Sexual response cycle, and common dysfunctions, 23
Sexuality, definition of, 24
and disability, 22–29
discussions of, with elderly, 274
Shoe modification, for elderly, 268
Shortwave diathermy, 65
Shoulder, abduction and adduction of, 52f
capsule, 229f
disarticulation, prosthesis in, 89
glenohumeral motion, 53f
injuries, in sports, 252
Shoulder impingement syndrome, 39–40, 40f
Shoulder-hand syndrome, hemiplegic, after stroke, 108
treatment of, 103f–104f, 108, 108f
Skeletal instability, orthosis in, 82
Skin, pressure, in elderly population, 267
in spinal cord injury, 187
Skin care, in traumatic brain injury, 120
Sling(s), shoulder, 161f, 162f
Sobue, segmental spinal muscular atrophy of, 153
Social worker, role of, after traumatic brain injury, 122
in prosthetic prescription, 92
Soft tissue(s), mobilization of, in

athletic injuries, 256
Spasticity, in amyotrophic lateral sclerosis, 154, 157
control, electrical stimulation in, 67
gait impairment in, 72
in multiple sclerosis, 176–177, 179
in neuropathic disease, 151
in spinal cord injury, 190
Speech disorders, after stroke, 107
after traumatic brain injury, 121
Speech therapy, in parkinsonism, 173
Spinal cord, injury, 182–193
acute management of, 184–185
areas of increased risk in, 185–191
depression in, 13
follow-up in, 192, 193t
hospitalization in, 191
patient education in, 191
residual functional capacities in, 192t
sexual concerns in, 25–26
suicide after, 13
terminology in, 182
zone of, 182–184
muscles of, motor level classification of, 183t
Spinal osteoporosis, etiology of, 215–216, 216t
medical treatment in, 223, 223t
physical therapy measures in, 218–223
preventive measures in, 223–224
symptoms of, 217, 219f
Spinal shock, 190
Spine, as bony landmark for goniometry, 62
motion, measurement of, 36–37, 37f, 38f
Splint(s), hand, in claw-hand deformity, 160f
in hand injury, 243f, 242–244
resting-hand, 103, 105f
thumb-shell, 158f
wrist-extension, with thumb–shell, 158f
and finger-extension device, 159f
Splinting, in cerebral palsy, 132–133
Spondylitis, ankylosing, 238–239, 238f
Sports fitness, measurement of, 263
Sports injuries, cardiovascular endurance, maintenance in, 261–262
care and treatment in, 254–263
causes of, 251–252
comprehensive rehabilitation program in, 254
to head, back, and trunk, 252, 252t
to lower extremity, 253–254, 253t
motor skills refinement in, 262
prevention of, 263
psychologic support in, 262–263
restoration and maintenance of motion, strength, and endurance in, 257–261
to upper extremity, 252–253, 253t
Step, forward, single, analysis of, 82–83, 82f
Steroids, in multiple sclerosis, 180
Stimulation, exteroceptive and proprioceptive, after stroke, 107
Stimulator, muscle, in athletic injuries, 258, 259f
nerve, 69
in athletic injuries, 256f
Straining, in lumbar disk problems, 208
Strength training, in athletic injuries, 258–259
Stretching, in athletic injuries, 257, 257f
in hand injury, 242
Stroke, causes of, 101–102
complications of, 103t
depression in, 13
dismissal planning in, 114
psychometric tests after, 114
rehabilitation after, 101–115
conditions complicating, 102
early phase, 102–106, 103t
evaluation of patients' potential in, 102, 102t
late phase, 103t, 107–111
survival after, 101t
with hemiplegia, orthoses in, 111–114, 111f, 112f, 113f, 114f, 157f
Subluxations, articular, 34
Substance abuse, 17–18
Substantia nigra, in parkinsonism, 165
Suicide, after spinal cord injury, 13
Surgery, of lower extremity, gait impairment after, 72
Synovial fluid, 34
Synovium, 34
Systems, review of, 5–6

T

Tarsals, as bony landmarks for goniometry, 62
Tendinitis, pain in, 37–39
Tendon(s), procedures, in cerebral palsy, 133
in rheumatoid arthritis, 229–230
"Tennis elbow", 39

Tension myalgia, diagnostic criteria for, 247
  differential diagnosis of, 247
  etiology of, 246
  pathophysiology of, 247
  pelvic floor, diagnosis of, 249
    initial complaints in, 248
    synonyms for, 248
    treatment of, 249
      goals of, 249–250
  symptoms of, 246–247
  synonyms for, 246
  treatment of, 248
Tetraparesis, 184
Tetraplegia, 184
  in cerebral palsy, 126
Thalamic pain, after stroke, 108–109
Therapists, role of, in prosthetic prescription, 91
"Thoracic pump", lymph and, 97
Thrombosis, deep venous, in acute polymyositis, 146
    prevention of, after spinal cord injury, 186–187
      after stroke, 105–106
Thumb, abduction, 46f
  flexion, 49f
  hyperextension and extension, 47f
  opposition, 48f
Tibia, as bony landmark for goniometry, 62
Tilt board, 262
Toxemia of pregnancy, cerebral palsy in, 125
Traction, in neck pain, 213
Transcutaneous electrical nerve stimulation, high-frequency, 69
  low-frequency, 69
  in neuropathic disease, 150
Tremor, in parkinsonism, 166–167
Trunk, sports injuries to, 252, 252t

U

Ulna, as bony landmark for goniometry 61
Ultrasound therapy, 65
  in stroke, 108
Urinary retention, in parkinsonism, 168
Urinary tract, care of, after stroke, 104, 106
  in spinal cord injury, 187–188

V

Valsalva maneuver, in bladder retraining, 202–204, 202f
  in multiple sclerosis, 180
Vision, impairment of, in elderly population, 267
Vocational and avocational skills, in cerebral palsy, 129–130

W

Walkers, 75f, 76–77, 77f
Weakness, gait impairment in, 72
Werdnig-Hoffman disease, 153
Wheelchair(s), 129f, 130f, 131f
  adaptive equipment, 114, 114f
  in primary muscle disease, 140, 141f
  in rheumatoid arthritis, 238
Whirlpools, in athletic injuries, 255–256
Wrist, deformities, in rheumatoid arthritis, 234
  injuries, in sports, 253

Z

Zimmer sling, 112
Zimmer strap, 112